Diagnosis & Treatment of Prevalent Diseases of North American Indian Populations: I

A Volume in MSS' Series on American Indian Health

Papers by
Melvin Lee, J. A. Birkbeck, I. D. Desai et al.

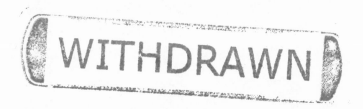
MSS Information Corporation
655 Madison Avenue, New York, N.Y. 10021

Library of Congress Cataloging in Publication Data

Main entry under title:

Diagnosis and treatment of prevalent diseases of North
    American Indian populations.

        1. Indians of North America--Diseases and hygiene.
[DNLM: 1. Indians, North American--Collected works.
2. Public health--North America--Collected works.
WA300 D536]
RA801.D5   616   74-4438
ISBN 0-8422-7215-1 (V. 1)
ISBN 0-8422-7216-X (V. 2)

TABLE OF CONTENTS

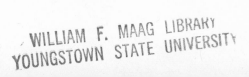

CREDITS AND ACKNOWLEDGEMENTS

Adams, Morton S.; Kenneth S. Brown; Barbara Y. Iba; and Jerry D. Niswander, "Health of Papago Indian Children," *Public Health Reports*, 1970, 85:1047-1061.

Bartha, Gregory W.; Thomas A. Burch; and Peter H. Bennett, "Hyperglycemia in Washoe and Northern Paiute Indians," *Diabetes*, 1973, 22: 58-62.

Bennett, Peter H.; Thomas A. Burch; and Max Miller, "Diabetes Mellitus in American (Pima) Indians," *The Lancet*, July 17, 1971, pp. 125-128.

Birkbeck, J.A.; Melvin Lee; Gordon S. Myers; and Braxton M. Alfred, "Nutritional Status of British Columbia Indians. II. Anthropometric Measurements, Physical and Dental Examinations at Ahousat and Anaham," *Canadian Journal of Public Health*, 1971, 62:403-414.

Birt, A.R.; and R.A. Davis, "Photodermatitis in North American Indians: Familial Actinic Prurigo," *International Journal of Dermatology*, 1971, 10:107-114.

Blodi, Frederick C.; and William S. Hunter, "Norrie's Disease in North America," *Docum. Ophthal.*, 1969, 26:434-450.

Comstock, George W.; Laurel M. Hammes; and Antonio Pio, "Isoniazid Prophylaxis in Alaskan Boarding Schools: A Comparison of Two Doses," *American Review of Respiratory Disease*, 1969, 100:773-779.

Desai, I.D.; and Melvin Lee, "Nutritional Status of British Columbia Indians. III. Biochemical Studies at Ahousat and Anaham Reserves," *Canadian Journal of Public Health*, 1971, 62:526-536.

Jeanes, C.W.L.; O. Schaefer; and L. Eidus, "Inactivation of Isoniazid by Canadian Eskimos and Indians," *Canadian Medical Association Journal*, 1972, 106:331-335.

Lee, Melvin; Rejeanne Reyburn; and Anne Carrow, "Nutritional Status of British Columbia Indians. I. Dietary Studies at Ahousat and Anaham Reserves," *Canadian Journal of Public Health*, 1971, 62:285-296.

Leichter, Joseph; and Melvin Lee, "Lactose Intolerance in Canadian West Coast Indians," *The American Journal of Digestive Diseases*, 1971, 16:809-813.

Levine, Stephen B.; Richard E. Sampliner; Peter H. Bennett; Norman B. Rushforth; Thomas A. Burch; and Max Miller, "Asymptomatic Parotid Enlargement in Pima Indians: Relationship to Age, Obesity, and Diabetes Mellitus," *Annals of Internal Medicine*, 1970, 73:571-573.

Lowry, R.B., "Sex-Linked Cleft Palate in a British Columbia Indian Family," *Pediatrics*, 1970, 46:123-128.

Nelson, Bruce D.; John Porvaznik; and John R. Benfield, "Gallbladder Disease in Southwestern American Indians," *Archives of Surgery*, 1971, 103:41-43.

Oakland, Lynne; and Robert L. Kane, "The Working Mother and Child Neglect on the Navajo Reservation," *Pediatrics*, 1973, 51:849-853.

Reid, Jeanne M.; Sandra D. Fullmer; Karen D. Pettigrew; Thomas A. Burch; Peter H. Bennett; Max Miller; and G. Donald Whedon, "Nutrient Intake of Pima Indian Women: Relationships to Diabetes Mellitus and Gallbladder Disease," *The American Journal of Clinical Nutrition*, 1971, 24:1281-1289.

Rimoin, David L., "Ethnic Variability in Glucose Tolerance and Insulin Secretion," *The Archives of Internal Medicine*, 1969, 124:695-700.

Rushforth, Norman B.; Peter H. Bennett; Arthur G. Steinberg; Thomas A. Burch; and Max Miller, "Diabetes in the Pima Indians: Evidence of Bimodality in Glucose Tolerance Distributions," *Diabetes*, 1971, 20: 756-765.

Scott, Edward M., "Genetic Disorders in Isolated Populations," *Archives of Environmental Health*, 1973, 26:32-35.

Sievers, Maurice L.; and Margaret E. Hendrikx, "Two Weight-Reduction Programs among Southwestern Indians," *Health Services Reports*, 1972, 87:530-536.

Steinberg, Arthur G.; Norman B. Rushforth; Peter H. Bennett; Thomas A. Burch; and Max Miller, "Preliminary Report on the Genetics of Diabetes among the Pima Indians," *Advances in Metabolic Diseases*, *1 Suppl.*, 1970, 1:11-21.

Thistle, Johnson L.; and Leslie Schoenfield, "Lithogenic Bile among Young Indian Women: Lithogenic Potential Decreased with Chenodeoxycholic Acid," *The New England Journal of Medicine*, 1971, 284: 177-181.

Wallace, Helen M., "The Health of American Indian Children," *American Journal of Diseases of Children*, 1973, 125:449-454.

Wallace, Helen M., "The Health of American Indian Children: A Survey of Current Problems and Needs," *Clinical Pediatrics*, 1973, 12:83-87.

Wood, Corinne S., "A Multiphasic Health Screening of Three Southern Californian Indian Reservations," *Social Science and Medicine*, 1970, 4:579-587.

PREFACE

The American Indian population is relatively small. There were 561,000 Amerinds or 0.3 percent of the total population of the United States in 1968. The health problems of this ethnic group are numerous and may be attributed to social, economic, geographic as well as genetic factors. In 1955, the United States Public Health Service was assigned the responsibility of providing health care to American Indians and Eskimos. In the intervening years, reports on USPHS findings accumulated in the course of health care delivery and studies supported by various public and private organizations in the United States and Canada have considerably increased the pool of knowledge and interest in this ethnic group. This collection of articles provides an introduction to the more commonly diagnosed ailments among North American Indians.

The first three comparative studies on nutrition provide data on two tribes, one inland and the other coastal, which are in an interim state of acculturation. Their contemporary diets combine the traditional spoils of gathering, hunting and agrarian societies with processed foods purchased at prices ten to thirty percent higher than the rates charged in the nearest metropolitan areas. Peanut butter, candy and vitamin biscuits share the menu with sealion oil, bannock and fried moose meat. Unbalanced diets with a high intake of carbohydrates have resulted in the common occurrence of obesity and concurrently activated a genetically probable pre-disposition in some tribes to diabetes mellitus and gall bladder disease. While the exact etiology of these maladies is not known, it is suggested that careful evaluation of these defined communities may provide the necessary insights to the causative components.

Interest in the health of children has been stimulated by their increasing numbers. In 1969, 55.2 percent of the American Indians were under twenty years of age and the birth rate was twice that of non-Indians in the United States. Although the health problems of children and adults may be generally attributed to environmental conditions, two tuberculosis studies in Alaska reveal that a genetic trait hampers the successful treatment of TB. Along with Japanese, Thais, Koreans, Soame Lapps and Eskimos, pure Indians seem to be fast inactivators of isoniazid. Other genetically related disorders are described and attributed to the closed societies and resultant intramarriage of distant relatives.

This volume is part of MSS' four-volume series on Indian health.

Nutrition

Nutritional Status of British Columbia Indians

1. DIETARY STUDIES AT AHOUSAT AND ANAHAM RESERVES[1]

MELVIN LEE , PH.D., REJEANNE REYBURN , M.SC.,
and ANNE CARROW , M.A.

Changing patterns of Indian life, many of which have direct implications for nutritional status, have stimulated interest in the dietary habits of British Columbia Indians. The diminishing isolation of Indian communities and the increasing exposure of Indians to non-Indian cultural patterns have been recognized. One consequence of this has been a gradual shift from traditional diets to a dependence on purchased manufactured foods, a change often effected without the benefit of nutrition education programs to assist in the establishment of new food habits. As well, a high rate of population growth (approximately 2.5% per year until recently) has resulted in a "young" population, a high dependency ratio, and a relatively large number of children under six years of age, an age category considered to be nutritionally at risk.

In view of the lack of published information on the dietary habits and nutritional status of British Columbia Indians, and the potential value of such information for the establishment of nutrition education programs, it was decided to carry out a series of comprehensive nutritional status studies. Two reserves, one dependent on fishing and marine resources and the other on hunting, were selected for initial study and comparison. The dietary information is presented here; anthropometric, physical, dental, and biochemical results will be reported in subsequent papers to be published in this journal. Detailed description of the populations and the survey samples, and more complete survey data have appeared in a report of the Division of Human Nutrition, School of Home Economics (1).

Nutritional status studies were carried out at Ahousat, a Nootka Indian fishing community, and at Anaham, a Chilcotin Indian hunting community. Nutrient intakes were computed from 24-hour recall records and compared with Canadian Dietary Standards. Calcium intakes were low in certain age groups at both reserves, and vitamin A and iron intakes tended to be low at Anaham, the latter particularly among teenage girls and adult women.

Diets were more varied at Ahousat than at Anaham, but the consumption of milk and milk products at both reserves was low, compared with the rest of the Canadian population. The Indian diets were remarkable in that a large proportion of the ascorbic acid

1. Supported in part by: Dept. of National Health and Welfare, research grant #609-7-236, University of British Columbia research grant #26-9666, Public Health Research Grant (Project #605-7-368) of National Health Program, and assistance from the Pacific Region Office, Medical Services Branch, Department of National Health and Welfare.

10

was supplied by fortified evaporated milk.

Traditional food patterns make an important contribution to nutrient intakes, particularly of protein, but also of calcium, iron, and vitamin A. A problem may exist for those persons unable to fish or hunt, such as the disabled, widowed, and elderly.

AHOUSAT is a Nootka Indian community located on an isthmus in the southeast corner of Flores Island, just west of Vancouver Island. Anaham reserve is a Chilcotin Indian community located 70 miles west of Williams Lake, on the road to Bella Coola in the interior of the province. Some salient features of the two survey sites are compared in Table I.

The general level of formal education is greater at Ahousat than at Anaham, and a larger proportion of the labour force at Ahousat would be classified as "skilled." Almost all Ahousat residents speak English whereas many of the older people at Anaham, particularly older women, have difficulty with English, and speak Chilcotin in the home. The general level of income appears to be higher at Ahousat than at Anaham although the range of incomes is greater at Anaham. The degree of isolation, particularly with regard to the availability of health services and emergency facilities, as well as day to day interaction with non-Indians, is noticeably greater at Ahousat than at Anaham.

In 1968 a total of 644 registered Indians were listed on the Ahousat band list. Approximately 260 persons were residing on the reserve at the time of the survey and of this number, 248 took part in the study. At the time of the Anaham survey 594 persons were listed on the official band list, although not all were residing on the reserve. The number of residents was not known, but was estimated to be not more than 300 persons. Of this number, 266 persons took part in the study.

The age and sex compositions of the registered band populations and of the survey samples are shown in Figure 1.

Collection and Analysis of Dietary Data

Despite its recognized shortcomings, the 24-hour recall method was used for dietary data collection. This method was deemed most suitable because of the difficulty in obtaining dietary records from native popula-

Table I: Comparison of Survey Sites and Populations.

	Ahousat	Anaham
Location	On an island 10 miles across the sound from nearest urban community (Tofino).	On a provincial road 7 miles from Alexis Creek, 70 miles from Williams Lake.
Weather	Relatively mild most of year; much rain.	Below freezing for most of winter.
Access to urban centers	By boat, plane, or radio-telephone.	By motor vehicle.
Schools	Elementary school on reserve.	Elementary school on reserve.
Health facilities	Community health worker on reserve; other facilities and personnel in Tofino.	Community health worker and teacher-nurse on reserve, public health nurse in Alexis Creek; other facilities in Williams Lake.
Utilities, conveniences	Diesel generators for electricity, indoor water taps, community sewage system.	Commercial electrical service, indoor water taps, no central sewage disposal system.
Most important source of earned income	Commercial ocean fishing; sale of lumber rights.	Guiding hunters, ranch labour, logging, etc.

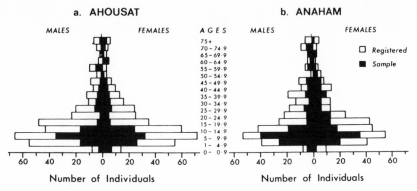

Figure 1: Age, Sex Population Tree for Ahousat and Anaham Reserves.

tions, the anticipated lack of variety in meal patterns, and the limitations in time. In essentially all cases the matriarchal head of the household was interviewed and asked to recall all food consumed by each member of the family during the preceding 24 hours. If other adults or older children were present they were interviewed also. Food models, fresh fruits and vegetables, cups, glasses, bowls, and measuring spoons were used to aid in establishing portion size. Because reported intakes of candy, ice cream, chips, popcorn, cheezies, carbonated beverages, and beer may have been incomplete, the intakes of those foods may be underestimated. In all, 189 records were obtained at Ahousat and 216 at Anaham.

Initial data processing was carried out by Dr. G. S. Beaton and Miss H. Milne, Department of Nutrition, University of Toronto, using computer programs developed by Miss E. P. McClinton. Daily intakes of nine nutrients were computed using modified U.S. Department of Agriculture food composition tables. Subsequently, programs were developed to compute daily intakes of total fat, polyunsaturated fat, carbohydrate, and Vitamin E. Calculation of Vitamin E intakes was based on unpublished food composition tables developed by Dr. I. D. Desai. Computer programs were developed for sorting and analyzing dietary data.

In addition to the 24-hour recalls, information was collected regarding weekly food purchases, seasonal food availability and consumption, and methods of preserving and preparing foods. This information served as a cross check on the recall data and offered a broader picture of dietary patterns.

Results

Many of the Nootkan food habits described by Drucker (2) have been retained, at least by some families at Ahousat. This is particularly apparent in the marked dependence on fish and other marine resources. Several varieties of salmon (Pinks, Cohoe, Sockeye, Spring, and Chum) are obtained at various times of the year and eaten fresh, smoked, dried, or canned. Many families have smokehouses and most preserve, by smoking or canning, sufficient salmon to last until late winter. Red snapper, halibut, and herring are popular and important food fish; the latter three are often dried for storage. Fish roe (fresh, dried, or salted) is still well liked by many. Several marine invertebrates, including clams, sea urchins, chitons and, rarely, sea cucumbers and crabs, are seasonal or occasional items in the diet. Seal and sea lion are not as common in the diets as in the past, but the oils are sometimes obtained and are highly regarded by some families, particularly for use with dried fish.

Food Sources, Selection and Prices

Non-marine food sources include deer (less common than at Anaham) and several varieties of wild duck. Some families collect sea-gull eggs. In the late spring and summer several kinds of wild berries are gathered (salmon berries, salal berries, red huckleberries and blackberries) and eaten fresh or made into preserves. Many families purchase fresh fruit for canning or bottling.

Ahousat residents indicated that there had at one time been orchards, gardens, and chickens on the reserve, but that all forms of food production had been discontinued.

Food is purchased at one of two large markets at Tofino, at a general store on Flores Island, or at two or three small stores on the reserve. The stores on the reserve have extremely limited selections, and are important primarily as sources of soft drinks, candy, ice cream, and a few staples. A typical shopping list would contain more grain products, sugars, oils, and canned products, and less fresh vegetables and meats than would be expected in a less isolated community — perhaps reflecting the lack of cold storage facilities and the availability of marine resources. Fresh milk rarely appears on the shopping lists, but large quantities of canned milk (24-144 cans per month per family) are purchased.

Meal patterns generally follow those of other Canadians, with three meals per day. One dish, top-of-the-stove meals (hashes, stews, soups) are popular. In addition, mid-morning, mid-afternoon, and late evening snacks, usually consisting of bread or pilot biscuits with margarine or jam, and coffee or tea, are common. Children often have, as well, apples, peanut butter, candy, chips, popcorn, or vitamin biscuits.* Snack foods are usually left on the table all day. Most

*Vitamin biscuits were distributed at the school and contained:

Nutrients/Biscuit	
Protein	3 gm
Calcium	53 mg
Iron	4.4 mg
Vit. A	1,200 I.U.
Thiamine	.36 mg
Riboflavin	.62 mg
Calories	120 C

families bake bread; a few without ovens make bannock. About half of the homemakers include some milk in the recipes. Sample food records are shown in Table II.

Selected food prices obtained at the two stores in Tofino were generally about 10 per cent higher than those in Vancouver, and the local store was found to be approximately 30 per cent more expensive than stores in Tofino.

When the cost of feeding a family was calculated according to the method used by the B.C. Provincial Government Departments of Health, and Trade and Industry, employing standardized food lists and costing procedures, it became apparent that collected and preserved foods represent an important factor in family food economics.

At Anaham there is a variety of food sources. Although fish is an important item in the diet, with salmon available in August and trout in winter, it is not as important as it is at Ahousat. It was estimated that, in 1969, 80 Anaham families obtained 96 moose, 480 deer, and 3,500 pounds of fish. Most families grow potatoes and several families grow beets, corn, peas, turnips, cabbage, onions and lettuce — all for family consumption. In addition, several kinds of wild berries are available locally.

Most food purchases are made at the two stores in Alexis Creek or at the supermarkets in Williams Lake. The list of food purchases differed from that of Ahousat in that the variety is less, and meats, fruits and vegetables are less prominent. Fruits, vegetables, frozen meats, chicken and canned products are available in the stores in Alexis Creek but are purchased more often by non-Indian members of the community. Purchased refined and processed foods (breads, cookies, cereals, candies, soft drinks, sugar, flour, etc.) contributed 48 per cent of the calories for adults and 40-60 per cent for children.

Bannock, a home-made fried bread containing enriched flour, salt, lard, baking powder and water (occasionally small amounts of milk, sugar, and eggs) is a staple in the diet.

13

Table II: Sample Menus, Taken From 24-Hour Recall Forms: Ahousat and Anaham Reserves

	Ahousat		Anaham	
	1	2	1	2
Early Morning	3 oz. smoked dried salmon, 3 tbsp. sealion oil, oatmeal with milk and sugar, coffee with milk and sugar	orange, oatmeal, milk, sugar, homemade bread, toasted, and margarine	toasted bannock, jam — margarine, fried moose meat, boiled potatoes	mush, powdered skim milk, sugar, bannock — margarine, tea
Mid-Morning	1 tbsp molasses, bannock with sealion oil, tea and sugar			apple
Noon	3 oz. dried halibut, 3 tbsp. sealion oil, 2 c. duck soup, 3 canned plums	clam chowder, carrots and cabbage, orange freshie, bread and margarine	salmon — boiled, rice, bannock — margarine, tea — sugar	roast salmon, mashed potatoes, bannock head — margarine, carrots, tea — sugar, white cake and icing
Mid-Afternoon	1 tbsp. molasses, bannock with sealion oil, tea and sugar		apple, candy (jelly beans)	tea — sugar, 2 cookies with cream filling
Evening	1 strip smoked seal meat, 3 tbsp sealion oil, 2 c. corned beef soup	deer meat stew with carrots, onions, and potato, bread and margarine	moose meat stew (potatoes, carrots, onions, turnips), tea — sugar	boiled moose, macaroni, rice, gravy, ketchup, tea — sugar
Late Evening	1 c. pork and beans, 1 tbsp. molasses, bannock with sealion oil	tea with sugar, bread, margarine, canned peaches		crackers, peanut butter

Most cooking is done on a wood stove, although about one-fourth of the families own electric ranges, hot plates, or propane stoves. Food is usually prepared on top of the stove, fried in lard, beef fat, or moose fat, or simmered, boiled, or stewed. Ovens, when available, are not commonly used.

In some families the food is prepared once daily and kept warm so that food can be taken as desired. Within a single day, meals would be of little variety. Bannock, jam, margarine, coffee, and tea are available at all times. Sample food records are shown in Table II. These records are not necessarily "representative" or "typical" but are chosen to illustrate the variety of food patterns encountered. Some families still depend heavily on traditional food items, while others have shifted to more processed and purchased foods. The menus also illustrate the lack of variety in some diets.

Market prices of 19 food items were compared. Williams Lake prices averaged only .72% higher than those in Vancouver, but the prices at the two stores in Alexis Creek were 13.6% and 18.6% higher than those in Williams Lake.

Nutrient Intakes

The average daily nutrient intakes for several age categories at the two reserves are shown in Tables III and IV. Table V shows the number of persons with nutrient intakes less than two thirds of the Canadian Dietary

Table III: Daily Nutrient Intakes of Ahousat and Anaham Children. Means and Standard Deviations are Given. Figures in parentheses are numbers of individuals.[1]

	2-4 Years, M+F		4-6 years, M+F		6-9 Years, M+F		9-13 Years, M+F	
	Ahousat (19)	Anaham (19)	Ahousat (25)	Anaham (32)	Ahousat (30)	Anaham (29)	Ahousat (32)	Anaham (27)
Calories	1448±355	1232±593	2154±886	1278±505	2340±708	1613±738	2796±830	1724±615
Protein	51±19	54±27	75±36	53±19	84±30	67±30	103±95	69±28
Calcium	680±342	794±502	786±381	756±422	963±510	886±579	1331±2940	907±574
Iron	7.7±4.4	5.2±3.0	11.9±5.3	6.0±3.8	14.4±6.2	7.6±5.1	13.5±5.3	8.7±4.6
Vitamin A	3035±2280	2670±2250	4273±3670	2565±2461	4748±3554	2970±3315	5818±6935	3123±3248
Thiamine	0.80±0.56	0.77±0.27	1.34±0.97	1.05±1.02	1.95±1.43	1.44±1.23	1.59±1.19	1.52±1.34
Riboflavin	1.16±0.56	1.40±0.69	1.55±1.03	1.59±1.19	2.20±1.55	1.98±1.55	2.44±4.12	2.02±1.69
Niacin	9.5±4.8	13.6±6.5	16.0±9.2	14.6±5.6	17.3±7.5	19.8±8.9	21.4±12.0	20.4±7.9
Ascorbic acid	73±76	43±33	73±56	35±22	73±47	41±21	113±152	44±21
Vitamin E	20.6±15.5	15.8±24.0	52.4±74.7	17.7±22.0	41.8±34.3	13.1±8.9	45.3±58.0	19.5±15.7

[1] For this and following tables, units are Protein (gm), Vitamin A (International Units), all others (mg).

Table IV: Daily Nutrient Intakes of Ahousat and Anaham Adolescents and Adults. Means and Standard Deviations are Given. Figures in parentheses are numbers of individuals.

	13-20 Years, Males		13-20 Years, Females		20+ Years, Males		20+ Years, Females	
	Ahousat (6)	Anaham (13)	Ahousat (11)	Anaham (18)	Ahousat (23)	Anaham (29)	Ahousat (29)	Anaham (45)
Calories	3035±847	1950±1189	2081±722	1590±534	2805±1077	2180±808	1748±519	1772±623
Protein	105±34	71±32	63±31	64±25	111±50	95±46	65±24	76±30
Calcium	930±405	871±572	671±486	727±438	804±451	997±646	514±275	802±441
Iron	15.3±4.4	8.3±4.1	10.1±3.4	8.2±4.4	14.6±6.2	9.2±3.8	9.7±4.0	7.6±3.1
Vitamin A	5884±5786	2320±2227	4500±4027	2124±2559	5885±3108	4060±5550	4934±6441	4960±5194
Thiamine	1.86±0.75	1.48±0.88	1.00±0.49	1.43±0.83	1.38±0.69	1.54±0.76	1.05±1.03	1.21±0.43
Riboflavin	2.00±0.93	1.93±1.27	1.08±0.61	1.76±1.14	1.65±0.75	2.16±1.24	0.99±0.36	1.68±0.74
Niacin	27.4±11.4	20.3±8.2	14.4±7.8	20.4±7.9	24.3±12.8	28.1±14.9	16.3±11.7	23.2±9.8
Ascorbic acid	77±52	42±25	69±53	40±18	73±55	58±30	46±38	47±26
Vitamin E	67.1±63.7	17.3±12.0	44.2±46.2	15.4±24.3	55.2±56.5	24.6±24.4	42.6±46.9	25.0±29.5

Standard (3). Although the selection of two thirds CDS as a standard for dietary comparison is arbitrary, it was based on the assumption that nutrient intakes of less than that level are clearly undesirable and where they occur in a large proportion of the population attention should definitely be given to improving or correcting the situation.

At all ages from two to 13 years average calorie intake at Ahousat was equal to or greater than the CDS, while those at Anaham were consistently below. Approximately 50 per cent of the Anaham children failed to achieve intakes equal to two thirds of the CDS. Calorie intakes of adults were, in most cases, below the CDS — usually less at Anaham than at Ahousat. The largest single source of calories at both reserves was grains and cereals (28-43%) but fats, oils, and sugars supplied 20-35% of the calories. In general, the contributions of the various food groups to calorie intakes were similar at the two reserves — the differences in total calories reflecting smaller intakes of all food groups at Anaham.

Average protein intakes exceeded the standards in every age category of both populations, but those at Ahousat were generally higher than at Anaham. Few individuals failed to obtain at least two thirds of the CDS for protein, except teenage girls. Approximately one-half of all the protein was derived from meat, fish, poultry, eggs, and legumes. At Ahousat this consisted chiefly of beef, fish, eggs, and legumes, while at Anaham beef was replaced by moose, eggs were less frequent, and legumes were absent.

Average calcium intakes for each sex/age group were similar at the two reserves and approximated the CDS except those of Anaham teenagers which were below that level. However, at every age significant numbers of persons failed to obtain two thirds of the CDS standard.

At all ages milk and milk products supplied a notable percentage of the calcium, although the proportion was greater among the children and teenagers than among adults. However, much of the calcium was contributed by fish, meat, and poultry, and 5-30% came from grains and cereals. In general, the absolute differences in calcium intakes at the two reserves are a reflection of the greater intake of milk and milk products at Ahousat, the amounts of calcium contributed by the other food groups being similar.

Up to the age of nine years, mean iron intakes at both reserves were equal to or greater than the CDS, although mean intakes were higher at Ahousat at every age. This situation also prevailed in all male groups over nine years of age except for Anaham boys 9-13 and 13-20 years of age, in which cases intakes were below CDS. Intakes were below CDS for teenage girls (13-20 years, both reserves) and for Anaham adult women. It is noteworthy that 11 of the 18 Anaham girls 13 to 20 years of age failed to attain iron intakes equal to two thirds of the CDS.

At all ages the primary sources of dietary iron were meat, fish, poultry, legumes, and grains and cereals. Meat, fish and poultry contributed more iron at Ahousat and grains and cereals contributed more iron at Anaham.

All adults had mean vitamin A intakes of 1.5 to 4 times the recommended standards. However, the range was so great that 15-70% of the Anaham residents had intakes below two thirds of the CDS. In general, the number of persons with low vitamin A intakes (less than two thirds CDS) was greater among females than males.

Food group contributions to vitamin A were similar at the two reserves, except that for some age groups vegetables (carotenes) contributed more vitamin A at Anaham than at Ahousat, and fats and oils (preformed vitamin A) made a disproportionate contribution (42%) to the intakes of teenage boys at Anaham.

Using the U.S. recommended dietary allowances (4) for vitamin E as standards, marked differences between the two reserves

Table V: Numbers of Individuals, by Age and Sex, with Daily Nutrient Intakes Less than Two Thirds of the Canadian Dietary Standards. Under 13 Years of Age, Males and Females are Considered Together. Figures in parentheses are total numbers of individuals in each group.

	2-4 Years AH (19)	AN (19)	4-6 Years AH (25)	AN (32)	6-9 Years AH (30)	AN (29)	9-13 Years AH (32)	AN (27)	13-20 Years Male AH (6)	AN (13)	13-20 Years Female AH (11)	AN (18)	20+ Years Male AH (23)	AN (29)	20+ Years Female AH (29)	AN (45)
Calories	2	8	0	14	1	15	2	13	0	10	3	12	6	11	15	22
Protein	1	0	0	0	0	2	0	2	0	2	4	4	1	1	1	4
Calcium	7	6	6	7	8	9	19	16	3	7	9	10	1	6	8	7
Iron	3	5	0	4	0	4	5	1	1	7	4	11	1	2	4	20
Vitamin A	1	3	2	5	1	13	3	9	1	7	4	13	4	18	13	21
Thiamine	2	0	1	0	0	2	3	0	0	0	2	0	3	1	3	3
Riboflavin	2	0	3	1	0	0	3	3	1	5	5	3	3	6	12	8
Niacin	1	0	0	0	0	0	1	0	0	0	0	0	3	1	1	1
Ascorbic acid	1	3	4	5	4	2	3	2	1	2	2	2	3	3	8	7

AH = Ahousat
AN = Anaham

Table VI: Percentage Contribution of Food Groups to Calories and Nutrients

Food Group	Calories AH*	AN**	CAN***	Protein AH	AN	CAN	Calcium AH	AN	CAN	Iron AH	AN	CAN	Vitamin A AH	AN	CAN	Thiamine AH	AN	CAN	Riboflavin AH	AN	CAN	Niacin AH	AN	CAN	Ascorbic Acid AH	AN	CAN
I (Milk, milk products)	13	9	14	18	14	11	33	54	80	3	5	4	15	10	15	6	4	14	36	20	52	3	1	4	25	22	8
II (Meat, fish, poultry, eggs, legumes)	21	18	20	47	59	59	18	15	5	34	16	38	18	8	14	21	27	26	20	43	23	44	60	48	7	2	1
III (Vegetables)	6	8	5	4	5	5	19	19	7	9	15	12	37	59	49	10	14	13	4	4	5	11	11	12	30	70	48
IV (Fruits)	7	3	3	1	2	2	2	1	1	6	4	7	17	19	17	5	1	5	1	3	3	3	3	5	34	5	42
V (Grains, cereals)	32	34	22	28	24	25	19	5	4	42	59	33	14	2	2	57	53	39	34	30	16	32	22	30	—	—	—
VI (Fats, oils)	10	15	16	1	—	—	—	—	—	4	4	4	—	—	—	1	1	1	1	1	2	—	—	—	—	—	—
VII (Sugars)	10	13	17	—	—	—	—	—	—	2	—	—	—	—	—	—	—	—	—	—	—	7	6	—	3	—	—
VIII (Misc.)	2	1	—	—	—	—	—	—	—	—	—	—	—	—	—	1	1	—	2	—	—	—	—	—	—	—	—

*AH=Ahousat
**AN=Anaham
***CAN=Canadians (4)

are seen. In the 2-4 year age group, intakes are 1.5 to 2 times the RDA at both reserves. At Anaham intake remains relatively constant with increasing age, so that by 9-13 years they approximate the RDA and above that age are somewhat below the RDA, except in the case of the adult women. At Ahousat the intakes continue to increase with age, and all groups were well above the RDA.

In most age groups at both reserves average intakes of thiamine and riboflavin were in excess of the CDS, although the intakes of both vitamins were usually greater at Ahousat than at Anaham. The number of persons in each age category with intakes below two thirds of the CDS, although variable, was small. The largest proportion of dietary thiamine (40-70%) was contributed by grains and cereals, with the next most important source being meats, fish, poultry and legumes. No clear differences were seen between the two reserves.

Milk and milk products contributed much of the dietary riboflavin, although at some ages the contribution was greater at Ahousat than at Anaham. Meat, fish, poultry, and legumes were important contributors, but the contribution was greater at Anaham than at Ahousat. Most of the remainder of the riboflavin came from cereals and grains.

Niacin intakes exceeded the CDS by a factor of 3-5 for all age groups, and the proportion of the populations with intakes below two thirds of the CDS was negligible. Among children the intakes were similar at the two reserves, but among teenagers and adults Ahousat females had lower intakes than did Anaham females. The major contributor to dietary niacin was the meat, fish, poultry, and legumes group, and the second most important contributor was the cereal and grain group.

Ascorbic acid intakes were in excess of the CDS for every age group, but tended to be greater at Ahousat than at Anaham. At most ages the number of persons failing to obtain two thirds of the CDS was small, with the exception of adult women, in which case 15-25% were below that level.

It is striking that 20-40% of the dietary ascorbic acid intake of children was contributed by milk and milk products. (Canned evaporated milk contains 14 mg/100 ml). Fruit contributed negligible amounts of ascorbic acid (5-9%) to the diets of Anaham children but larger amounts (29-45%) to Ahousat diets, and vegetables contributed larger amounts of ascorbic acid at Anaham than at Ahousat. Rather similar patterns were seen for teenage and adult diets, except that milk was a less important contributor.

In general, with obvious exceptions and variations, calorie, calcium, vitamin A, and iron intakes reflect the differences in use of the meat, fish, poultry, and legume group, the relative lack of milk and milk products at Anaham, and the almost complete absence of fruits in Anaham diets.

Table VI shows the contribution of each food group to nutrient intakes at Ahousat and Anaham, as well as for the Canadian population as a whole (5). Group I (milk and milk products) makes a smaller contribution to the Indian intakes of all nutrients except ascorbic acid, and in general contributes less to Anaham diets than to Ahousat diets. Although Group II foods (meat, fish, poultry, legumes) contribute about one fifth of the calories at each reserve, they contribute more protein and very much more calcium to Indian diets than to national diets. The contribution of Group II foods to iron, riboflavin, and niacin intakes at Ahousat corresponds to the national situation. However, the contribution of Group II foods to intakes at Anaham is about half as great for iron and twice as great for riboflavin and niacin as the Canadian average. Vegetables (Group III) contribute more vitamin A and ascorbic acid to Indian diets than to national diets. For example, at Anaham they supply 70 per cent of the ascorbic acid intake. Fruits (Group IV) make a relatively minor contribution only to ascorbic acid intakes at Ahousat. Grains and cereals (Group V), on the other hand, make a greater contribution to the intakes of most nutrients at Ahousat and Anaham than to those of national diets. The three remaining food groups (fats and oils, sugars and sweets, and the miscellaneous category) make lesser contributions to all nutrients.

The lack of variety in the diets is more pronounced at Anaham than at Ahousat. At Anaham, for example, only eight Group I foods (milk and milk products) were recorded in 189 records, and canned evaporated milk accounted for 75-85% of the servings from this group. Similarly, 50% of the servings of Group II foods (meat, fish, poultry, eggs, legumes, nuts) consisted of moose and 75-85% of the vegetable intake consisted of potatoes.

Whereas Ahousat diets contained 35, 21, 27, and 30 items of foods from Groups II, III, IV, and V, respectively, Anaham diets contained only 16, 14, 11, and 20 different foods from each of the groups. This difference illustrates that although the average number of servings of foods (from each food group) may not have differed markedly at the two reserves, the variety at Ahousat was greater than at Anaham.

Discussion

Several investigations of diet and nutritional status of Canadian Indians were carried out in the 1940s and 1950s, primarily in Manitoba, Saskatchewan, and Ontario (6, 7, 8, 9, 10, 11). Although few instances of classical deficiency signs were recorded, the dietary data suggested that intakes of vitamin A, riboflavin, and possibly ascorbic acid, were less than adequate. In general, records of food purchases tended to emphasize flour, sugar, and fats, with lesser amounts of milk and milk products, fruits and vegetables. Some of the studies included dietary and biochemical evaluations, as well as physical examinations, but none were comprehensive nutritional status surveys, in the sense that the term is currently used.

With respect to the nutritional status of British Columbia Indians, less information is available. Hawthorn, et al. (12) refer to the inclusion of large quantities of staple, manufactured foodstuffs in the contemporary diets, but present no quantitative data, and it is apparent that much regional variation exists. Dong and Feeny (13) studied Indian and non-Indian children at Alert Bay, British Columbia, and concluded from the dietary survey information that intakes of vitamin A were low (approximately two thirds of the Canadian Dietary Standard) for many Indian children. Both vitamin A and ascorbic acid intakes were lower for Indian than for non-Indian children, but no measurements of plasma levels of either nutrient were carried out. There appear to have been no other recent studies of nutritional status of British Columbia Indians, although health surveys (14) have made reference to poor dietary habits as contributing factors in the occurrence of health problems.

Before discussing the dietary results, some comments need to be made regarding the 24-hour recall as an instrument for the collection of dietary information. Pilot studies at Ahousat demonstrated that dietary records would not be a suitable means of collecting information in the populations under study. However, full co-operation was obtained from the subjects in the eliciting of recall data. When the recall data were examined against the weekly shopping lists and the seasonal food usage forms, the correspondence was good, allowing for expected seasonal differences in food availability. No attempt was made to compute average daily nutrient intakes from the weekly or seasonal lists, but they did not appear to be at variance with the kinds of food patterns appearing in the recalls. The recalls do not necessarily represent usual or typical food patterns, but they do have the advantage of representing, within the limits of technique, the actual food intake at a particular point in time. The physical, dental, anthropometric, and biochemical data (to be reported subsequently) were collected at the same point in time.

In analyzing the dietary data by age and sex categories the sample sizes were reduced to smaller numbers than would ordinarily be desirable. However, the age and sex categories were selected for their relationship to nutrient requirements, and to combine them in order to increase sample sizes would make the data more difficult to interpret and would tend to obscure some of the findings. It should be noted that the sample populations, at both reserves, represented virtually the entire resident populations at the time (although only a part of the registered populations) and the dietary data refer to more than three fourths of the resident population, not to a limited subsample.

In the study reported here, low intakes (defined as less than two thirds of the Canadian Dietary Standards) were frequent only for calories, vitamin A, calcium, and iron. The lower calorie intakes at Anaham than at Ahousat suggest differences in interviewing techniques, but the absence of correspondingly low intakes of several nutrients at Anaham is not necessarily consistent with that interpretation.

Calcium intakes are inadequate when compared with the CDS, at both reserves, particularly for males and females 9-20 years old. This reflects the inadequate milk intakes during periods of rapid growth and elevated requirements. Were it not for the large intakes of Group II foods, the calcium intakes would be a more serious problem. Recent studies on the distribution of lactase deficiency in populations, including northern native populations (15, 16), as well as studies documenting a high incidence of lactose intolerance in British Columbia Indians (17), cast some doubt on the advisability of nutrition education programs directed toward increasing milk consumption, and suggest that more extensive investigations are in order. Nevertheless, the results of the dietary investigations raise questions as to the ability of present-day native diets to supply sufficient calcium. Some consideration must be given to whether currently accepted recommendations and requirements are realistic (18, 19).

Vitamin A intakes may be a matter for concern at Anaham, because of a greater dependence on carotenoids as a source of dietary vitamin A. At Ahousat, on the other hand, a greater proportion of this nutrient is supplied by preformed vitamin A. Increased milk consumption at Anaham would ameliorate the problem, but the possibility of lactase deficiency, as noted, must again be considered.

Other studies have focused attention on teenagers, particularly girls, as an "at risk" group with respect to iron intakes (20), and it has been suggested that this is at least in part a result of increased requirements and a tendency to subscribe to fad diets. The frequency of low iron intakes at Anaham was approximately 50 per cent for teenagers and for adult women. The small teenage populations available at the time of the surveys leaves the significance of these data in question, but the need for additional studies is indicated.

Although more than adequate by Canadian Dietary Standards, ascorbic acid intakes represent a very special problem. Unlike other Canadian populations, where ascorbic acid is obtained primarily from fruits and vegetables, the Indian populations studied are largely dependent on milk (as inadequate as the supply may be with respect to calcium intakes) for ascorbic acid. A shift either to fresh or to powdered skim milk would significantly decrease ascorbic acid intakes.

Examination of the dietary sources of nutrients makes it clear that those traditional food patterns which have been retained are of considerable importance in ensuring adequate dietary intakes. In the absence of locally obtained fish and meat it would be difficult to maintain adequate intakes of protein, calcium and iron, and in the case of Ahousat, vitamin A. Therefore, factors which adversely affect the availability of traditional foods or mitigate against their collection and incorporation into the diet may have a deleterious effect on nutritional status.

The availability of traditional foods, at this time, may be adequate for many families, but it merits some concern for those elderly, disabled, and widowed who are unable to hunt or to fish. For this group the relative inaccessibility of large food stores, the higher local prices, and the lack of storage facilities make adequate food supplies more of a problem, even with the availability of social assistance. It appears, on the basis of data obtained from the surveys at Ahousat and at Anaham that, in addition to the dietary problems characteristic of the entire populations, some distinctions may need to be made with respect to the dietary problems of particular subgroups within the native populations.

ACKNOWLEDGEMENTS

We wish to acknowledge the assistance of the following persons, primarily in the collection of dietary data: Miss Carolyn Ritchie, Mrs. Sharon Strachan, Miss Jan Bray, Miss Joan Henderson, Miss Joyce Nettleton, Mrs. Phyllis Macdonald, and Mrs. Beverly Lee. We are indebted to Mr. Bruce Graham for assistance in carrying out the field work and to Mrs. Pamela Fitzpatrick for data processing. Computer programs for analyzing survey data were developed by Mr. R. D. Meldrum.

We are particularly indebted to the chiefs and councillors of the Ahousat and Anaham Bands and to the personnel of Medical Services Branch (Pacific Region) for their co-operation in this study.

REFERENCES

1. Lee, M., Alfred, B. M., Birkbeck, J. A., Desai I. D., Myers, G. S., Reyburn, R. G., and Carrow, A.: "Nutritional Status of British Columbia Indian Populations I. Ahousat and Anaham Reserves." Report, Division of Human Nutrition, School of Home Economics, University of British Columbia, 1971, pp. 1-216.
2. Drucker P.: "The northern and central northern tribes". Bureau of American Ethnology, Smithsonian Institution, Washington, D.C., 1951, Bulletin 144.
3. Canadian Council on Nutrition: "Dietary Standards for Canada". Canad. Bull. Nutr., 1964, 6:1.
4. Food and Nutrition Board, National Research Council: "Recommended dietary allowances". Publication 1964 of the National Academy of Sciences, Washington, 1968.
5. Sinclair, D.: "Canadian food and nutrition statistics 1935 to 1965". Canad. Nutr. Notes, 1969, 25:109.
6. Moore, P. E., Kruse, H. D., Tisdall, F. F., and Corrigan, R. S. C.: "Medical survey of nutrition among the Northern Manitoba Indians". Canad. Med. Ass. J., 1946, 54:223.
7. Corrigan, C.: "Scurvy in a Cree Indian". Canad. Med. Ass. J, 1946, 54:380.
8. Vivian, R. P., McMillan, C., Moore, P E., Robertson E., Sebrell, W. H , Tisdall, F. F.,, and McIntosh, W. G.: "The nutrition and health of the James Bay Indians". Canad. Med. Ass. J., 1948, 59:505.
9. Pett, L. B. "Signs of malnutrition in Canada". Canad. Med. Ass. J., 1950, 63:1.
10. Best, S. C., and Gerrard, J. W.: "Pine House (Saskatchewan) nutrition project". Canad. Med. Ass. J., 1959, 81:915.
11. Best, S. C., Gerrard, J. W., Irwin, A. C., Kerr, D., Flanagan, M., and Black, M.: "The Pine House (Saskatchewan) nutrition project II". Canad. Med. Ass. J., 1961, 85:412.
12. Hawthorn, H. B., Belshaw, C. S., and Jamieson, S. M.: "The Indians of British Columbia". University of Toronto Press, 1960.
13. Dong, A., and Feeney, M. C.: "The nutrient intake of Indian and non-Indian School Children". Canad. J. Public Health, 1968, 59:115.
14. Cambon, K., Galbraith, J. D., and Kong, G.: "Middle-ear disease in Indians of the Mount Currie Reservation, British Columbia." Canad. Med. Ass., J., 1965. 93:1301.
15. Davis, A. E., and Bolin, T.: "Lactose intolerance in Asians". Nature, 1967, 216, 1244.
16. Gudmand-Hoyer, E., and Jarnum, S.: "Lactose malabsorption in Greenland Eskimos". Acta. Med. Scand., 1970, 186:235.
17. Leichter, J., and Lee, M.: "Lactose intolerance in Canadian West Coast Indians". Amer. J. Dig. Dis. In press.
18. Hegsted, D. M.: "Present knowledge of calcium, phosphorus, and magnesium." Nutr. Rev., 1968, 62:63.
19. FAO-WHO: "Calcium Requirements." WHO Technical Report, 1961, Series No. 230.
20. Committee on Iron Deficiency: "Iron deficiency in the United States". JAMA, 1968. 203:407.

Nutritional Status of British Columbia Indians

II. ANTHROPOMETRIC MEASUREMENTS, PHYSICAL AND DENTAL EXAMINATIONS AT AHOUSAT AND ANAHAM[1]

J. A. BIRKBECK , M.B., CH.B., MELVIN LEE , PH.D., GORDON S. MYERS ,.D.D.S., PH.D., and BRAXTON M. ALFRED , PH.D.

Anthropometric, physical and dental examinations on Ahousat and Anaham Indians revealed that stature and skeletal maturation for age in children was less than in Caucasian controls. Adults were also shorter and female obesity was prevalent. Physical findings were not striking, but dental and periodontal health was poor. Nutritional factors are probably of major causative significance.

IN A preceding paper (1) the results of a study of dietary habits and nutrient intakes of two British Columbia Indian populations were presented. During the survey, anthropometric measurements and physical and dental examinations were carried out. In this paper we present the results of those studies and attempt to relate the findings to the dietary data.

The studies were carried out at Ahousat, a Nootka Indian reserve on Flores Island, off the west coast of Vancouver Island, and at Anaham, a Chilcotin Indian reserve west of Williams Lake, British Columbia. The economy of Ahousat is largely dependent on commercial salmon fishing, and fish and other marine resources make a prominent contribution to the diets. Although the economy at Anaham is somewhat more varied, ranch work and guiding hunters are important sources of income. Wild game, particularly moose and deer, as well as fish, are important features of the diet.

The physical settings of the reserves, as well as the age and sex distributions of the resident populations and of the survey samples, are described elsewhere (1). Detailed data on all aspects of the surveys are presented in a report printed by the Department of National Health and Welfare (2).

Methods

Anthropometric measurements and physical and dental examinations were carried out on all persons who presented themselves for inclusion in the survey. This consisted of 248 subjects at Ahousat and 266 subjects at Anaham.

Anthropometry

The techniques follow those described in IBP Handbook No. 9 (3), and include standing height (without footwear), sitting height, weight (lightly clothed), arm circumference, head circumference, and triceps skinfold thickness (measured with Harpenden Skin

1. Supported in part by National Health Grant #609-7-263, University of British Columbia Research Grant #26-9666, and assistance from Pacific Region, Medical Services Branch, Department of National Health and Welfare.

Fold Calipers, Holtain Ltd., Pembrokeshire, Wales). For children too young to stand, supine length was substituted for standing height. Details of the methodology are not presented here as they are well described in the IBP reference cited.

A single posteroanterior radiograph of the left hand and wrist was obtained using portable equipment and non-screen film. Skeletal maturity was rated according to the method of Greulich and Pyle (4).

Physical Examinations

The examination was divided into (a) head and neck, (b) trunk, and (c) extremities and blood pressure, with one physician responsible for each area. This assured comparability within one survey, but not necessarily between surveys. Pre-survey instructions and frequent review of criteria minimized differences in judgement between surveys.

Interpretation of Data

Sorting and analysis of data was carried out with computer programs developed by Mr. R. D. Meldrum, using the University of British Columbia IBM 360/67 computer.

Results

Anthropometry

Standing heights and weights of Ahousat and Anaham residents 0-20 years of age, together with the Iowa standards (7), are shown in Figures 1 a-d, and 2 a-d. Table I shows standing heights, sitting heights, and weights for Ahousat and Anaham residents over 20 years of age.

Measurements of head circumference are not presented. Compared with the North American standards of Watson and Lowrey (8), all Ahousat residents under 20 years of age lie well within ±2 standard deviations of the mean. At Anaham males fall within the

Table I: Stature and Sitting Height of Ahousat and Anaham Residents 20 Years of Age and Over. Means and Standard Deviations are Given. Figures in Parentheses Indicate Numbers of Individuals Measured.

	Ahousat		Anaham	
	Men	Women	Men	Women
Stature (cm)	170.4±6.0 (36)	158.3±6.3 (45)	170.3±5.4 (36)	156.5±4.4 (55)
Sitting Height (cm)	92.3±3.3 (35)	85.7±3.3 (45)	90.2±4.7 (35)	83.6±3.1 (51)
Body Weight (kg)	79.61±10.58 (36)	65.60±13.37 (45)	70.67±15.70 (36)	65.83±11.33 (55)

Dental Examinations

All examinations at both reserves were carried out by two dentists. The condition of each tooth was recorded as deciduous or adult normal, decayed, missing, or filled, with the exception that the "missing deciduous" category was not used. Teeth and periodontal tissues were examined in order to assess debris, calculus, and periodontal condition. Illumination was by artificial light. The Simplified Oral Hygiene Index of Greene and Vermillion (5), and the Periodontal Index described by Ramfjord (6) were employed.

normal range, but younger females (under 6 years of age) lie below the mean, many by more than 2 standard deviations. In later childhood Anaham females are within the normal range.

Arm circumference data are not included here. When arm circumference is plotted against body weight (9) the regression lines follow the equations:

$Y = 0.216 \ x + 12.879$ (Ahousat males);
$Y = 0.196 \ x + 13.755$ (Ahousat females);
$Y = 0.217 \ x + 12.456$ (Anaham males);
$Y = 0.234 \ x + 12.253$ (Anaham females).

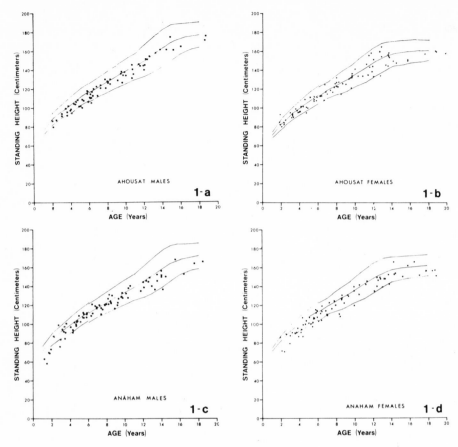

Figure 1a-d: Standing Height, 0-20 years. Standards (mean ± 2 standard deviations) Shown (7).

Table II presents the data for triceps skin fold thickness. Figures 3 a, b, show skeletal age plotted against chronological age for males and females at both reserves.

Physical Findings

Table III lists the frequency of occurrence of physical abnormalities at the two reserves.

Eye abnormalities were more frequent at Anaham, but in most cases were probably of environmental origin. One case of Bitot spots, and three cases of angular palpebritis were observed at Ahousat. All cases of Xanthelasma at both reserves had elevated cho-

lesterol levels, but several other individuals with equally elevated cholesterol levels did not exhibit Xanthelasma.

Lesions of the mouth and lips, and tongue changes were rare at Ahousat, but frequent at Anaham. Only 13 individuals at Ahousat (12 children, 1 adult) had tonsillar hypertrophy, but approximately half of the individuals at Anaham exhibited this condition. The influence of the seasons during which the surveys were carried out (early spring at Ahousat and early winter at Anaham) was not assessed.

No abnormalities of the nasolabial regions

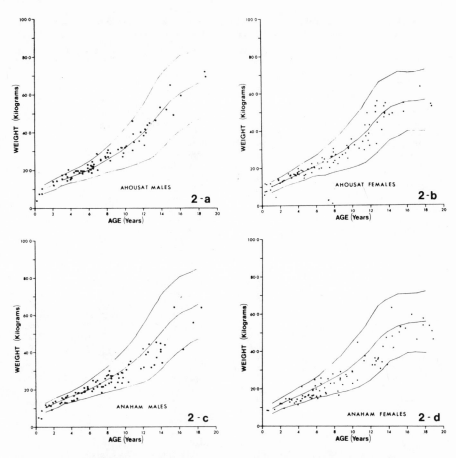

Figure 2a-d: Body Weight, 0-20 years. Standards (mean and 3rd and 97th centiles) Shown (7).

Table II: Triceps Skin Fold Thickness of Ahousat and Anaham Residents. Means and Standard Deviations are given. Figures in Parentheses Indicate Numbers of Individuals Examined.

Age (years)	Ahousat		Anaham	
	Males	Females	Males	Females
0-5	1.05±0.23 (20)	1.08±0.23 (31)	0.97±0.25 (28)	1.07±0.22 (21)
6-10	0.81±0.16 (33)	0.89±0.13 (32)	0.80±0.16 (36)	0.87±0.25 (35)
11-20	0.83±0.19 (21)	1.05±0.26 (31)	0.78±0.25 (23)	1.11±0.48 (27)
21-60	0.88±0.29 (29)	1.59±0.73 (32)	0.79±0.38 (26)	2.26±0.90 (46)
60+	0.81±0.18 (5)	1.16±0.64 (10)	0.84±0.46 (10)	2.23±0.66 (6)

Sign	Ahousat	Anaham	Sign	Ahousat	Anaham
1. Eyes			7. Neck		
Corneal scarring			Lymph glands:		
one eye	4	7	enlarged	86	2
both eyes	0	3	inflamed	0	0
Conjunctival:			Thyroid: palpable	1	0
injection	2	106	visible	0	0
pigmentation	2	25	8. Thorax		
thickening	8	14	Rib margins:		
Xerosis	0	12	beading	3	0
Bitot spots:			flaring	21	0
unilateral	0	0	Heart enlargement:		
bilateral	1	0	sounds:		
Xanthelasma	3	16	pathological	9	2
Angular palpebritis:			non-pathological	15	5
one eye	0	1	Lung field sounds:		
both eyes	2	1	abnormal	2	1
2. Lips			9. Abdomen and back		
Angular lesions:			Protuberant	58	5
mild	4	29	Hepatomegaly	4	1
severe	1	0	Splenomegaly:		
Angular scars	3	5	mild	0	0
Cheilosis	1	1	marked	0	0
			Scoliosis	7	0
3. Tongue			Kyphosis	0	0
Edema	0	0	Winged scapulae	42	1
Scarlet	2	2			
Purple	2	1	10. Extremities		
Atrophic papillae	2	17	Nails:		
Fissures:			spoon-shaped	1	0
mild	0	19	transverse lines	0	0
severe	0	0	Epiphyses:		
			enlarged	0	1
4. Throat					
Tonsils:			11. Skin		
hypertrophied	13	167	Hyperkeratosis	24	0
infected	0	0	Petechiae	0	0
Oropharynx:			Crackled	51	1
infected	0	27	Xerosis	12	7
			Infection	3	6
			Hyperpigmentation	1	7
5. Facial Skin			Acneiform eruption	1	3
Nasolabial seborrhea	0	0			
Xerosis	0	2	12. Lower limbs		
Pigmentation	2	15	Edema	0	0
Acne	0	0	Ankle jerk:		
			absent	3	0
6. Ears					
Infected: acute	3	0	13. Hair		
chronic	20	15	Easy pluckability	0	0

were seen. A few cases of chronic otitis were observed at each reserve. Cervical node enlargement was frequent at Ahousat, but not at Anaham. Visible thyroid enlargement was not seen at either reserve.

Rib flaring and beading were rarely seen at either reserve. A few cases of cardiomegaly were observed at both reserves, with only two or three cases at each reserve associated with pathological sounds. Abdominal enlargement

Table IV: Dental Findings at Ahousat and Anaham Reserves.

Means and Standard Deviations are given.

Age/Reserve Dentition	Males					Females				
	No.	Normal	Decayed	Missing	Filled	No.	Normal	Decayed	Missing	Filled
0-6										
Ahousat, Decid.	28	11.82 ± 6.85	5.00 ± 5.12		0	40	11.90 ± 6.67	3.92 ± 4.83		0
Perm.	28	0.36 ± 0.91	0.07 ± 0.26		0	40	0.35 ± 1.19	0.05 ± 0.32		0
Anaham, Decid.	36	11.61 ± 6.69	4.81 ± 5.62		0	33	12.97 ± 6.14	4.52 ± 4.48		0
Perm.	36	0.67 ± 2.28	0.22 ± 1.33		0	33	0.67 ± 1.47	0.09 ± 0.52		0
7-12 years										
Ahousat, Decid.	34	4.03 ± 4.91	5.26 ± 4.45		0.06 ± 0.24	36	2.39 ± 3.90	2.94 ± 3.48		0.06 ± 0.23
Perm.	34	10.74 ± 6.68	1.59 ± 2.18		0.85 ± 1.31	36	11.42 ± 4.91	3.17 ± 3.05		1.75 ± 2.10
Anaham, Decid.	33	4.28 ± 4.81	3.55 ± 2.93		0.27 ± 0.63	27	5.74 ± 4.58	4.07 ± 3.63		0.04 ± 0.19
Perm.	33	10.67 ± 5.42	1.06 ± 1.32		0.42 ± 0.90	27	11.52 ± 5.95	0.78 ± 1.19		0.59 ± 1.15
13-20 years										
Ahousat	14	16.50 ± 6.28	4.57 ± 5.65	1.29 ± 1.59	4.86 ± 3.51	20	14.00 ± 6.59	6.40 ± 4.85	2.90 ± 4.32	4.85 ± 2.76
Anaham	17	22.71 ± 3.12	1.65 ± 1.73	0.59 ± 0.80	1.24 ± 1.30	24	20.46 ± 4.35	3.54 ± 3.54	1.17 ± 1.20	2.92 ± 2.59
21-40 years										
Ahousat	18	9.38 ± 6.18	4.83 ± 3.78	15.94 ± 8.13	0.89 ± 1.23	24	4.79 ± 6.81	3.79 ± 4.54	20.92 ± 10.50	0.79 ± 1.61
Anaham	15	18.07 ± 8.95	4.33 ± 4.15	5.40 ± 6.82	1.47 ± 2.07	30	10.10 ± 8.19	9.33 ± 8.26	10.93 ± 10.71	1.00 ± 1.80
Over 40 years										
Ahousat	16	9.06 ± 7.21	1.69 ± 1.74	20.75 ± 8.54	0.50 ± 0.82	18	4.44 ± 5.46	1.44 ± 3.38	25.83 ± 7.14	0.28 ± 0.46
Anaham	20	15.75 ± 10.14	5.85 ± 5.17	9.85 ± 8.05	0.30 ± 0.66	23	7.70 ± 8.12	6.43 ± 7.77	16.00 ± 11.11	1.00 ± 2.98

27

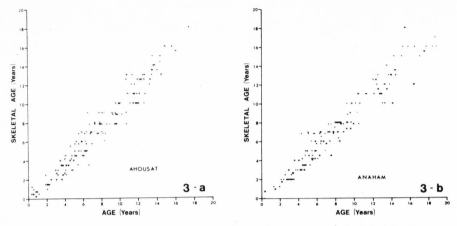

Figure 3a-b: Skeletal Maturity, 0-20 years. Standards (mean ± 2 standard deviations) Shown (4).

was infrequent at Anaham but common at Ahousat. As organomegaly was infrequent at both reserves, the abdominal protuberance was presumably due either to obesity or poor muscle tone. Scapular winging occurred in only one child at Anaham, but was very common at Ahousat. The nutritional significance of this finding is not clear. Skin changes, consisting of "crackled" skin and xerosis, were observed at both locations but more frequently at Ahousat than at Anaham. Rather than being of nutritional origin, they probably reflected poor cutaneous hygiene.

Blood pressure measurements were interpreted on the basis of WHO criteria (10) for "Probable Hypertension" (systolic pressure greater than 140 mm and diastolic pressure greater than 90 mm of mercury) and "Definite Hypertension" (systolic greater than 160 and diastolic greater than 100 mm of mercury). A few cases each of probable and definite hypertension were seen at each reserve, usually in older adults.

Dental Findings

Results of the dental examinations are shown in Table IV. Findings at the two reserves are not markedly different in the younger age groups (0-6 and 7-12 years of age). The relative infrequency of filled teeth in these groups, either deciduous or permanent, is apparent, as is the prevalence of decayed deciduous in the 7-12 year age group.

Among adult males the most striking feature is the very rapid increase, with age, in the numbers of missing teeth at Ahousat, a finding not paralleled at Anaham. A similar situation is observed among Ahousat females, who, by age 20-40 have an average of only 4.79 normal teeth each. Figure 4 shows the DMF indices at the two reserves, together with indices for Baltimore, Maryland, and for Blackfoot Indians from Montana (11). The DMF index at Anaham is similar to those of the reference populations, whereas the DMF index at Ahousat is distinctly higher, even at an early age.

Oral hygiene and periodontal indices are shown in Figures 5 and 6. It should be noted that Oral Hygiene Index increases rapidly among Anaham males and attains a value well in excess of those of Anaham females or of Ahousat males and females. Periodontal indices increase with age and are always higher for Anaham residents than for Ahousat residents. There is a marked deterioration of periodontal tissues among Anaham females during the early adult years.

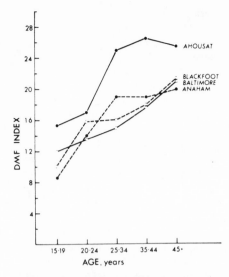

Figure 4: DMF Indices, Ahousat and Anaham Reserves. For Comparison, Indices are Shown for Residents of Baltimore, U.S.A., and for Blackfoot Indians, Montana, U.S.A. (10).

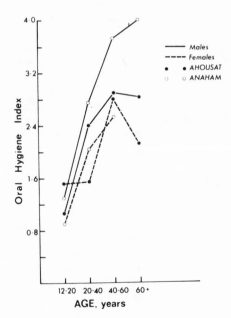

Figure 5: Oral Hygiene Indices, Ahousat and Anaham Reserves.

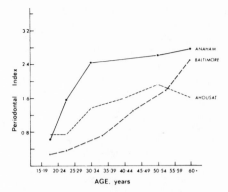

Figure 6: Periodontal Indices, Ahousat and Anaham Reserves. Baltimore Indices are Shown for Comparison.

Discussion

Anthropometry

Male children at Ahousat are taller for age than are male Anaham children, although both are shorter than would be expected from Iowa standards. The same trend is observed for female children, although the difference between the Indian females and the Iowa standards tends to diminish with increasing age. There is also a lag in skeletal maturity in the Indian children as compared to standards, and this, by prolonging the growth phase, might tend to lessen the potential difference in mature stature which would otherwise be anticipated from the data on children. However, it has recently been shown that notwithstanding this maturational lag, at adolescence skeletal maturity advances rapidly in such individuals and the statural deficit is not fully recovered (12).

Mean adult male statures at the two reserves were similar, but approximately 5 cm below the figure for North American Caucasians (13). Ahousat adult females were on the average 1.8 cm taller than their Anaham counterparts, although 6 cm below mean heights for North American Caucasian women.

On the basis of cross-sectional data, the delay in skeletal maturity does not appear to correct for their statural deficit. Although the ultimate mature stature of the Ahousat and Anaham children may be greater than that of the present adult population, this would only become apparent from longitudinal studies. There is no evidence that young adults in this study are taller than their predecessors. Any statural diminution with age is small and readily accounted for by the usual changes of aging alone (14,15).

Sitting height is a convenient measure of the relative contributions of the trunk and limbs to stature, and is best expressed as the ratio of sitting to standing height. There is evidence that increase in stature associated with improved environmental conditions is largely related to an increase in leg, rather than trunk, length. Unfortunately, suitable standards for sitting/standing ratio are not available. Both Indian groups showed sitting heights in children that were less than North American standards, although Ahousat values were proportionally greater in later childhood than in early childhood in both sexes. Adult values at Ahousat were larger, by approximately 2 cm, than those at Anaham.

Body weights of children lie within ±2 standard deviations of the Iowa mean. However, Ahousat weights, especially of females, are greater than those recorded at Anaham. Adult weight, in general, is not remarkable by North American standards, although a significant number of subjects are more than 2 standard deviations above the standard mean. No instances of serious underweight were observed.

Head circumferences of all children fell within expected limits, except for those of young Anaham females, where the values were low: the reason is not apparent. It is not justifiable to draw conclusions in the absence of longitudinal data, as skull growth is not complete by six years of age.

Although not the best criterion for estimating adipose tissue stores, triceps skinfold thickness is generally accepted as a useful measurement of adiposity, particularly in field studies. Values in Ahousat and Anaham

children are similar to those in the literature (16), although younger boys at Ahousat have larger values than do their counterparts at Anaham. In both communities older girls tend to lie below the expected mean.

Skinfold values of adults were similar to those of other North Americans (17,18). Ahousat men had higher values than did Anaham men, except among older subjects, where they were similar. Anaham women of all ages had substantially greater values than did Ahousat women, suggesting that notwithstanding weight data, adiposity is more prevalent among Anaham women.

These findings suggest that caloric excess, rather than insufficiency, may be a problem. The skinfold data are in agreement with the dietary data in that Ahousat males have a greater caloric intake than Anaham males, the reverse being the case for females. The small difference in skinfold thickness of males, despite a substantial difference in caloric intake, may be a consequence of greater energy expenditure at Ahousat. There is evidence then of a significant problem of obesity in certain segments of these populations. This is a significant problem, not only from the point of view of health, but also of physical performance. Nutrition education would be of value here.

Skeletal maturation of children was below the expected values for age. In boys the delay was greater at Anaham than at Ahousat, but in girls the delay was comparable. The delay appears to be proportionate at all ages, suggesting an origin in very early life. Unfortunately, too few teenagers were seen to establish the time of skeletal maturity.

The dietary data show that for most age groups protein intakes were substantially greater at Ahousat than at Anaham, although within acceptable limits (by Canadian standards) at both reserves. However, caloric intakes at all ages in childhood are lower at Anaham, often less than two thirds of the Canadian Dietary Standards, and dietary protein may be diverted to meet caloric needs rather than growth requirements. It is felt that this is the principal mechanism of the differences in growth patterns at Ahousat and Anaham, although genetic factors may also contribute to the differences. The two populations are genetically distinct, on the basis of blood groups and related data (19, 20). This problem will be examined more fully elsewhere (17).

While these child populations are not by current standards protein-deficient, it is undesirable that changes in their dietary pattern should be in the direction of more refined carbohydrate rather than improvement in the quality of the food and stabilization of fluctuating protein supplies.

In view of our evidence that the observed deficits in growth and skeletal maturation commence in early life, it is particularly unfortunate that breast feeding is rare in these populations, as this, particularly if associated with improved maternal nutrition during pregnancy, could have a salutary effect on child development.

Physical Findings

Physical signs commonly associated with nutritional deficiency or inadequacy were infrequently observed at both reserves and, when found, could reasonably be ascribed to non-nutritional conditions. This is not surprising in view of the dietary data (1) which show moderate frequencies of low nutrient intakes (less than two thirds of the Canadian Dietary Standards) only for calcium and vitamin A (and for iron among teenagers and adult females).

Physical signs indicative of nutrient deficiencies, are, in most cases, associated with relatively advanced degrees of the deficiency, conditions which do not appear to obtain at either Ahousat or Anaham. The absence of signs usually associated with either protein inadequacy or with deficiencies of B vitamins (thiamine, riboflavin, and niacin) is not unexpected, as the dietary and laboratory data document adequate intakes of these.

Signs suggestive of vitamin A or vitamin D deficiency were infrequently seen, and did not correlate with dietary or biochemical data on the same individuals.

General health status at Ahousat and Anaham was good; respiratory and skin infections, and other acute or chronic diseases, were uncommon.

Reliance on physical examinations as a method of assessing nutritional inadequacy where any deficiency is likely to be small, as was the case in this instance, is probably unwarranted. However, physical examinations may reveal the prevalence of conditions which might either be influenced by nutritional status, or may alter nutritional requirements or dietary patterns.

It must be recognized, however, that if "good health" is defined in the broader sense of well-being and ability to perform daily tasks without undue difficulty, and if "optimum nutrition" is defined as more than an absence of quantifiable nutritional deficiencies, then the lack of unusual physical findings in these communities does not necessarily indicate that poor nutrition is not present in the populations, but only that overt signs attributable to nutritional deficiencies were not present.

Dental Examinations

The dental and periodontal findings clearly demonstrate that early deterioration of teeth is extensive at Ahousat, even when compared with other native populations. Examination of individual data suggests that tooth loss begins at an earlier age at Ahousat than at Anaham, and is more pronounced at every age. This may, at least in part, reflect a tendency to remove rather than restore teeth even when damage is slight, instead of indicating early and extensive dental or periodontal deterioration. A contributing factor at Ahousat may be the relative isolation from urban centers where regular dental care is available. Poor dietary habits, as well as unsatisfactory oral hygiene and inadequate professional care, are important factors in the poor dental and periodontal situations observed in the two communities. The problem of decay and tooth loss at Ahousat is undoubtedly a reflection of the high consumption of refined carbohydrate and sugar as sweets and carbonated beverages; dietary recalls may well have underestimated the intake of these. These observations suggest that a combination of nutrition education and increased dental care services would be most beneficial in these communities.

Summary

Anthropometric measurements and physical and dental examinations were carried out at Ahousat and Anaham Indian reserves, as part of comprehensive nutritional status surveys. The principal findings were:

1. Among the children and adults at both reserves stature is less than would be expected from North American Caucasian standards, and there is a lag in skeletal maturity among the children. It is possible that these differences are related to differences in caloric and protein intakes. Underweight is not a serious problem. Triceps skinfold thicknesses indicated that adiposity is more prevalent among Anaham than Ahousat women. Other parameters tend to be within ±2 standard deviations of mean standard values.

2. Physical signs commonly associated with nutritional deficiency were infrequently observed at both reserves, and, when found, could reasonably be ascribed to non-nutritional factors. The usefulness of physical examination in nutritional status investigations of populations where dietary inadequacies are likely to be mild is considered.

3. Early dental deterioration is extensive at Ahousat but much less so at Anaham. On the other hand, poor oral hygiene and periodontal health appears to be more of a problem at Anaham than at Ahousat. Poor dietary habits, with an excessive intake of sweets and processed foods, may be one contributing factor although the excessive tooth loss at Ahousat may also reflect a lack of accessible dental care.

ACKNOWLEDGEMENTS

The authors are indebted to C. S. Gamble, M.D., L. Wyatt, D.D.S., N. L. Petrakis, M.D., and A. Thores, M.D. for assistance with the physical and dental examinations, and to Mrs. P. Fitzpatrick for assistance with the data processing.

We are particularly indebted to the Chiefs and Councillors of the Ahousat and Anaham Bands, and to the Pacific Region Office, Medical Services Branch, Department of National Health and Welfare, for co-operation and assistance with all aspects of the study.

REFERENCES

1. Lee, M., Reyburn, R., and Carrow, A.: "Nutritional status of British Columbia Indians. I. Dietary studies at Ahousat and Anaham." Canad. J. Public Health, 1971, 62:285.
2. Lee, M., Alfred, B. M., Birkbeck, J. A., Desai, I. D., Myers, G. S., Reyburn, R. G., and Carrow, A.: "Nutritional status of British Columbia Indian populations. I. Ahousat and Anaham reserves." Queen's Printer, 1971.
3. Wiener, J. S., and Lowrie, J. A.: *Human Biology, A Guide to Field Methods.* International Biological Programme Handbook No. 9, 1969, Blackwell Scientific Publ., Oxford.
4. Greulich, W. W. and Pyle, S. E.: *Radiographic Atlas of Skeletal Development of the Hand and Wrist,* 2nd edition. Stanford University Press, Stanford, 1959.
5. Greene, J. C. and Vermillion, J. R.: "The simplified oral hygiene index." J. Amer. Dent. Ass., 1964, *68*: 7.
6. Ramfjord, S. P.: "Indices for prevalence and incidence of periodontal disease." J. Periodont, 1959, *30*: 51.
7. Jackson, R. L., and Kelly, H. G.: "Growth charts for use in pediatric practice." J. Pediat., 1945, *27*: 215.
8. Watson, E. H., and Lowrey, G. H.: "Growth and Development of Children." 5th Edition, Year Book, Chicago, 1967.
9. Keet, M. P., Hansen, J. D. L., and Truswell,

A. S.: "Are skinfold measurements of value in the assessment of suboptimal nutrition in young children?". Pediat. 1970, *45*: 965.

10. World Health Organization: "Arterial Hypertension and Ischemic Heart Disease: Preventative Aspects." WHO Technical Report Series, No. 231, 1962, p. 97.

11. Interdepartmental Committee on Nutrition and National Defence: "Nutritional Survey of the Hashemite Kingdom of Jordan, 1962." Washington, D.C., ICNND, 1963.

12. Frisancho, A. R., Garn, S. M., and Ascoli, W.: "Childhood retardation resulting in reduction of adult body size due to lesser adolescent skeletal delay." Amer. J. Phys. Anthrop., 1970, *33*: 325.

13. Society of Actuaries: "Build and Blood Pressure Study." Society of Actuaries, Chicago, 1959, *1*: 255.

14. Trotter, M., and Gleser, G. C.: "The effect of ageing on stature." Amer. J. Phys. Anthrop., 1951, *9*: 311.

15. Miall, W. E., Ashcroft, M. T., Lovell, H. G., and Moore, F.: "A longitudinal study of the decline of adult height with age in two Welsh communities." Hum. Biol., 1967, *39*: 445.

16. Tanner, J. M., and Whitehouse, R. H.: "Standards for subcutaneous fat in British children. Percentiles for thickness of skinfolds over triceps and below scapula." Brit. Med. J., 1962, *1*: 446.

17. Parizkova, J., and Eiselt, E.: "Body composition and anthropometric indicators in old age, and the influence of physical exercise." Hum. Biol., 1966, *38*: 351.

18. Sloan, A. W., Burt, J. J., and Blyth, C. S.: "Estimation of body fat in young women." J. Appl. Physiol., 1962, *17*: 967.

19. Alfred, B. M., Stout, T. D., Birkbeck, J. A., Lee, M., and Petrakis, N. L.: "Blood groups, red cell enzymes, and cerumen types of the Ahousat (Nootka) Indians." Amer. J. Phys. Anthrop., 1969, *31*: 391.

20. Alfred, B. M., Stout, T. D., Lee M., Birkbeck, J. A., and Petrakis, N. L.: "Blood groups, phosphoglucomutase, and cerumen types of the Anaham (Chilcotin) Indians." Amer. J. Phys. Anthrop., 1970, *32*: 329.

Nutritional Status of British Columbia Indians

III. BIOCHEMICAL STUDIES AT AHOUSAT AND ANAHAM RESERVES[1]

I. D. DESAI , PH.D., and MELVIN LEE , PH.D.

The findings of the biochemical assessments of the nutritional status of British Columbia Indians indicate low hematological values among certain age groups which may be related to the insufficient intake of iron in their diet. Attention also needs to be drawn to the low levels of plasma vitamin C and vitamin E and to the high levels of plasma cholesterol which may reflect lack of certain essential food items and the quality and quantity of dietary fat and sugars consumed by these people.

I N THE course of carrying out comprehensive nutritional status studies at two British Columbia Indian reserves, blood and urine samples were collected for the assessment of biochemical parameters, employing currently acceptable methods. The biochemical measurements, when carried out together with dietary, anthropometric, clinical, and dental studies, offer an objective appraisal of nutritional status and general health.

The reserves selected for study were Ahousat, a Nootka Indian community on Flores Island, west of Vancouver Island, and Anaham, a Chilcotin community west of Williams Lake. The economy at Ahousat is largely dependent on marine resources, whereas the economy at Anaham, although more varied, is largely related to ranch work and guiding hunters.

Marine foods are prominent in Ahousat diets, whereas wild game, particularly moose and deer, makes an important contribution to Anaham diets.

The physical settings of the reserves, as well as the age and sex distributions of the resident and sample populations are described elsewhere (1), together with detailed survey data. The dietary studies and the anthropometric, physical, and dental findings appearing in the preceding two papers (2, 3) of this series will be considered wherever applicable for implications to the biochemical studies presented in this final paper.

Collection of Samples for Biochemical Analysis

Blood

Approximately 20 ml of blood was collected into vacutainer tubes containing an appropriate quantity of heparin. The tubes were gently shaken and placed in ice until the initial processing could be carried out.

Aliquots of whole blood were taken for hemoglobin and hematocrit determinations and the remainder of the sample was centrifuged immediately for separation of the plasma. After removing aliquots for ascorbic acid determination, plasma samples were placed in screwcap tubes, frozen immediately, and shipped to Vancouver by air express. Plasma samples were stored frozen, at −20°C until further analysis could be carried out.

1. Supported in part by: National Health Grant #609-7-263, University of British Columbia Research Grants #26-9666 and #26-9665, National Research Council Grant #67-4686 and assistance from Pacific Region, Medical Services Branch, Department of National Health and Welfare.

Urine

At the field laboratory, individual urine samples were collected in plastic cups. The volume was recorded and the sample was tested for pH, protein and glucose using Labstix.* Suitable aliquots were poured into collection bottles containing sufficient 1.0 N HC1 to bring acidity of the added specimens to a pH of 2 to 3. This was rechecked with pH paper after acidification. The urine samples were frozen and shipped to Vancouver where they were stored at $-20°$ C until ready for biochemical analyses.

Biochemical Methods

A summary of the biochemical methods used in this survey is presented in Table I.

centage distribution among Ahousat and Anaham subjects are presented in Figure 1. The mean plasma protein level for the Ahousat population was considerably lower (6.9 ± 0.4 g per 100 ml) than that for the Anaham population (7.5 ± 0.6 g per 100 ml). No difference was observed between males and females or between age groups zero to 13 and 13 and above in either of these populations. Although the incidence of deficiency in both populations was insignificant, the occurrence of "low" levels was frequent, especially among Ahousat subjects of all ages. Although the dietary data (2) are not consistent with the laboratory findings, the latter indicate that the overall state of protein nutriture at Ahousat is less than desirable but of Anaham

Table I: Summary of Biochemical Methods Used in the Indian Nutrition Survey.

Determination	Method
Total plasma protein	Biuret (4)
Hemoglobin	Cyanmethemoglobin (5)
Hematocrit	Micromethod (6)
Plasma iron and total iron-binding capacity	Modified Giovaniello et al. (4)
Plasma vitamin A and carotene	Macro Carr-Price (trifluoroacetic acid chromogen) (5)
Plasma vitamin E	Emmerie – Engel (7)
Plasma ascorbic acid	Semi-micro dinitrophenyl hydrazine (5)
Plasma cholesterol	Lieberman – Burchard (4)
Urinary creatinine	Picrate (4)
Urinary thiamine	Thiochrome (5)
Urinary riboflavin	Modified Slater – Morell (5)
Urinary N'-methylnicotinamide	Modified fluorometric (5)

Results and Discussion

The findings of the biochemical analyses of blood and urine samples are reported and discussed in the following section. Unless otherwise mentioned, the reference standards developed by the ICNND (5) were used for the interpretation of most of the biochemical measurements.

Evaluation of Protein Nutrition

Serum Protein

The mean plasma protein levels and per-

is satisfactory and reflects the contribution of their traditional diet consisting of fish and game meat.

Evaluation of Hematological Data

Hemoglobin

The mean hemoglobin levels and the percentage distribution among subjects at Ahousat and Anaham are summarized in Figure 2. In both populations the difference between males and females was obvious only in age groups 13 years and above, the females having lower hemoglobin values than the males. When compared with hemoglobin

---

*Ames Company, Division of Miles Laboratory, Rexdale, Ontario.

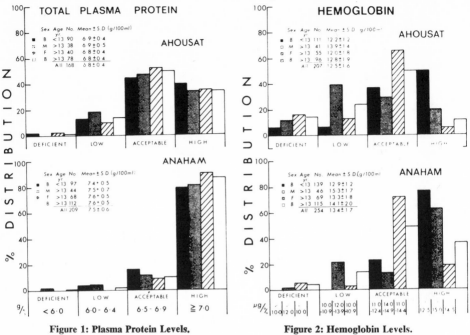

Figure 1: Plasma Protein Levels.

Figure 2: Hemoglobin Levels.

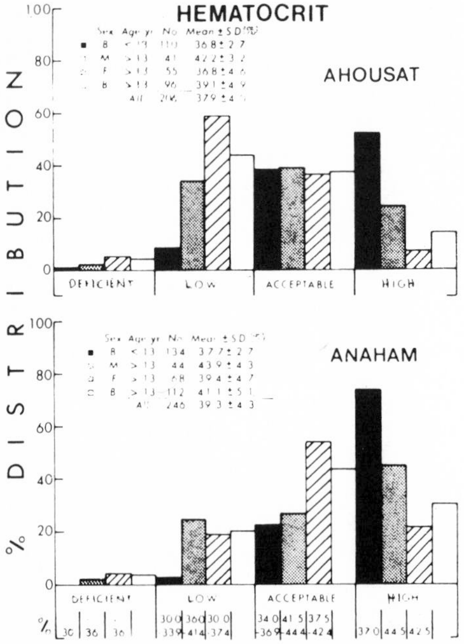

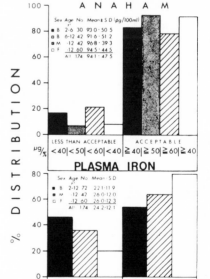

Figure 3: Hematocrit Levels.

Figure 4: Plasma Iron and
Transferrin Saturation.

values of 21,580 normal healthy Canadians, as compiled recently in a nationwide survey by Weatherburn *et al.* (8) it is noteworthy that for the most part the mean values for adult males and females at Anaham were similar to those quoted as "normal means" for average Canadians, but values at Ahousat were distinctly lower.

The percentage distribution as shown in Figure 2 further indicates that among the Ahousat population a large percentage of subjects, especially females above 13 years, had hemoglobin values which can be classified as "deficient" and/or "low", whereas among Anaham subjects no one below 13 years of age and only a small percentage of subjects above 13 years showed hemoglobin values in this range. It appears that the hemoglobin status of Ahousat subjects is less satisfactory than that of Anaham residents. A notable incidence of low levels of hemoglobin among Indian children in Ontario (9) and Saskatchewan (10, 11) has been reported in earlier Canadian studies.

Hematocrit

The mean hematocrit levels and the percentage distribution among Ahousat and Anaham subjects are presented in Figure 3. As in the case of hemoglobin, the mean hematocrits of Ahousat subjects, at all ages, were lower than those of Anaham subjects. In general the hematocrit values of both populations showed trends similar to those for hemoglobin, confirming the finding that hematologic indices of both Indian populations, and of Ahousat reserve in particular, are lower than those frequently quoted as "normal" for Canadians (8).

Plasma Iron and Transferrin Saturation

Plasma iron levels and transferrin saturation provide a relatively objective index of iron deficiency. Figure 4 shows the group means of plasma iron, total iron-binding capacity, transferrin saturation, and their percentage distribution among Anaham subjects.

The values for Ahousat subjects were, unfortunately, not available.

The percentage distribution of subjects into "less than acceptable" and "acceptable" categories was carried out according to the suggested guidelines of O'Neal *et al.* (12). It is apparent that although the group means for both plasma iron and transferrin saturation appeared "normal", there were many subjects with "less than acceptable" values. The percentages of "less than acceptable" levels of plasma iron were 16.7 for two to six year olds, 7.1 for six to 12 year olds, 21.4 for males above 12 years, and 8.3 for females above 12 years of age. The percentages of "less than acceptable" values of transferrin saturation were 45.8 for two to 12 year olds, 35.7 for males above 12 years, and 20.0 for females above 12 years of age. In considering these results, together with the hematologic data and the dietary results reported separately (2), it appears that a significant percentage of British Columbia Indians shows definite biochemical indications of anemia which may be related to low levels of dietary iron intake, resulting in low levels of plasma iron and transferrin saturation. It is difficult to state whether other factors, such as riboflavin deficiency (as suggested by Pett (9) for Indian children of Ontario), and/or vitamin E deficiency, or other vitamins related to hematopoesis may also be interrelated with the etiology of low hematological indices as seen among British Columbia Indians.

Evaluation of Vitamin Status
Plasma Ascorbic Acid

Mean plasma ascorbic acid concentrations and percentage distribution of values are presented in Figure 5. Means for the populations under study were 0.6 ±0.3 for Ahousat and 0.4 ± 0.3 for Anaham. Although the mean values were generally higher at Ahousat than at Anaham, averages for both populations were well within the "acceptable" or "high" ranges, according to the ICNND reference standard (5). This correlates very well with

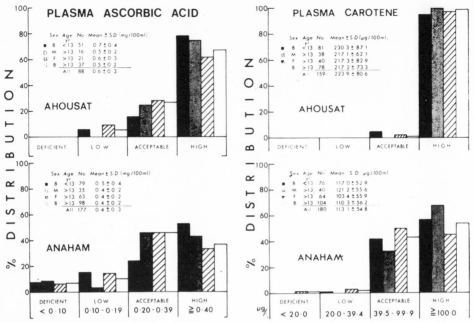

Figure 5: Plasma Ascorbic Acid.
Concentrations.

Figure 6: Plasma Carotene Values.

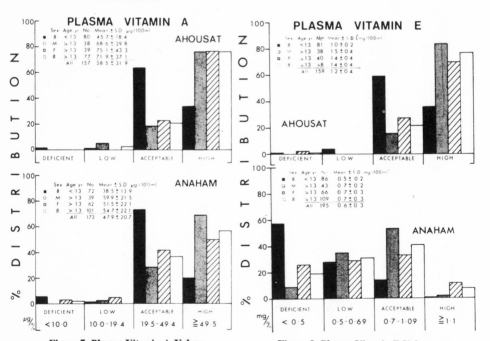

Figure 7: Plasma Vitamin A Values.

Figure 8: Plasma Vitamin E Values.

the dietary intakes which were found to be in excess of the Canadian Dietary Standards (13) for every group, the intakes at Ahousat being greater than those at Anaham (2).

At Ahousat there was no one in the "deficient" range and only about five per cent in the "low" range whereas at Anaham six to seven per cent were in the "deficient" range and 10 to 15 per cent in the "low" range. However, the overall status of plasma ascorbic acid in both of these Indian populations appears "normal". It is interesting to note that no definite signs of ascorbic acid deficiency were observed in similar studies with Alaskan Eskimos (14), Montana Indians (15), and Ontario Indians (9).

Plasma Carotene

Mean plasma carotene values and the percentage distribution of values among Ahousat and Anaham residents are presented in Figure 6. Most subjects were within the "acceptable" or "high" ranges as per the ICNND standard (5) and there appears no indication of any "deficient" or "low" levels of plasma carotene in either of these populations. Ahousat subjects on the whole have much higher plasma carotene levels than do Anaham subjects. Similar findings were observed among Fort Belknap Indians (15) where all plasma carotene levels were in the "acceptable" or "high" range. It is obvious, therefore, that the nutritional status with regard to plasma carotene among British Columbia Indians is satisfactory.

Plasma Vitamin A

In recent years there has been a considerable interest in assessing the plasma levels and body reserves of vitamin A among Canadians (16). Mean plasma vitamin A values and the percentage distribution of values in the two populations under consideration are presented in Figure 7. The mean plasma vitamin A concentrations, in μg per 100 ml, for Ahousat and Anaham were 58.5 ± 31.9 and 47.9 ± 20.7 respectively and are well within the "ac-

ceptable" or "high" ranges of the ICNND reference standard (5). Although the values for age groups below 13 years were slightly lower than for subjects over 13 years of age, there were no major differences between males and females at the two reserves.

The percentage distribution, as shown in Figure 7, further indicates that the incidence of plasma vitamin A deficiency in either population is of no great consequence. Ahousat had only 1.2 per cent and Anaham 5.6 per cent of the subjects under 13 years of age in the "deficient" range. Among those over 13 years of age, no one at Ahousat and only 4.0 per cent at Anaham had levels of plasma vitamin A within "deficient" range. The percentage of subjects with "low" plasma vitamin A concentrations was insignificant. These findings are in agreement with the dietary intakes of vitamin A which were equal to or greater than the Canadian Dietary Standards (13.) It appears that, except for a few individuals, the overall vitamin A status of the two populations is satisfactory.

Plasma Vitamin E

The percentage distribution of subjects into "deficient", "low", "acceptable" and "high" categories was based on information from population surveys (17-20), from human experiments (21) and on interpretations of Dr. I. D. Desai. The classification into these categories should be considered as reflections of dietary intake and as working guidelines to be modified as better evidence justifies. The mean plasma vitamin E levels and the percentage distribution of values are summarized in Figure 8. The overall mean at Ahousat was "high" (1.2 ± 0.4 mg per 100 ml) but at Anaham was "low" (0.6 ± 0.3 mg per 100 ml), one half that at Ahousat. These marked differences between the two reserves correlate well with their dietary intake of vitamin E (2). Plasma vitamin E levels increased with age but there is no difference between the levels of males and females at either reserve.

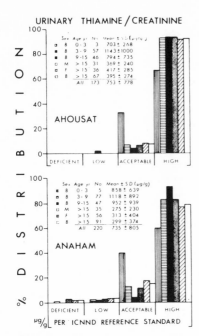

Figure 9: Urinary Thiamine Excretion.

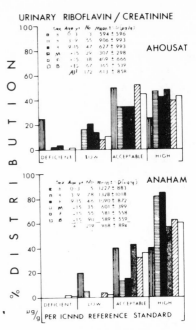

Figure 10: Urinary Riboflavin Excretion.

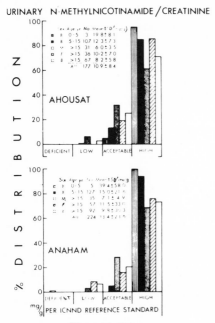

Figure 11: Urinary
N'methylnicotinamide Excretion.

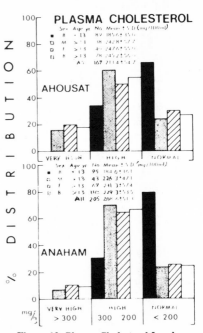

Figure 12: Plasma Cholesterol Levels.

It can be seen that while Ahousat had only about one per cent of all subjects in the "deficient" group, and four per cent under 13 years in the "low" category, Anaham had 57 per cent below 13 years, and 19 per cent above 13 years in the "deficient" group, and 38 per cent below 13 years and 31 per cent above 13 years in the "low" category of plasma vitamin E concentration. Whether this high incidence of low levels of circulating vitamin E (plasma concentration less than 0.5 mg per 100 ml), especially among Anaham children, has any relationship to dietary availability or some metabolic peculiarities, needs to be investigated. It is interesting to note that varying degrees of plasma vitamin E deficiency have also been observed in certain segments of the populations studied in England (22), Rochester (23), Holland (24), East Pakistan (18) and Central America (25).

These findings clearly point to the importance of extensive population surveys to establish more accurately the actual intake of both vitamin E and polyunsaturated fatty acids, in order to assess the adequacy and dietary requirement of vitamin E for Canadians in general and Canadian Indians in particular.

Urinary Thiamine

The mean urinary thiamine excretion per g of creatinine and the percentage distribution of values are presented in Figure 9. The mean values for Ahousat and Anaham populations were 753 ± 778 and 735 ± 805 mg respectively; very high by any standards. This correlates with the mean dietary intakes of thiamine which were two to four times the Canadian Dietary Standards (13) for every age group at both reserves (2). None of the values of Ahousat Indians was "low" or "deficient" by ICNND reference guidelines (5). A very small percentage (3-4 per cent) of the values was "low" or "deficient" at Anaham. As expected, the level of thiamine excretion in urine decreased with age. It ap-

pears from these results that the status of thiamine nutriture among these Indians is satisfactory.

Urinary Riboflavin

Mean values of urinary riboflavin excretion per g of creatinine and the percentage distributions are presented in Figure 10. Mean values at Ahousat and Anaham reserves were 613 ± 858 and 968 ± 894 mg respectively; "acceptable" or "high" by ICNND standards. This is understandable since mean dietary riboflavin intakes at both reserves (2) were one to three times the Canadian Dietary Standards (13). However, a comparison of percentage distributions indicates that 25 per cent of Ahousat subjects zero to three years of age had riboflavin excretion within the "deficient" range whereas none of the Anaham subjects in the same age group showed "deficient" urinary riboflavin excretion. Among subjects over 13 years of age only about one to 1.5 per cent showed "deficient" excretions. The percentage of subjects of various ages showing "low" excretions ranged from 10 to 21 per cent at Ahousat and two to 20 per cent at Anaham. Similar results were reported for Montana Indians (15).

Urinary N'Methylnicotinamide

In Figure 11 are presented the mean levels of urinary N'methylnicotinamide excretion per g of creatinine and the percentage distribution of values, according to the ICNND classification. Mean values for Ahousat and Anaham residents were 10.9 ± 8.4 and 13.4 ± 23.6 mg respectively; "acceptable" or "high" by any of the published standards. The dietary data documented mean niacin intakes of greater than the Canadian Dietary Standards in every group at both reserves by factors of three to five (2). As was the case for thiamine, the urinary N'-methylnicotinamide excretion decreased with age. The percentage distribution of values from both of these populations indicates that most if not all persons excreted "acceptable" or "high" levels of N'-methylnicotinamide; none were in the "deficient" category and very few (two to eight per cent) in the "low" category. These results are similar to those reported for Montana Indians (15) and Alaska Eskimos (14).

Evaluation of Plasma Cholesterol Levels

It is impossible to establish a single set of criteria for the interpretation of cholesterol levels in plasma. Levels in apparently normal people vary widely from place to place, depending on the dietary habit (26-30). In North America the average cholesterol concentration of men and women in the third decade is approximately 200 mg per cent. Consequently for the purposes of this report 200 mg per cent and values below that are defined as "normal", values between 200 and 300 mg per cent are defined as "high" and values above 300 mg per cent are defined as "very high". Although there may be differences of opinion as to the range of "normal" values, these categories will serve for analysis of the data.

Mean plasma cholesterol levels and the percentage distribution by age group are presented in Figure 12. Mean plasma cholesterol concentrations for all subjects at Ahousat and Anaham were 213.4 ± 54.7 and 208 ± 51.3 mg per 100 mg respectively. Those for children (below 13 years) were slightly lower than those for young adults and adults (above 13 years). The differences between male and female were very small. No one below 13 years at either reserve had "very high" levels (above 300 mg per 100 ml). Among subjects above 13 years, 18 per cent at Ahousat and about half of that (nine per cent) at Anaham had "very high" levels of plasma cholesterol. Furthermore, there were more subjects above than below 13 years showing higher than "normal" levels of plasma cholesterol at both reserves. The high concentration of plasma cholesterol may be a reflection of the high intake of animal fats

(2,29). Whether this has any correlation with coronary heart disease in these populations needs to be investigated. The only significant correlation of plasma cholesterol levels with other biochemical indices was with plasma vitamin E level. The significance and importance of the relationship between plasma cholesterol and plasma vitamin E is under active investigation in this laboratory.

Public Health Implications and Suggestions

The results of the biochemical studies reported in this paper have important implications which may need consideration from the public health aspect of some of the dietary and nutritional problems of the British Columbia Indians. The low hematological indices, as observed in certain age groups especially the teenage girls at both reserves and the adult women at Anaham reserve, provide biochemical and clinical evidence of iron deficiency anemia among these populations. The plasma iron and transferrin saturation values substantiate these possibilities. The dietary data presented in an earlier paper of this series (2) further confirm these findings in that the groups which showed low hematological indices also showed low iron intakes in their diet.

It is imperative that attention should be focused on increasing the iron intake of the teenage girls and adult women by dietary means (increased use of organ meats and legumes) as much as possible within the customary dietary habits of the Indians and by special iron supplements in form of dietary fortifications (enriched flour) or oral supplements. It should, however, be recognized that insufficient dietary intake of iron among certain age groups is also a public health problem of wide magnitude, among many non-Indian populations of North America today, and that it is becoming increasingly difficult to attain the recommended dietary allowances of iron through traditional diets.

Attention needs to be drawn to the low levels of vitamin C and vitamin E observed among Anaham subjects. In addition, high levels of blood cholesterol also warrant serious considerations to be given to the types of food items and the amounts of fat and refined sugars consumed in these communities. These are some of the areas in need of public health programs such as child feeding services and school luncheon for children; review of possible dietary fortification and enrichment practices; increasing the availability of fresh fruits and vegetables; and implementation of many phases of nutrition education to achieve improved overall health in these communities.

Summary

Biochemical assessments of nutritional status were carried out as part of comprehensive nutritional status surveys at Ahousat and Anaham Indian reserves in British Columbia. The principal findings are as follows:

Mean plasma protein concentrations of Ahousat and Anaham populations were 6.9 ± 0.4 and 7.5 ± 0.6 g per 100 ml respectively, indicating that the overall status of protein nutriture at Ahousat is less than desirable, while that at Anaham is "acceptable" by ICNND reference standard.

The hematologic indices of both Indian populations, and of Ahousat reserve in particular, are lower than those frequently quoted as "normal" for Canadians.

Although the overall biochemical indices with respect to plasma iron and transferrin saturation appeared "normal", at Ahousat a significant percentage of subjects had values which may be considered as "less than acceptable".

Although Ahousat subjects had higher levels of plasma ascorbic acid than did Anaham subjects, the overall status of plasma ascorbic acid in both Indian populations appears "normal" by currently accepted (ICNND) criteria.

Vitamin status with respect to plasma carotene, plasma vitamin A, and urinary excretion of thiamine and N'-methylnicotinamide appears normal and satisfactory at both reserves.

The urinary riboflavin excretion data indicate that there may be some incidence of ariboflavinosis among Ahousat children below three years of age. About 25 per cent of Ahousat subjects zero to three years of age were "deficient" and about two to 21 per cent of subjects above 13 years of age at both reserves were "low", according to the ICNND reference standard.

A large number of Anaham residents had levels of plasma vitamin E below 0.5 mg per 100 ml (low or deficient by our criteria). The overall plasma vitamin E status of Ahousat population is superior to that of Anaham.

A large number of residents above 13 years of age, at both reserves, had higher than "normal" (above 200 mg per 100 ml) levels of plasma cholesterol. Approximately 18 per cent of the people at Ahousat and nine per cent at Anaham had "very high" plasma cholesterol levels (above 300 mg per 100 ml). A significant correlation between plasma cholesterol concentration and plasma vitamin E level was observed.

ACKNOWLEDGEMENTS

The authors wish to acknowledge gratefully the competent technical assistance of Miss Ilse Borgen, Mrs. Charlott Myers, Mrs. Wendy Baldwin and Mr. Bruce Graham for laboratory analyses and of Mrs. Pamela Fitzpatrick for data processing. Computer programs for analyzing laboratory data were developed by Mr. R. D. Meldrum. Urinary creatinine and urea nitrogen analyses were kindly carried out by Mr. E. J. Hamilton, Laboratory of Hygiene, Department of National Health and Welfare, Ottawa.

The kind co-operation of the chiefs, councillors and volunteers of the Ahousat and Anaham Bands and of the personnel of Medical Services Branch (Pacific Region) is also greatly appreciated and acknowledged.

REFERENCES

1. Lee, M., Alfred, B. T., Birkbeck, J. A., Desai, I. D., Myers, G. S., Reyburn, R. C., and Carrow, A.: "Nutritional status of British Columbia Indian populations. I. Ahousat and Anaham reserves". A Report Printed by Medical Services Branch, Department of National Health and Welfare, 1970.

2. Lee, M., Reyburn, R., and Carrow, A.: "Nutritional status of British Columbia Indians. I. Dietary studies at Ahousat and Anaham reserves." Canad. J. Public Health, 1971, 62: 285.

3. Birkbeck, J. A., Lee, M., Myers, G. S., and Alfred, B. T.: "Nutritional status of British Columbia Indians. II. Anthropometric measurements, physical and dental examinations at Ahousat and Anaham." Canad. J. Public Health, 1971, 62: 403.

4. "Technicon Auto Analyzer Methodology." Technicon Instruments Corporation, Ardsley, N.Y.

5. "Manual for Nutrition Surveys", 2nd ed., Interdepartmental Committee on Nutrition for National Defence, Dept. of Defence, Washington, D.C., 1963.

6. Wintrobe, M. M.: Clinical Hematology, 6th ed., Lea & Febiger, Philadelphia, 1967.

7. Quaife, M. L., and Harris, P. L.: "The chemical estimation of tocopherols in blood plasma." J. Biol. Chem., 1944, 156: 499.

8. Weatherburn, M. W., Stewart, B. J., Logan, J. E., Walker, C. B., and Allen, R. H.: "A survey of hemoglobin values in Canada." Canad. Med. Ass. J., 1970, 102: 493.

9. Pett, L. B.: "Signs of malnutrition in Canada." Canad. Med. Ass. J., 1950, 63: 1.

10. Best, S. C., Gerrard, J. W.: "Pine House (Saskatchewan) nutrition project." Canad. Med. Ass. J., 1959, 81: 915.

11. Best, S. C., Gerrard, J. W., Irwin, A. C., Kerr, D., Flanagan, M., and Black, M.: "The Pine House (Saskatchewan) nutrition project II". Canad. Med. Ass. J., 1961, 85: 412.

12. O'Neal, R. M., Johnson, O. C., and Schaefer, A. E.: "Guidelines for classification and interpretation of group blood and urine data collected as part of the National Nutrition Survey." Pediat. Res., 1970, 4: 103.

13. Canadian Council on Nutrition: "Dietary standards for Canada." Canad. Bull. Nutr., 1964, 6: 1.

14. "An Appraisal of the Health and Nutrition Status of the Eskimo: Alaska." Interdepartmental Committee on Nutrition for National Defence. Dept. of Defence, Washington, D.C., 1959.

15. "Nutrition Survey, Blackfeet and Fort Belknap Indian Reservations." Interdepartmental Committee on Nutrition for National Defence and the Division of Indian Health. U.S. Public Health Ser., DHEW, 1961.

16. Hoppner, K., Phillips, W. E. J., Murray, T. K., and Campbell, J. S.: "Survey of liver vitamin A stores of Canadians." Canad. Med. Ass. J., 1968, 99: 983.

17. Bieri, J. G., Teets, L., Belavady, B., and Andrews, E. L.: "Serum vitamin E levels in a normal adult population in the Washington, D.C., Area." Proc. Soc. Exp. Biol. Med., 1964, 117: 131.

18. Rahman, M. M., Hossain, S., Talukdar, S. A., Ahmad, K., and Bieri, J. G.: "Serum vitamin E levels in the rural population of East Pakistan." Proc. Soc. Exp. Biol. Med., 1964, 117: 133.

19. Harris, P. L., and Embree, N. D.: "Quantitative consideration of the effect of polyunsaturated fatty acid content of the diet upon the requirements for vitamin E." Amer. J. Clin. Nutr., 1963, 13: 385.

20. Desai, I. D.: "Plasma tocopherol levels in normal adults". Canad. J. Physiol. Pharmacol., 1968, 46: 819.

21. Horwitt. M. K.: "Interrelations between vitamin E and polyunsaturated fatty acids in adult men." Vitamins and Hormones, 1962, 20: 541.

22. Leitner, Z. A., Moore, T., and Sharman, I. M.: "Vitamin A and vitamin E in human blood. 2: Levels of vitamin E in the blood of British men and women, 1952-7." Brit. J. Nutr., 1960, 14: 281.

23. Harris, P. L., Hardenbrook, E. G., Dean, F. P., Cusack, E. R., and Jensen, J. L.: "Blood tocopherol values in normal human adults and incidence of vitamin E deficiency." Proc. Soc. Exp. Biol. Med., 1961, 107: 381.

24. Engel, C.: "Vitamin E in human nutrition." Ann. N.Y. Acad. Sci., 1949, 52: 292.

25. Guzman, M. A., Arroyave, G., and Scrimshaw, N. S.: "Serum ascorbic acid, riboflavin, carotene, vitamin A, vitamin E and alkaline phosphatase values in Central American school children." Amer. J. Clin. Nutr., 1961, 9: 164.

26. Keys, A.: "Epidemiological aspects of coronary heart disease." J. Chron. Dis., 1957, 6: 552.

27. Epstein F. H.: "Epidemiology of coronary heart disease." J. Chron. Dis., 1965, 18: 735.

28. Brown, H. B., and Page, I. H.: "Lowering blood lipid levels by changing food patterns." JAMA, 1958, 168: 1989.

29. Hegsted, D. M., McGandy, R. B. Myers, M. L., and Stare, F. J.: "Quantitative effects of dietary fat on serum cholesterol in man." Amer. J. Clin. Nutr., 1965, 17: 281.

30. McGandy, R. B., Hegsted, D. M., Myers, M. L., and Stare, F. J.: "Dietary carbohydrate and serum cholesterol levels in man." Amer. J. Clin. Nutr., 1966, 18: 237.

Lactose Intolerance in Canadian West Coast Indians

Joseph Leichter, PhD and Melvin Lee, PhD

Lactose tolerance tests were performed on 30 healthy Canadian West Coast Indians and 16 non-Indians of Northern European extraction. Among the Indians, there were 7 males and 23 females, aged 14–24 years, with only 1 above 20 years of age (mean 15.8 years). The non-Indians consisted of 3 males and 13 females, aged 15–26 years, with only 2 above 18 years of age (mean 17.4 years). The tests revealed that of the 30 Indians, 19 (63.3%) were lactose intolerant on the basis of maximal blood glucose rise of less than 20 mg/100 ml above the fasting level after the lactose load. Gastrointestinal symptoms during or after the test were observed in 68.4% of the subjects with a flat blood glucose curve and in 18.2% of those with normal curves. In contrast, of the 16 non-Indians, only 1 (6.3%) was lactose intolerant, and none experienced abdominal discomfort during or after the test. Milk consumption among most of the Indian subjects seems to be low by North American standards, as judged by their past milk-drinking habits. The results suggest a high incidence of lactose intolerance among West Coast Indians during adolescence.

Within the past few years, several investigators have reported marked ethnic variability in the prevalence of lactase deficiency. Lactase deficiency seems to be particularly common among African and United States Negroes (1–6), Orientals (7–12), East Indians (7, 11–13), Greek Cypriots (14), Eskimos (15), Jews (16, 17), Filipinos (9), Australian Aborigines (18) and South American Indians (19). The incidence in these groups was found to be over 70% in adult populations. On the other hand,

Northern Europeans and persons of Northern European extraction exhibit a low incidence of adult lactase deficiency, probably not greater than 10% (4, 20–24). Most of the published studies on the incidence of lactose intolerance were on adults, but very few were on children and adolescents (4, 18). The results of Huang and Bayless (4) suggest a gradual increase in lactase deficiency in Negroes, with age, after weaning. The etiology of lactase deficiency in adults is unclear, and various possibilities have been discussed extensively by Simoons (25, 26). Gilat et al (16) have recently reported a high incidence of lactase deficiency in Jewish communities in Israel. They found no difference in lactase deficiency among the three major communities of European, Mediterranean and Oriental extraction, despite their obvious dietary and environmental differences over many centuries. Their findings therefore suggest a genetic etiology.

The incidence of lactose intolerance

Supported by National Health Grant 609-7-236 and NRC Grant A6249, Canada.

The authors wish to thank Father T. Lobsinger and the students at the Cariboo Student Residence, Williams Lake, British Columbia for their cooperation; and Dr. J. A. Birkbeck and Miss Ilse Borgen for their assistance.

among Canadian Indians has so far not been studied. The only published study on North American Indians was that of Welsh et al (5). However, only 3 adult Indians were included in the group.

The purpose of this study was to determine the incidence of lactose intolerance in Canadian Indian teenagers and to compare them with non-Indian teenagers of Northern European extraction.

MATERIALS AND METHODS

The studies were performed on 46 healthy subjects. There were 30 Canadian West Coast Indians (7 males and 23 females) and 16 non-Indians (3 males and 13 females) of Northern European extraction. The ages of the Indians ranged from 14 to 24 years, with only 1 above 20 years of age (mean 15.8 years). They were volunteers from the Cariboo Student Residence in Williams Lake, British Columbia. Most of the Indians included in this study originally were from the reserves near Williams Lake, BC. About 50% were from the Anaham reserve, the rest being from Soda Creek, Alkali Lake, Nazko, Canim Lake, Skwah and Kluskus. The ages of the non-Indians ranged from 15 to 26 years, with 2 above 18 years of age (mean 17.4 years). These were volunteers living in Vancouver, British Columbia. All subjects were free of gastrointestinal disorders and diabetes.

Lactose tolerance tests were performed in the morning, after an overnight fast. Venous blood samples were taken while the subjects were fasting, and at 15, 30, 60 and 90 minutes after oral administration of 50 g lactose dissolved in 330 ml of water with lemon flavoring. The subjects were asked if they experienced any symptoms from the administration of lactose during or after the test. A rise in blood glucose level of less than 20 mg/100 ml over the fasting blood glucose level was considered to indicate lactose intolerance. Blood glucose was determined by the glucose oxidase method (27). Analyses were performed within a few days after the lactose tolerance test.

RESULTS

Lactose tolerance tests (Fig 1) revealed that of the 30 young Canadian West Coast Indians, 19 (63.3%) were lactose intolerant on the basis of maximal blood sugar rise of less than 20 mg/100 ml above the fasting level after the oral lactose load. The lactose load produced symptoms in 13 (68.4%) of the 19 Indians with flat sugar curves, and in 2 (18.2%) of the 11 with normal curves. The symptoms included distension, abdominal cramps and, in 4 cases, diarrhea.

In contrast, only 1 (6.3%) of the 16 young non-Indians was lactose intolerant (Fig 1). None of the non-Indians, including the 1 individual with a flat glucose curve, experienced any abdominal discomfort during or after the lactose tolerance test.

Curves of the mean blood glucose rise over the fasting level at the various time intervals are given in Fig 2. The peak blood glucose levels occurred in the

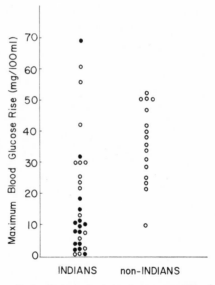

Fig 1. Maximum rise in blood glucose (mg/100 ml) over fasting levels during lactose tolerance tests (● — subjects reporting gastrointestinal symptoms during study, ○ — no symptoms reported).

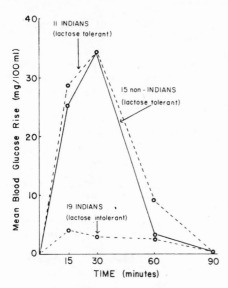

Fig 2. Mean blood glucose rise (mg/100 ml) over fasting levels during lactose tolerance tests. Indians are divided into lactose tolerant (glucose rise > 20 mg) and lactose intolerant (glucose rise < 20 mg). Non-Indian lactose intolerant individual is not included. Numbers refer to number of subjects.

30-minute sample and were identical (34 mg/100 ml) for both the lactose tolerant Indians and the non-Indians. In the 19 lactose intolerant Indians, the mean rise in blood glucose was 4.3 mg/100 ml (range 2.8–17.6) over the fasting level, and occurred in the 15-minute sample. The difference in the mean blood glucose rise over the fasting level between the lactose tolerant group (both Indians and non-Indians) and the lactose intolerant group was highly significant ($P < 0.001$).

The maximum blood glucose rise occurred within 60 minutes in all but 1 subject. Therefore, the omission of the 90-minute sample would have had no effect on the results.

An attempt was made to estimate past and present milk-drinking habits, but difficulty was experienced in obtaining accurate information. Recently, Lee et al (28) studied the nutritional status of Anaham Indians and concluded from the dietary survey information that intakes of milk were low compared with the rest of the Canadian population. It is, therefore, probable that the consumption of milk and milk products by the British Columbia Indians in this study was significantly lower than that of the non-Indian subjects.

DISCUSSION

The criteria for diagnosis of lactase deficiency include lactase activity of intestinal biopsies and the lactose tolerance test. Published results (1, 2, 16) indicate that there is a good correlation between the lactose tolerance test and lactase activity of the intestinal biopsy samples. Gilat et al (16) report that the peak glucose rise showed a better correlation (90%) with lactase levels than the presence or absence of symptoms due to the lactose load (80%). Therefore, the orally administered lactose intolerance test is reliable in the determination of lactase deficiency.

The results of this study indicate that there is a high incidence of lactose intolerance (63.3%) among adolescent British Columbia Indians and, in contrast, a low incidence of lactose intolerance among adolescent non-Indians of Northern European extraction. This is in agreement with the published study of lactose intolerance in 2 of 3 adult North American Indians (5), and with the low incidence of lactose intolerance among young and adult Northern Europeans and their descendants (4, 5, 20–24). The results of this study, together with other reports (1, 4, 18), indicate that the prevalence of lactose intolerance among certain populations is not restricted to adult individuals, but also occurs earlier in life. Huang and Bayless (4) reported that the incidence of lactase deficiency in healthy Negroes increases linearly with age. They found no lactose intolerance in 5 children who were less than 6 years old; in 15 children, 6–12 years of age, about 47% were lactose intolerant; in 18 subjects in the 18–24 years age group, about 70% were lactose intolerant; and in 10 subjects who were over 24 years, 100% were ·lactose intolerant. In contrast, the incidence of lactose intolerance in 34 whites remained reasonably constant over the corresponding age groups, averaging 17%. The incidence of lactose intolerance among the Canadian Indian teenagers and their Negro counterparts of the same age, in the study of Huang and Bayless (4), is strikingly similar. It would be interesting to find out whether this similarity also holds for the other age groups.

None of the lactose intolerant Indians in this study associated milk consumption with gastrointestinal disturbances. This is probably due to the fact that lactase content among lactose intolerant subjects is greatly reduced but is rarely completely absent, and that milk intake among the subjects studied rarely exceeded one glass at any one time. The incidence of lactose intolerance seemed to be equally common among males and females.

The studies of lactose intolerance among the various ethnic groups are not only of theoretical importance but have also some practical value in relation to public health nutrition education programs, as the condition is recognized to be common in some populations and uncommon in others.

It is interesting to note that the survival rations recommended by the Survival at Sea Sub-Committee of the British Royal Naval Personnel Research Committee (29) contain condensed sweet milk. In lactase deficient subjects, this may cause diarrhea and, as a result, dehydration where water is so essential for survival at sea.

Condon et al (30) recently investigated the effect of lactose on calcium and phosphorous balance in lactose tolerant and intolerant patients. Their results suggest that lactose may induce a negative calcium balance in lactase deficient subjects. This may become a factor in the production of osteoporosis.

REFERENCES

1. Bayless TM, Rosensweig NS: A racial difference in incidence of lactase deficiency. JAMA 197:968–972, 1966
2. Cook GC, Kajubi SK: Tribal incidence of lactase deficiency in Uganda. Lancet 1: 726–729, 1966
3. Cuatrecasas P, Lockwood DH, Caldwell JR: Lactase deficiency in the adult. Lancet 1: 14–18, 1965
4. Huang SS, Bayless TM: Lactose intolerance in healthy children. New Eng J Med 276: 1283–1287, 1967
5. Welsh JD. Rohrer V, Knudsen KB, et al: Isolated lactase deficiency. Arch Intern Med 120:261–269, 1967
6. Littman A, Cady AB, Rhodes J: Lactase and other disaccharidase deficiencies in a hospital population. Israel J Med Sci 4: 110–116, 1968
7. Davis AE, Bolin T: Lactose intolerance in Asians. Nature 216:1244–1245, 1967
8. Chung MH, McGill DB: Lactase deficiency in Orientals. Gastroenterology 54:225–226, 1968
9. Huang SS, Bayless TM: Milk and lactose intolerance in healthy Orientals. Science 160:83–84, 1968
10. Calloway DH, Murphy EL, Bauer D; Determination of lactose intolerance by breath analysis. Amer J Dig Dis 14:811–815. 1969
11. Bolin TD, Davis AE: Asian lactose intolerance and its relationship to intake of lactose. Nature 222:382–383, 1969
12. Bryant GD, Chu YK, Lovitt R: Incidence

and etiology of lactose intolerance. Med J Austral 1:1285–1288, 1970

13. Murthy MS, Haworth JC: Intestinal lactase deficiency among East Indians. Amer J Gastroent 53:246–251, 1970

14. McMichael HB, Webb J, Dawson AM: Jejunal disaccharidases and some observations on the cause of lactase deficiency. Brit Med J 2:1037–1041, 1966

15. Gudmand-Hoyer E, Jarnum S: Lactose malabsorption in Greenland Eskimos. Acta Med Scand 186:235–237, 1969

16. Gilat T, Kuhn R, Gelman E, et al: Lactase deficiency in Jewish communities in Israel. Amer J Dig Dis 15:895–904, 1970

17. Rozen P, Shafrir E: Behavior of serum free fatty acids and glucose during lactose tolerance tests. Israel J Med Sci 4:100–109, 1968

18. Elliot RB, Maxwell GM, Vawser N: Lactose maldigestion in Australian Aboriginal children. Med J Austral 1:46–49, 1967

19. Alzate H, Gonzalez H, Guzman J: Lactose intolerance in South American Indians. Amer J Clin Nutr 22:122–123, 1969

20. Newcomer AD, McGill DB: Disaccharidase activity in the small intestine: prevalence of lactase deficiency in 100 healthy subjects. Gastroenterology 53:881–889, 1967

21. Gudmand-Hoyer E, Dahlqvist A, Jarnum S: Specific small-intestinal lactase deficiency in adults. Scand J Gastroent 4:377–386, 1969

22. Jussila J, Isokoski M, Launiala K: Prevalence of lactose malabsorption in a Finnish rural population. Scand J Gastroent 5:49–56, 1970

23. Haemmerli UP, Kistler H, Ammann R, et al: Acquired milk intolerance in the adult caused by lactose malabsorption due to a selective deficiency of intestinal lactase activity. Amer J Med 38:7–30, 1965

24. Bolin TD, Morrison RM, Steel JE, et al: Lactose intolerance in Australia. Med J Austral 1:1289–1292, 1970

25. Simoons JF: Primary adult lactose intolerance and the milking habit: a problem in biologic and cultural interrelations. I. Review of medical research. Amer J Dig Dis 14:819–836, 1969

26. Simoons JF: Primary adult lactose intolerance and the milking habit: a problem in biologic and cultural interrelations. II. A culture historical hypothesis. Amer J Dig Dis 15:695–710, 1970

27. Raabo E, Terkildsen TC: On the enzymatic determination of blood glucose. Scand J Clin Lab Invest 12:402–407, 1960

28. Lee M, Reyburn R, Carrow A: Nutritional status of British Columbia Indians. I. Dietary studies at Ahousat and Anaham reserves. Canad J Public Health (in press)

29. Nicholl GWR: Survival at Sea. London, Aldrad Coles Limited, 1960, p 142

30. Condon JR, Nassim JR, Millard FJC, et al: Calcium and phosphorous metabolism in relation to lactose tolerance. Lancet 1:1027–1029, 1970

49

A MULTIPHASIC HEALTH SCREENING OF THREE SOUTHERN CALIFORNIAN INDIAN RESERVATIONS

CORINNE S. WOOD

Abstract—A multi-phasic health screening study on 96 Indians from southern California reservations is reported. Blood samples were run through a sequential multiple analyzer to determine 12 biochemical levels. Complete blood counts and urinalyses were performed and preliminary nutritional data were collected.

Twelve elevated levels of true glucose, 16 abnormal lactic dehydrogenase, 4 alkaline phosphatases and 3 total bilirubins were found. A high rate of eosinophilia, a slight leucocytosis, and a significant degree of urinary tract infections is reported. Nutritional data revealed an absence of Vitamin C in the diet, plus an excessive commitment to starches with a correspondingly high degree of obesity.

NINETY SIX Cauhilla and Luiseno Indians, residents of the Morongo, Soboba and San Manuel Indian Reservations of Southern California participated in a multiphasic health screening study conducted by members of the Anthropology Department of the University of California, Riverside. The population examined consisted of 35 males and 61 females with a diverse age distribution.

The initial requests for screening came from concerned members of the reservations. Their primary interest was to discover hidden cases of diabetes mellitus, a condition believed by many Indians to be present to a marked degree and reported as extremely high in studies made of other Indian groups [4, 6, 8].

On each of the volunteers screening was conducted for hyperglycemia; the initial tests employed one drop of whole blood and "Dextrostix"* plus urine tests with "Clinistix".† In addition, approximately three ml whole blood were collected in fluoride-treated tubes from all adults and one-half of the children. These specimens were tested within six hours using a modified Somogyi–Nelson chemical procedure (see Appendix 1).

Thirty-five larger (20 ml) blood samples were collected and subsequently processed through a Sequential Multiple Analyzer‡ to determine the following data: cholesterol, calcium ion, inorganic phosphorus, total bilirubin, serum albumin, uric acid, blood urea nitrogen, blood glucose, lactic acid dehydrogenase, alkaline phosphatase, total protein and serum glutamic oxalacetic transaminase. Thus in effect, heart, liver, kidney, bone, muscle and other body functions were chemically screened.

On all but two of the subjects, complete blood counts were performed. These included hemoglobin and micro-hematocrit determinations, total leucocyte count, differential of

---

*Dextrostix and †Clinistix Reagent Strips. The Ames Company, division of Miles Laboratories, Inc., Elkhart, Indiana.
‡SMA 12/60: Technicon Corp., Tarrytown, N.Y.

100 white blood cells and platelet and erythrocyte examinations. Through this facet of the study it was possible to obtain indications of the presence of anemias, allergies, parasitic infestations and systemic infections as well as of hematological dyscrasias.

Eighty-six of the participants submitted urine samples which were examined for albumin, glucose, acetone content and the specific gravity and pH measured. The urinary sediment obtained by five minutes centrifugation at 1800 rpm was examined microscopically, 10 fields under low (10×) and 10 under high (44×) powers.

Each person was interviewed to elicit information concerning age and marital status; women were questioned as to the number of living children as well as known pregnancies; height, weight and blood pressure were measured. Nutritional data were gathered by requesting reports of the total food consumption for the 24 hr which preceded the testing.

RESULTS—BIOCHEMICAL ANALYSES

Twelve elevated levels of true glucose were found, two in children under ten years of age. A familial tendency toward hyperglycemia may have been operating in the cases of these two boys who are brothers and whose maternal grandmother and granduncle also revealed elevated glucose levels.

Lactic dehydrogenase (LDH) levels above normal range (described in Appendix 2) were found in 16 of the adults, out of a total of 33 analyses. The causes of these findings cannot be determined at this point; however, elevations of this nature are often a result of excessive red cell degradation, most commonly failure to separate cells from serum promptly, hemolysis and hemolytic anemias. Frequently, heart or liver damage may be the underlying cause.

Further suggestion of liver distress was indicated by concomitant elevated total bilirubin levels in three participants. The abnormal levels ranged from 1·1 to 16·0 mg per cent. In addition, four subjects had elevated alkaline phosphatase levels ranging from 18·2–28·0 King-Armstrong units. Levels of this degree are frequently associated with high lipid content, bone growth in youth or bone anomalies in adults and other conditions. Normal ranges for all the biochemical tests are listed in Appendix 2.

Two of the adults were found to have uric acid levels of 9·1 and 9·3 mg per cent, ranges which may accompany gout, diabetes, and many other conditions. Finally, there was one sub-normal calcium level, 7·6mg per cent and one elevated cholesterol level, 320 mg. per cent (See Appendix 2).

HEMATOLOGICAL FINDINGS

The chief finding revealed by the hematological examinations was a high degree of eosinophilia. Thirteen young people were found to have counts ranging from 8 to 24 eosinophils per 100 white blood cells (normal range: 0–7 eosinophils/100WBC). Eosinophils in the proportions found in these participants often correlate with minor parasitic infestations and/or allergic reactions.

Hemoglobin and hematocrit determinations as well as morphological examinations of the blood smears revealed no indication of any frank anemias. Each slide was examined under oil immersion (1000×) until 100 leucocytes were differentiated. Except for an occasional anisocytosis and a rare suggestion of target cells, erythrocytes and platelets were essentially normal. Three subjects exhibited occasional basophilic stippling—a not uncommon occurrence in Southern California—which could not be correlated with any further morphological anomalies.

51

Leucocyte studies revealed 13 slightly elevated counts (normal: 5–10,000 WBC/cc) with an occasional proportional increase of neutrophils in the differential analysis of 100 white cells. Half of these leucocyte elevations were found in conjunction with abnormal urinary findings. Urine analyses are discussed below. In addition, three of the differentials disclosed lymphocytes of aberrant appearance and two of the older participants showed questionable "smudge" cells, both of which conditions warrant more extensive hematological investigation.

RESULTS OF URINE ANALYSES

The macroscopic examinations of the 86 urine specimens gave results unremarkable except for six slight elevations of protein content and two positive glucose tests. The latter findings, incidentally, indicate the relatively greater sensitivity of blood testing for the presence of hyperglycemia; had the screening been limited to the urine "dipstick" technique usually employed in mass screenings, all but two of the actual and potential diabetic states discovered in this survey would have been missed.

The microscopic examinations of urinary sediment disclosed 20 persons, including six children under 12 yr old with conditions of their urinary tract requiring medical attention as indicated by the presence of more than 10 white blood cells in every high power field, varying amounts of red blood cells, occasional casts and increased numbers of bacteria [3]. Blood content in potentially menstruating women was discounted. As indicated above, many of these abnormal urine findings were correlated with elevated blood leucocyte levels.

Measurements of blood pressure levels were conducted on 60 of the Indian participants. Four adults were found to have slight elevations ranging from 150/130 to 178/120. Three of these subjects had been advised in the past by physicians that a degree of hypertension was present; however, during the period in which this study was being conducted, none of the participants was under medical care.

RESULTS OF THE NUTRITION STUDY

Nutrition information based on 24 hr total recall revealed a diet based largely on starchy staples and low grade meats but strikingly deficient in fruit and vegetable content. The luxury of the balance urged by nutritionists does not seem to be a part of the life of these people.

Since the majority of the participants live within a very limited income, with food supplies available only at a considerable distance from the reservations, the tendency is to purchase foods which "keep", "go far" and can be purchased in large quantities. These foods inevitably turn out to be beans, rice, macaroni, tortillas, etc. The high calorie content results in part from the use of multiple starch elements at one sitting—a typical meal consists of macaroni, cheese, beans and cornbread or tortillas, rice and beans. There is a marked tendency to repeat the same meal for lunch and dinner.

Variety over the period of a day is quite limited, 5 or 6 solid items constitute the average number of foods consumed for most of the people reporting. Starches represent 60–75 per cent of all foods eaten. In contrast with the starch items, total fruit and vegetable consumption averaged 5 per cent.

Fortunately, protein is eaten in large amounts, particularly in bean-based dishes. Meat is almost invariably ground beef served as hamburgers, tacos, tortillas, etc., plus frequent utilization of bacon, sausages, frankfurters and lunch meats. No participants reported having eaten fish; similarly, roast, steaks and other higher priced cuts of meat are conspicuously absent. Nevertheless, the high rate of protein consumption, such as it is, may be a relevant factor in maintaining the high hemoglobin level in what might otherwise be an anemia-producing diet.

The scarcity of fruit and vegetable items is particularly striking. No fruit whatever was reported by 71 persons, while a large number of the fruit which was reported was eaten by children who had purchased school lunches. The absence of a source of Vitamin C with no concomitant presence of physiological signs of a deficiency is difficult to explain. One possible source may be the consumption of large amounts of beer by many adults. A more extensive survey might reveal some factors acting as Vitamin C sources which are not disclosed in the brief time encompassed by this study.

The heavy dependency on starchy foods correlates with a high degree of obesity found in the adults. No obese children were seen. Using the Metropolitan Life Insurance Company scale for optimum weight-height-age-sex relationship, 45 adults, 86 per cent of those measured, were obese, ranging from 2–82 pounds overweight with the mean for women 37 pounds and for men 35 pounds above the maximum of the optimum range.

DISCUSSION

Unfortunately, it was beyond the scope of this study to investigate the cultural components of the diet described. That there is a strong emotional element was made obvious by remarks from several Indians who had been ordered in the past by their physicians to change their diets. Added to these were reports from members of the study who had been subjected to other diets in hospitals or other institutions. All had found the white man's diet intolerable.

An intensive study, such as that conducted by Cook [2] to investigate the role which food plays in the lives of the reservation-based Indian today would be extremely rewarding. Moreover, the possible correlations of the diet reported here with the high incidence of obesity, hyperglycemia, elevated lactic dehydrogenase levels and other conditions suggest that such a study should be done.

The high rate of hyperglycemia (12·5 per cent) discovered in this survey, compares favorably with the rates found by the studies listed on page 579 which deal with other Indian groups. In contrast, the authoritative text by Stanbury et al. [9] describes as "the most accurate attempt to evaluate the over-all incidence of diabetes mellitus the studies of Wilkerson and Krall [11] who tested 77 per cent of 4983 inhabitants of a New England community with an age distribution closely approximating that of the United States as a whole". They found a prevalence of 2 per cent, or a projected 1·7 per cent of the entire population of the town.

Additional references [7, 10] cite even lower projected incidences of diabetes for non-Indian U.S. populations. Whether there be a genetic factor operating among the Indians may be disclosed by more extensive studies. Certainly the wide discrepancy bears further investigation.

CONCLUSION

Subsequent to the completion of this study, it was found by the author and associates that no medical agencies were prepared to offer medical treatment satisfactory to reservation residents for the conditions which the survey had revealed. This is largely the result of the unique position of the California reservation Indian who exists in a medical limbo, having been severed in 1954 from Federal health facilities, yet having little or no replacement given by the agencies of the state to whom the health responsibilities were delegated.

Those conditions which warranted urgent medical attention had to be directed to the county hospital facilities which were often as far as 35 miles from the reservation, always required long hours in waiting lines and in innumerable ways exuded an atmosphere, humiliating to the Indian patients, of condescending charity. Consequently, contact was established with numerous governmental agencies and nominally responsible individuals, all of whom deplored the conditions disclosed by this study, admitted a need for remedial action and all of whom in turn suggested another agency or person to whom the information should be supplied.

As a result of the serious medical findings and the dearth of meaningful medical response, it is felt by the author as well as by many of the Indians involved that this report be considered a pilot study which points up the need for further screening and particularly reveals the need for critical reassessment of the responsibility of the medical community and concerned government agencies toward the Indian population of southern California.

Acknowledgements—The author wishes to express grateful acknowledgement to Lowell J. Bean, assistant professor of anthropology, Hayward State College for his invaluable advice and support; to Vivienne Jordan, R.N., Fidelia Salgado, L.V.N. and Dollie Sosa, L.V.N. for giving so generously of their time at all hours on the reservations; and to Diane Kagan, Judith Scher, Richard Lando and Robert Bettinger for technical assistance.

APPENDIX 1

Somogyi–Nelson method for determination of blood glucose*

(a) 1·0 ml whole blood mixed with an anti-coagulant lysed in 5 ml distilled water in large tube.

(b) 2·0 ml barium hydroxide (0·3N) added, mixed well by inversion.

(c) 2·0 ml 5 per cent zinc sulfate added; tube stoppered and shaken vigorously.

(d) After 5 min, solution filtered or centrifuged.

(e) Add 2 ml alkaline copper tartrate to water blank, glucose standard and unknown.

(f) Place each tube in boiling water for 7 min.

(g) Add 2 ml phosphomolybdic acid.

(h) Place in cold water for 3 min.

(i) Dilute to 25 ml with distilled water.

(j) Read per cent transmittance at 420μ

APPENDIX 2

Sequential Multiple Analyzer (Technicon Corp., Ardsley, N.Y.)
The Sequential Multiple Analyzer-12 channel (SMA-12) survey model is a system which automatically and sequentially analyzes an individual serum sample for the following:

---

*Modification of original method which appeared in *J. Biol. Chem.* 195 19, 1952.

Analysis	Normal range
Cholesterol	150 –300 mg%
Calcium ion	8·5– 11 mg%
Inorganic phosphorus	2·5– 4·5 mg%P
Total bilirubin	0·2– 1·0 mg%
Albumin	3·0– 5·0 mg%
Total protein	5·8– 8·0 mg%
Uric acid	2·5– 7·5 mg%
Blood urea nitrogen	10·0– 20·0 mg%
Glucose	65 –110 mg%
Lactic dehydrogenase	30 –120 Wacker units
Alkaline phosphatase	4 – 17 King Armstrong units
Serum glutamic oxalacetic transaminase	15 – 45 Karmen units

The analysis rate is 30 samples/hr. Blood serum samples of 2·5–3·0 ml. are used. Results are reported on a moving strip of pre-calibrated, tear-off recorder chart paper which is directly readable in concentration units. The entire system is calibrated by means of a standard solution containing all twelve of the components being analyzed (see Figs. 1 and 2).

APPENDIX 3

Desirable weights for men and women according to height and frame, ages 25 and over. Metropolitan Life Insurance Company: Statistical Bulletin, 40 3, 1959.

Men			
Height, in shoes (in.)	Weight in pounds (indoor clothing)		
	Small frame	*Medium frame*	*Large frame*
62	112–120	118–129	126–141
63	115–123	121–133	129–144
64	118–126	124–136	132–148
65	121–129	127–139	135–152
66	124–133	130–143	138–156
67	128–137	134–147	142–161
68	132–141	138–152	147–166
69	136–145	142–156	151–170
70	140–150	146–160	155–174
71	144–154	150–165	159–179
72	148–158	154–170	164–184
73	152–162	158–175	168–189
74	156–167	162–180	173–194

58	92– 98	96– 98	104–119
59	94–101	98–110	106–122
60	96–104	101–113	109–125
61	99–107	104–116	112–128
62	102–110	107–119	115–131
63	105–113	110–122	118–134
64	108–116	113–126	121–138
65	111–119	116–130	125–142
66	114–123	120–135	129–146
67	118–127	124–139	133–150
68	122–131	128–143	137–154

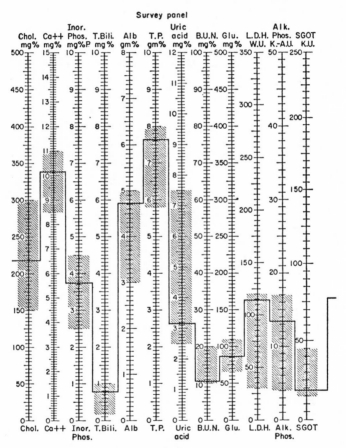

FIG. 1.   Example of normal SMA.

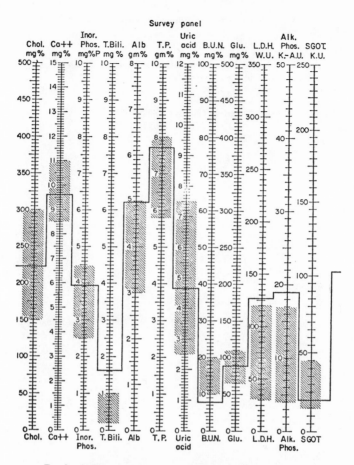

Fig. 2. SMA example demonstrating several abnormal values.

REFERENCES

1. BEAN, L. J. and WOOD, C. S. Crisis in Indian health. *Ind Hist.*, **2**, 29–32, 1969.

2. COOK, S. F. *The Mechanism and Extent of dietary adaptation among Certain Groups of California and Nevada Indians.* University of California Press, 1941.

3. DAVIDSOHN, I. and HENRY, J. B. *Clinical Diagnosis by Laboratory Methods*, pp 30–97. W. B. Saunders, Philadelphia, 1969.

4. JOHNSON, J. E. and MCNUTT, C. W. Diabetes mellitus in an American Indian population isolate. *Texas Rep. Biol. Med.* **27**, 110–125, 1964.

5. LEAVELL, B. S. and THORUP, J. *Fundamentals of Clinical Hematology.* W. B. Saunders, Philadelphia, 1966.

6. MILLER, M., BENNETT, P. H. and BURCH, T. A. Hyperglycemia in Pima Indians: a preliminary appraisal of its significance. Scientific Publication No. 165, W.H.O., 1968.

7. REMEIN, Q. R. A current estimate of the prevalence of diabetes mellitus in the United States. *Ann. N.Y. Acad. Sci.* **82**, 229, 1959.

8. REICHENBACH, D. D. Autopsy incidence of disease among southwestern American Indians. *Arch. Path.* **84,** 81–86, 1967.

9. STANBURY, J. B., WYNGAARDEN, J. B. and FREDERICKSON, D. S. *The Metabolic Basis of Inherited Diseases.* McGraw-Hill, New York, 1960.

10. THORNE, G. W. and FORSHAM, *Diabetes Mellitus in Principles of Internal Medicine,* edited by HARRISON, T. R., McGraw-Hill, New York, 1951.

11. WILKERSON, H. L. C. and KRALL, L. P. Diabetes in New England town: study of 3516 persons in Oxford, Mass. *J. Am. Med. Ass.* **135,** 209, 1947.

12. WINTROBE, M. *Clinical Hematology,* 4th ed. Lea & Febiger, Philadelphia, 1956.

58

Two Weight-Reduction Programs Among Southwestern Indians

MAURICE L. SIEVERS, M.D., and MARGARET E. HENDRIKX, R.D.

OBESITY is extremely prevalent among most American Indians. More than half of those over 15 years old from southwestern desert tribes—65 percent of women and 39 percent of men —exceed their ideal weights (*1*) by more than 25 percent. Since obesity is also considered a widespread health hazard in the general population, numerous methods of medically supervised weight reduction have been proposed. None has been highly successful, although most evaluations have extended for only a few months to a few years from the start of therapy.

This report compares the long-term results of two weight-reduction programs for overweight patients at the Phoenix Indian Medical Center. One group received conventional low-calorie therapy, and the other received an initial fasting program with subsequent conventional therapy.

The Phoenix Indian Medical Center is a referral hospital for more than 55,000 southwestern Indians from Arizona, California, Nevada, and Utah. It also is the primary medical facility for Indians from nearby reservations or communities. The tribal distribution of the patients at the center is Pima 35 percent, Apache 21 percent, Navajo 10 percent, Papago 9 percent, Hopi 6 percent, other southwestern tribes 16 percent, and nonsouthwestern Indians 3 percent.

Methods

Patients attending the diabetic or medical clinics of the center during 1963–68 who exceeded 125 percent of their ideal weights were offered an in-patient, weight-reduction program consisting of medically supervised fasting in a minimal-care unit for variable periods. Most of these patients entered the program during the early part of the investigation. The minimum study period was 18 months, and the maximum was 90 months. Selection was based on acceptance by the patients and availability of hospital space.

The duration of starvation was individualized. Although most of the patients in the fasting program (FP) participated for 2 or 3 weeks, a few fasted longer. Some interrupted the program

59

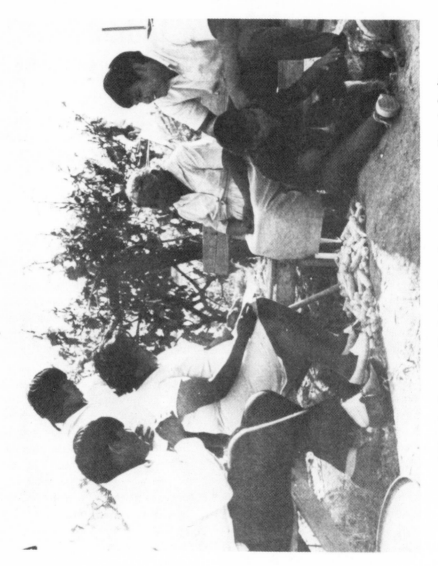

A typical Pima family group, illustrating the early onset and generality of obesity briefly with low-calorie meals, and a small number underwent repeated fasts. Following starvation, the patients were placed on conventional low-calorie therapy.

Most of the patients in the conventional management (CM) program were given dietary instructions for 1,500 calories a day or less. Anorectogenic agents were seldom prescribed; when given, they were generally used only for brief periods.

The patients were weighed, wearing their street clothes, at each clinic visit. Weights recorded during pregnancy, fluid accumulation, or debility, and, for the FP group, during fasting and the following 2 months, were excluded from the evaluation.

Patients were matched for the FP and CM study groups in order to evaluate the relationship of sex, age, initial weight, diabetic status, and treatment program to the long-term results. Criteria for the diagnosis of diabetes mellitus were those of most authorities, as described in a previous publication (2). The data were analyzed by the paired t test.

Results

Sufficient long-term information for this comparative study was available for 51 (12 men and 39 women) of the 71 patients who fasted, and they were matched with 51 CM patients. The average followup period for the CM group (71.5 months)

was 15 months longer than for the FP group (56.5 months). The diabetic patients had a longer mean evaluation (FP 65.2 months, CM 75.2 months) than the nondiabetics (FP 44.2 months, CM 66.3 months). The mean number of formal instructions per patient for diets of 1,500 calories or less was slightly more for the FP group (2.2) than for the CM group (1.6).

The two study groups were statistically similar in age and sex and identical in number of diabetics. However, since most of the extremely obese patients attending the clinics elected the FP, few patients of comparable weight were available for matching in the CM group. There were only three CM patients. in contrast to the 20 FP patients, who weighed 250 pounds or more. To exclude the influence of weight variations, data were compared for the 31 FP and 48 CM patients whose initial weights were less than 250 pounds, as well as for the 32 pairs whose disparity of initial matched weights was less than 10 percent (table 1). In both evaluations of patients with similar beginning weights, the final mean weights remained almost unchanged for the CM group but were significantly less for the FP group.

In table 2, the long-term weight changes are compared in three separate initial weight categories. The CM differences are insignificant in each weight

Table 1. Comparison between the fasting and conventional management programs of long-term weight changes among patients with similar initial weights

Program	Number patients	Mean weight (pounds)		Percent change
		Initial	Final	
Initial weight ≤249 pounds				
Fasting.................	31	212.7±33.4	197.1±31.9	[1] −7.3
Conventional............	48	208.1±29.7	208.6±30.0	+0.2
Matched pairs [2]				
Fasting.................	32	220.2±32.9	199.8±32.0	[1] −9.3
Conventional............	32	218.6±31.7	216.5±30.8	−0.9

[1] $P<0.05$; all other values not significant at 95 percent confidence level.
[2] <10 percent initial weight disparity.

Table 2. Comparison of long-term proportionate weight changes in the fasting and conventional management programs in relation to initial weights of patients

Initial weight (pounds) and program	Number patients	Mean weight (pounds)		Percent change
		Initial	Final	
≥250:				
Fasting................	20	272.3±16.5	241.0±30.2	[1] −11.5
Conventional..........	3	281.3±27.1	289.7±23.7	+3.0
200–249:				
Fasting................	24	222.4±12.9	206.3±25.1	[1] −7.2
Conventional..........	33	220.4±12.5	220.8±18.8	+0.2
≤199:				
Fasting................	7	183.1±11.1	174.3±15.7	−4.8
Conventional..........	15	181.1± 9.9	181.6±10.9	+0.3

[1] $P<0.05$; all other values not significant at 95 percent confidence level.

Table 3. Relationship of age to long-term weight change in the reduction programs

Age group (years)	Number patients	Mean weight (pounds)		Percent change
		Initial	Final	
≤29.....................	19	222.2±33.1	226.0±35.7	+1.7
30–49...................	67	227.3±32.5	212.6±35.2	[1] −6.5
≥50....................	16	213.9±35.7	206.0±25.2	−3.7
All ages.............	102	224.2±32.9	212.9±37.1	[1] −5.0

[1] $P<0.05$; other values not significant at 95 percent confidence level.

group. However, the FP percentage of weight loss was disproportionately greater for the highest (11.5 percent) than for the intermediate (7.2 percent) or the lowest (4.8 percent) weight category.

The yearly changes of mean weights are shown in figure 1. For each of the 7 years a much larger percentage of FP than CM patients weighed at least 5 percent less than initially. The long-term weight decrease was significantly greater for the 60 diabetics (5.9 percent) than for the 42 nondiabetics (2.6 percent). During the study, a progressively larger percentage of the diabetic patients weighed at least 5 percent less than originally, while the pattern for the nondiabetics was more variable (fig. 2).

As shown in table 3, a significantly larger proportionate weight loss ($P < 0.05$) occurred in the intermediate age group (30–49 years) than among the younger or older age groups. Additionally, about three-fourths of the age group 30–49 years had a long-term weight reduction compared with about one-half of the younger and older age groups (table 4).

Of the 51 FP patients, 42 attained long-term weight losses, while only 26 of the 51 CM patients achieved this result. Twenty pounds or more were gained by nine of the CM patients but only by two of the FP patients. In contrast, 23 FP and nine CM patients had lost 20 pounds or more. Nine FP patients sustained weight reductions of more than 45 pounds; one of these patients had lost 91 pounds and another, 83 pounds.

Although 41 percent of the FP patients attained a long-term reduction of 10 percent or greater, this result occurred among only 14 percent of the CM patients (fig. 3). One FP patient sustained a 40 percent weight reduction. A long-term gain of 10 percent or more occurred in 20 percent of the CM group but in only 4 percent of the FP group.

Table 4. Percentage of patients with long-term gain or loss of weight in each age group

Age group (years)	Number Patients	Long-term gain [1]		Long-term loss	
		Number	Percent	Number	Percent
≤29........................	19	9	47.4	10	52.6
30–49........................	67	17	25.4	50	74.6
≥50........................	16	8	50.0	8	50.0
All ages................	102	34	33.3	68	66.7

[1] Includes 1 patient with weight unchanged.

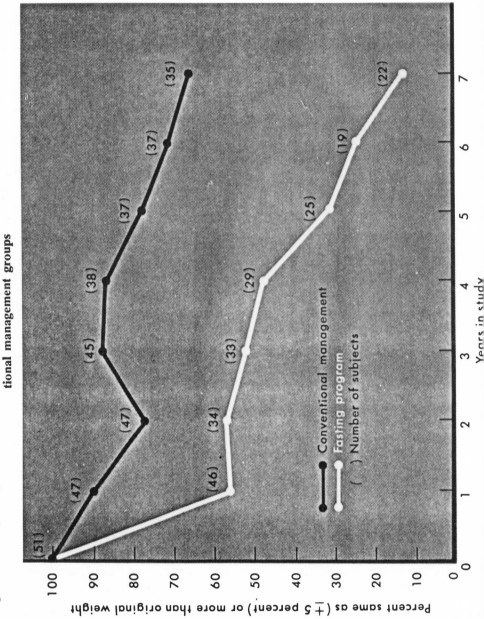

Figure 1. Yearly comparison of the proportionate weight change between fasting program and conventional management groups

Figure 2. Yearly comparison of proportionate weight changes in the diabetic and nondiabetic patients in the weight-reduction programs

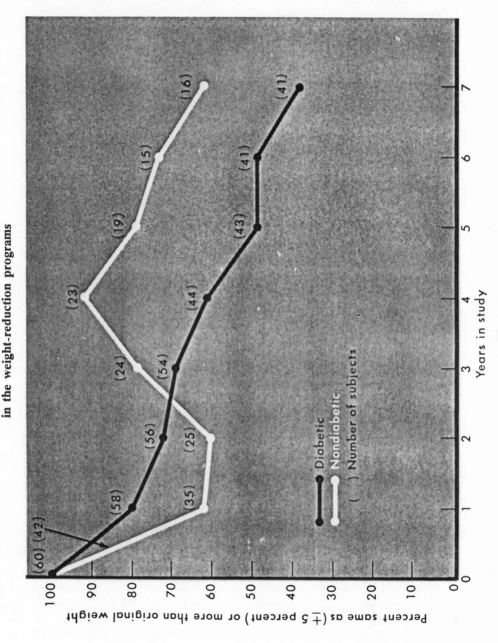

Discussion

In 1959 Bloom (3) reported that short periods of fasting at the start of treatment for obesity were effective and well tolerated. The risks are small if adequate selection criteria (4,5) are followed. Few clinicians used therapeutic starvation until Duncan and associates (6,7) published their dramatic results in 1962 and 1963. Thereafter, enthusiastic endorsement (4,5,8,9) was soon followed by reports that fasting removed less adipose tissue than protein (10,11). A recent study (12), however, found that man tolerates prolonged starvation by markedly attenuating protein catabolism, while deriving 95 percent of the caloric requirement from fat tissue. Although some limited brief followup studies of persons who had fasted were unfavorable (13,14), no long-term evaluations were reported.

In a 1959 review of nine studies of the conventional management program for obesity (15), 27 percent of the 1,468 subjects achieved an initial weight loss of 20 pounds or more. However, followup of 299 overweight persons in the evalautions by Stunkard and McLaren-Hume (15) and by Glennon (16) revealed that only 10 percent maintained a weight loss of 20 pounds or more beyond 1 year. Thus, conventional management of obesity attains limited success with the initial reduction and even less for the subsequent maintenance.

In the present investigation, 18 percent of the CM patients and 45 percent of the FP group had a weight loss of 20 pounds or more at an average followup period of 64 months. Therefore, the long-term results of conventional management among southwestern Indians were similar to those reported for other overweight groups, but the FP patients achieved a sustained weight loss of 20 pounds or greater about two and a half times as often as CM patients. Furthermore, the extent of long-term weight reduction was much greater for the FP patients than the CM patients.

Most of the FP patients—37 of the 51—underwent only one initial fast, which was usually concluded and its effects dissipated several years before final weight determinations were made. The major impact was short term. Most patients regained 15 to 30 percent of the lost weight within a few days or weeks of refeeding, and a few regained most of it within a few months. However, their subsequent weight pattern was generally more favorable than that of the CM patients. Perhaps fasting produced a durable physiological or psychological effect.

Hollifield and associates (17) demonstrated that prolonged fasting decreased the ability of human beings to synthesize fat, as shown by reduced incorporation of C^{14} labeled glucose into the

Figure 3. Comparison of percentage of long-term weight change between the fasting program and conventional management

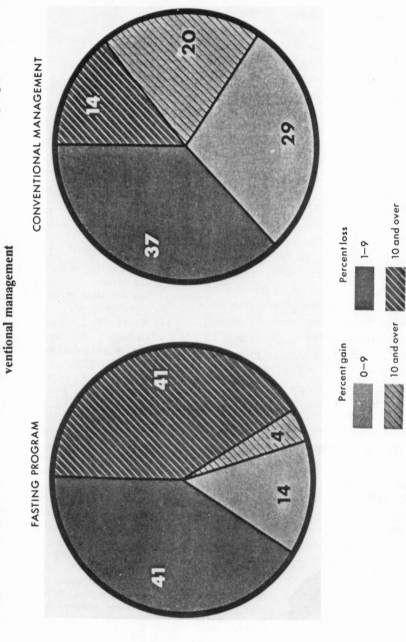

FASTING PROGRAM

CONVENTIONAL MANAGEMENT

Percent gain

0–9

10 and over

Percent loss

1–9

10 and over

NOTE: Figures in sectors are percentages of subjects.

lipids of adipose tissue. This reduced fat synthesis appears to result from an "atrophy" of the enzymes of the hexosemonophosphate shunt, since lowered activity of both glucose-6-phosphate (G6PD) and 6-phosphogluconic dehyrdrogenase (6PGD) were found in adipose tissue after fasting. If these fasting effects persist, they might relate to the long-term superiority of results from initial fasting compared with conventional therapy in the present investigation. However, in animal studies (18) refeeding restored the enzyme activity of G6PD and 6PGD as well as the lipogenetic capacity of fat tissue; and the periods of fasting and refeeding produced no apparent change in the number of fat cells.

After fasting, the amount of food intake required to produce a sense of satiety is smaller than previously (17). The hypothalamic satiety centers may become more sensitive or the appetite center may be depressed. Whether these effects of fasting on the satiety response are lasting or only temporary has not been established.

Perhaps the long-term potentiality of the FP may counterbalance its expense and inconvenience. The findings of this study suggest that the fasting program is most successful in the intermediate age group (30–49 years) of diabetic men who weigh 250 pounds or more. Therefore, clinicians may be justified in emphasizing the fasting program for such diabetics, as well as considering it for other well-motivated overweight patients.

REFERENCES

(1) Society of Actuaries: Build and blood pressure study. Chicago, 1959, vol. 1.

(2) Sievers, M. L.: A study of achlorhydria among southwestern American Indians. Am J Gastroenterol 45: 99–108, February 1966.

(3) Bloom, W. L.: Fasting as introduction to treatment of obesity. Metabolism 8: 214–220, May 1959.

(4) Stewart, W. K., Fleming, L. W., and Robertson, P. C.: Massive obesity treated by intermittent fasting. Am J Med 40: 967–986, June 1966.

(5) Mayer, J.: Reducing by total fasting. Postgrad Med J 35: 279–282, March 1964.

(6) Duncan, G. G., Jenson, W. K., Fraser, R. I., and Cristofori, F. C.: Correction and control of intractable obesity. JAMA 181: 309–312, July 28, 1962.

(7) Duncan, G. G., Jenson, W. K., Cristofori, F. C., and Schless, G. L.: Intermittent fasts in the correction and control of intractable obesity. Am J Med Sci 245: 515–520, May 1963.

(8) Drenick, E. J., Swendseid, M. E., Blahd, W. H., and Tuttle, S. G.: Prolonged starvation as

treatment for severe obesity. JAMA 187: 100–105, Jan. 11, 1964.

(9) Thomson, T. J., Runcie, J., and Miller, V.: Treatment of obesity by total fasting for up to 249 days. Lancet No. 7471: 992–996, Nov. 5, 1966.

(10) Laszlo, J.: Changes in the obese patient and his adipose tissue during prolonged starvation. South Med J 58: 1099–1108, September 1965.

(11) Benoit, F. L., Martin, R. L., and Watten, R. H.: Changes in body composition during weight reduction in obesity. Balance studies comparing effects of fasting and a ketogenic diet. Ann Intern Med 63: 604–612, October 1965.

(12) Felig, P., Owen, O. E., Morgan, A.P., and Cahill, G. F.: Utilization of metabolic fuels in obese subjects. Am J Clin Nutr 21: 1429–1433, December 1968.

(13) Ball, M. F., Canary, J. J., and Kyle, L. H.: Comparative effects of caloric restriction and total starvation on body composition in obesity. Ann Intern Med 67: 60–67, July 1967.

(14) Parsons, W. B.: Changes in serum cholesterol, beta-lipoproteins, cholesterol and triglyceride levels in hospitalized patients on zero-calorie diets. Circulation (supp. III) 33, 34: 24, October 1966.

(15) Stunkard, A., and McLaren-Hume, M.: The results of treatment for obesity. Arch Intern Med 103: 79–85, January 1959.

(16) Glennon, J. A.: Weight reduction—an enigma. Arch Intern Med 118: 1, 2, July 1966.

(17) Hollifield, G., Owen, J. A., Jr., Lindsay, R. W., and Parson, W.: Effects of prolonged fasting on subsequent food intake in obese humans. South Med J 57: 1012–1016, September 1964.

(18) Anderson, J., and Hollifield, G.: The effects of starvation and refeeding on hexosemonophosphate shunt enzyme activity and DNA, RNA and nitrogen content of rat adipose tissue. Metabolism 15: 1098–1103, December 1966.

Nutrient intake of Pima Indian women: relationships to diabetes mellitus and gallbladder disease

Jeanne M. Reid, M.S., Sandra D. Fullmer, M.S., Karen D. Pettigrew, M.A.,

Thomas A. Burch, M.D., M.P.H., Peter H. Bennett, M.B., M.R.C.P.,

Max Miller, M.D., and G. Donald Whedon, M.D.

Previous studies have shown that there is an extremely high prevalence of diabetes mellitus (1, 2) and gallbladder disease (3, 4) among the Pima Indians living on the Gila River Indian Reservation in Arizona. Diabetes in this populace is 10 to 15 times as frequent as in the general population of the United States and diabetes prevalence increases from approximately 3% in females aged 5 to 14 years to nearly 69% in those aged 55 to 64. In males, diabetes prevalence is somewhat lower, 3% in the 15 to 24 age group and 46% in those aged 65 to 74 years (1). Gallbladder disease is also much more prevalent in this population than in the predominantly Caucasian community of Framingham, Massachusetts (5). Prevalence of gallbladder disease is also higher in females than in males; at ages 15 to 24 the prevalence among women is 13% and increases to 73% in those aged 25 to 34. In males, the prevalence is 4% beginning at ages 25 to 34 and reaches a maximum of 68% among those 65 years and over (4).

The only previous published report on nutrient intake of southwestern Indians is that of Hesse (6); in that study, no attempt was made to determine relationships between nutrient intake and prevalence of diabetes mellitus and gallbladder disease. A preliminary diet study by Alice Hoover (unpublished observations) showed no significant differences in nutrient intakes of diabetics and non-diabetics.

A detailed diet survey of Pima and Papago Indian women was undertaken with the following objectives: *a*) to determine whether there is an association between dietary intake of selected nutrients and prevalence of either diabetes mellitus or gallbladder disease, and *b*) to ascertain whether dietary intake of some nutrient(s) changes with age among patients with and without diabetes mellitus or cholelithiasis in the following 10 years.

Methods

Study population

The Pima and Papago Indians have resided in the region of the Gila River in south-central Arizona for at least several centuries. This region is typical of the hot, dry Sonoran Desert of the southwestern United States. The Pima and Papago Indians are believed to be the direct descendents of the Hohokams, whose culture dates back to the beginning of the Christian era (7). These people are agricultural, as were their forebears who made an amazing adjustment to an unfavorable environment through the use of an extensive canal system for irrigation (8, 9). Pimas and Papagos are related tribes who speak different, but mutually understandable, dialects of the Piman language.

Before the arrival of the Spanish in 1687, the aboriginal crops were beans, maize, squash, and pumpkins. The cultivated crops comprised 50 to 60% of the total food supply, wild plants and animals constituting the remainder; thus, food gathering was absolutely necessary to supplement the inadequate crops. It is generally agreed that the predominant ancient food was mesquite beans, followed in order by saguaro fruit and cholla buds. Wild game constituted a valuable source of food and included javalina, deer, quail, dove, rabbit, and fish from the Gila River. Historical data show quite conclusively that tepary beans (white and brown) were grown by the Pimas at the time of the Spanish arrival. The earliest foreign crop to be

71

introduced was wheat. The principal crops today are cotton, barley, sorghum and grains, alfalfa, tepary beans, and more recently sugar beets and safflower. Melons, cabbage, pumpkins, onions, and carrots are grown in small quantities for home consumption (8). The scarcity of water is a limiting factor for family gardens. Water is not piped into all homes and often has to be carried 10 to 12 miles.

Damming the Gila River and periods of drought around the turn of the century resulted in a definite shortage of water on the Reservation, resulting in variable intervals of undernutrition. It was not until the 1930's, upon completion of the Coolidge Dam and the formation of the San Carlos Irrigation Project, that adequate food supplies have been available to all on the Reservation.

The older people still prepare traditional foods used by their ancestors, but younger people are eating more contemporary foods. Pinole, for example, a beverage from ground parched wheat, is consumed almost exclusively by the older people. The most marked changes in Pima food habits probably occurred in the past 20 years, principally when men left the Reservation to join the Armed Forces and acquired the food habits of the white man. When they returned to the Reservation, these newly acquired food habits influenced changes in family eating patterns.

The study population included all Pima and Papago women between the ages of 25 and 44 years living on the Sacaton Service Unit portion of the Gila River Indian Reservation. This age group would not have been affected by the periods of famine and drought. Limiting the study to women took advantage of the facts that females have a higher incidence of both diabetes mellitus and cholelithiasis, which would facilitate cross-sectional analysis and, as the survey was to be carried out by home visits made by the dietitians, women would be more readily accessible than men.

Dietary survey techniques

In our study, a method that would assess individual food consumption had to be used because we wished to determine if there was an association between an individual's dietary intake and the presence or absence of diabetes mellitus or gallbladder disease. We used a modification of the dietary interview technique developed earlier by Burke (10).

A short letter was written to each subject prior to a home visit to make them aware of our interest. Two Pima women assisted with the interview and served as guides and interpreters when necessary. Because they were well known members of the community, their help was invaluable in establishing rapport between interviewers and subjects.

Before the study began, several visits were made to the Reservation trading posts and to nearby grocery stores to determine what foods were available in the area and those most likely to be involved in the survey. Although prices are lower in the off-reservation stores than at the Reservation trading posts, the latter are a necessity for those families lacking transportation; and they are patronized almost exclusively by Indians.

Each subject was interviewed by one of two dietitians, neither of whom had prior knowledge of the subject's clinical status as to diabetes or gallbladder disease. As a background to more specific questions relative to actual intake, information was first obtained regarding food purchases, use of surplus food commodities, fuel used in cooking, physical activity, and other factors relative to nutrition. This information proved helpful in eliciting more specific data. Food models were used routinely to assist in determining the size and amount of each food eaten by the subject. The women were asked specific questions regarding food preparation. A valuable "crosscheck" was a food intake record of the previous 24-hr period.

Coding rules (assignment of arbitrary but logical food quantities) were established for use when subjects did not know the exact amounts of sugar, fats, milk, jelly, and syrup added to foods. These rules permitted the dietitians to interpret indefinite answers consistently. For example, addition of cream and sugar to coffee may be recorded in varying amounts by different interviewers; coding rules eliminated this possibility. Coding rules were also necessary for recording amounts and kinds of fats used in frying, an important procedure as fried foods were usually eaten daily. Because many of the dishes eaten are characteristic of these people, dietitians, with the assistance of Indian women, prepared these characteristic foods. In this way, the amounts and kinds of fats used in frying and of other ingredients used in food preparation were determined.

Twenty-eight subjects, a 10% random sample of the five districts of the Reservation, were re-interviewed independently by each of the two dietitians in order to assess reliability of the diet interview method. Signed-rank tests were used to evaluate differences between the initial and repeat interviews for 18 nutrients. Eleven of the repeat interviews were done by the dietitian who had not done the initial interview. Significant differences were found in 5 of the 72 comparisons made. Animal protein and magnesium intakes were significantly lower at the 5% level of probability in the repeat interviews by different dietitians. The remaining 17 subjects were re-interviewed by the same dietitian who had completed the initial interview. For one dietitian, fat intake ($P < 0.05$) and potassium intake $(P < 0.01)$ were significantly lower in the repeat interviews. For the second dietitian, the only significant difference was a lower starch intake $(P < 0.05)$ for the repeat interviews. As the number of significant signed-rank tests was small relative to the number of comparisons made, the interviews were judged reliable and consistent.

Two-hundred-seventy-seven subjects or 91% of the total population of women in the selected age group were interviewed. Of the 26 subjects not interviewed, three could not be located and 23 refused to be interviewed.

Data processing and statistical analysis

The individual dietary intakes were calculated with a digital computer. Intake of each food had been recorded in terms of frequency of consumption, i.e., how many times per day, week or month it was eaten; therefore seasonal variation in dietary patterns could be computed for each subject. For example, prepared cereal may have been eaten daily during the hot summer months, whereas hot cereal may have been eaten three times a week during the winter months. Provisions were made in the computer program to convert these items to a daily intake. Seasonal items such as fruits, vegetables, and desert foods were also converted to a daily figure.

Foods were divided into the following classes for ease of interviewing and coding:

1) Meats	8) Juices
2) Dairy products	9) Beverages
3) Fats	10) Soups
4) Breads and cereals	11) Desert vegetables
5) Desserts and sweets	12) Desert fruits
6) Vegetables	13) Dried beans
7) Fruits	14) Mixed dishes

Food groups were then subdivided so that a total of 216 items in the food table were coded and each item identified by a three-digit code. Intake from foods not included in the food table was hand-calculated and included with the input data for computation. Nutrient values of foods were obtained from Agriculture Handbook No. 8 (11), Food Values of Portions Commonly Used (12) and Home Economics Research Report No. 7 (13). For the many unfamiliar dishes, Pima women who worked in the clinic and the two guides were helpful in supplying recipes from which necessary calculations were made.

Calculations and summaries were made for nutritional components and their interrelationships. Statistical comparisons were made between subgroups of individuals by using t-tests and analyses of variance.

74

Clinical diagnosis of diabetes mellitus
and gallbladder disease

Records of the Sacaton Indian Hospital and the National Institute of Arthritis and Metabolic Diseases Southwestern Field Studies Section (NIAMD) were examined for evidence of diabetes and gallbladder disease. The diagnosis of diabetes was considered established if the individual had a venous plasma glucose levels of ≥ 160 mg/100 ml 2 hr after an oral 75-g glucose equivalent carbohydrate load. Only those individuals with either a hospital record of gallbladder surgery, a patient's history of having gallbladder surgery, or a hospital or NIAMD record of an abnormal cholecystogram (stones or a nonvisualizing gallbladder) were considered to have "definite" gallbladder disease. Those individuals without records were omitted from any analyses concerned with the presence of diabetes and gallbladder disease.

Results

General findings

Surplus food commodities are available to most who live on the Reservation, although they are not widely used; these include canned meat, white beans or split peas, peanut butter, raisins, rolled wheat, rice, yellow cornmeal, powdered skim milk, and lard. White beans, rolled wheat and cornmeal are generally unpopular items. The two most widely used foods in the Pima diet are beans (generally pinto) and tortillas; the latter are made from white flour, lard, salt, and water. They are either baked on an ungreased grill or deep-fat fried and called "popovers." Corn tortillas, popular with other southwestern tribes and Mexicans, are not consumed in significant amounts by the Pimas. Corn is eaten as a vegetable or is used for masa harina (ground corn paste) in making tamales. Other dried beans are teparies (brown and white), pinks, whites, limas, black-eyed peas, and garbanzos; kidney beans are generally disliked.

The most popular meats are beef, pork, and chicken; lamb and veal are never eaten. Organ and variety meats are considerably more popular than among white populations. Quail, dove, and rabbit are significant additions to the meat group if hunting is done by a member of the family. More oils and margarine are being used now than previously, but lard is still the predominant fat in use.

Fruits and vegetables are not consumed in large quantities. The most commonly used vegetables are green beans, corn, spinach, carrots, onions, and fried potatoes. During the fall and winter, citrus fruit is popular as well as economical. In the summer, melons are plentiful and popular. Canned fruits and vegetables are used more frequently than either fresh or frozen items.

Cakes, sweet rolls, and soft drinks make large caloric contributions to the Pima diet. Bread and rolls are purchased when tortillas are not available. Both enriched and unenriched flour are sold in large quantities; Pima women say that unenriched flour makes the best tortillas. Cake, pancake, and various other mixes are widely used. Self-rising flour is also sold in large quantities. Convenience foods such as instant potatoes, macaroni and cheese dinners, and gelatin desserts are popular.

Due to lack of refrigeration in many homes, milk is often of the canned evaporated type. Eggs are popular and are usually eaten at least once a day. Mild yellow cheese (Longhorn) is a frequent accompaniment of beans at the meal; consequently, this provides a valuable addition to calcium intake.

Desert fruits and vegetables, although well liked, do not make any significant contribution to the diet in the age groups of this study. For a short time in spring, if rain has been sufficient, "wild spinach" may be eaten by a few. Saguaro cactus fruit, cholla buds, mesquite beans, and squawberries are among the desert foods that are well liked but eaten infrequently.

Chili peppers, fresh, dried, powdered, canned and pickled, are a staple of the Pima diet. They are eaten separately as one would eat pickles or are included in a variety of dishes such as beans, stews, rice, or on tortillas. Only a few families grow them at present.

Nutrient intake

The mean nutrient intakes and interrelationships are shown in Tables 1 and 2. The mean caloric intake was 3,164 kcal/day. This is in excess of the allowances recommended by the National Research Council (16). The recommended calorie requirements for women in these age groups would vary between 1,600 and 2,300 kcal. Although the caloric intake was more than adequate, the percent of calories derived from protein, carbohydrate, total fat, saturated and polyunsaturated fat was comparable to the percent of calories available for consumption in the retail market in the United States in 1965 (Tables 1 and 2). The degree of saturation of

TABLE 1

Comparison of nutrient intakes of 277 Pima Indian women and the United States general population

Nutrients	Indians Mean ± SE	United States[a] Mean
Calories[b]	3,163.7 ± 55.8	3,160.0
Protein, total, g	89.4 ± 1.4	96.0
Animal	42.2 ± 0.9	65.3
Vegetable	47.2 ± 1.0	30.6
Fat, total, g	155.0 ± 2.9	145.0
Saturated	55.9 ± 1.1	53.9
Monounsaturated	70.0 ± 1.4	58.8
Polyunsaturated	19.7 ± 0.4	19.1
Carbohydrate, total, g	349.9 ± 6.8	374.0
Sucrose	64.3 ± 2.3	191.5
Starch	219.2 ± 4.7	182.5
Other	66.4 ± 2.3	
Calcium, mg	770.6 ± 18.9	961.0
Phosphorus, mg	1,393.2 ± 24.8	
Iron, mg	18.9 ± 0.3	16.5
Potassium, mg	3,790.1 ± 67.2	
Magnesium, mg	416.4 ± 8.0	340.0
Fluoride, mg[c]	2.36 ± 0.06	
Cholesterol, mg	489.2 ± 11.6	600.0

[a] See references 14 and 15. [b] Components may not add to total, due to rounding. [c] From water intake only. Fluoride content of foods is extremely uncertain, and no analyses of foods were made. Mean North American fluoride intake from foods is estimated to be 0.3 to 0.5 mg daily (18, 19).

TABLE 2

Percent of calories obtained from protein, fat, and carbohydrate among Pima Indians and the United States general population

Nutrients	Indians	United States[a]
Percent of calories from[b]		
Protein	11.5	12.1
Fat, total	44.1	41.0
Saturated	15.9	15.2
Monounsaturated	19.9	16.6
Polyunsaturated	5.7	5.4
Carbohydrate, total	44.0	47.0
Sucrose	8.0	24.2
Starch	27.6	23.1
Other	8.4	
Percent of carbohydrate from		
Sucrose	17.9	51.2
Starch	62.9	48.8
Percent of protein from		
Animal source	47.2	68.0
Vegetable source	52.8	31.9
Ratios		
Polyunsaturated/saturated	0.35	0.35
Calcium/phosphorus	0.55	0.64

[a] See references 14 and 15. [b] Components may not add to total, due to rounding.

dietary fat may be expressed as the P/S ratio, the proportion of polyunsaturates (P) to saturates (S). The P/S ratio (0.35) found was the same as that in the general United States population, although considerably lower than the recommended P/S ratio of either 1.0 or 2.0 (17).

The mineral content of the diets met the recommended daily intake for calcium and phosphorus. The adequate calcium intake was due mainly to consumption of Longhorn cheese and beans. Beans make a significant contribution to the calcium intake because they are eaten in large quantities. Milk is being used more now than in the past but is still not a favorite item. Fluoride intake was determined from estimated water consumption. The values for fluoride content of water were obtained by analysis by the Public Health Service. Fluoride content varied from 0.99 to 2.00 ppm. There are approximately

20 to 30 sources of water available on the Reservation. About one-half are community systems whereby water is piped into the homes; the remaining watering points are wells that necessitate transportation of water. Sixty-six percent of the subjects interviewed had water piped in from various community systems. These families had a consistent source of fluoride, whereas the remaining people obtained their water from different wells. One area had four wells to choose from, each well differing in fluoride content. The mean estimated fluoride intake from water of 2.36 mg daily was considerably higher than most household water supplies in the rest of the country (fluoride not added) where fluoride concentration ranges from a trace to 0.2 ppm (18). Standard food composition tables do not include fluoride content, as it varies widely in plants, even between samples of the same kind of food, due to air contamination, type of soil, season, and numerous other environmental conditions. Meat fluoride is low; in animals most fluoride accumulates in the skeleton. Most foods, with the exception of sea fish, contain only small amounts of fluoride (19). Normal mixed North American diets contribute about 0.3 to 0.5 mg fluoride daily (20, 21).

The mean magnesium intake was 416 mg/day, as compared with the recommended allowance of 300 mg/day. Beans are an excellent source of magnesium and iron, and it was not unusual to see beans served at two meals of the day. The iron requirements were met by an intake of 18.9 mg daily.

The cholesterol intake of 489 mg was not surprising; eggs, a popular item, were frequently eaten at a second meal of the day. The mean serum cholesterol of this group was 179 mg/100 ml (SD ± 46). Sievers (22) reported comparable serum cholesterols in Pima women of these ages, whereas Caucasian female controls had significantly higher serum cholesterol levels.

It was not possible to obtain an estimate of sodium intake. Although sodium content of water in this area is relatively high, the majority of women stated that they added salt to food after it was cooked. In our experience, less salt is used when it is added to cooked food as opposed to adding it during food preparation.

Subgroups determined by presence of diabetes, employment status, and district of residence were compared on selected nutrients by two-way analyses of variance. No first order interactions were found to be significant and no significant differences were found between the five districts for any of the selected nutrients.

There were 79 diabetics and 169 non-diabetics. The remaining 29 subjects had not been investigated and were therefore omitted from Table 3 and from any analyses con-

TABLE 3

Comparison of nutrient intakes of Pima Indian diabetics and non-diabetics

Nutrients	79 Diabetics	169 Non-diabetics
Calories[a]	3,070.8 ± 97.1	3,237.0 ± 74.2
Protein, total, g	90.0 ± 2.4	89.6 ± 1.8
Animal	42.5 ± 1.5	41.5 ± 1.2
Vegetable	47.6 ± 2.0	48.0 ± 1.3
Fat, total, g	153.4 ± 5.3	157.3 ± 3.8
Saturated	55.0 ± 2.0	57.2 ± 1.4
Monounsaturated	69.7 ± 2.6	70.8 ± 1.8
Polyunsaturated	19.5 ± 0.7	20.0 ± 0.5
Carbohydrate, total, g	328.9 ± 11.2	363.2 ± 9.1
Sucrose	48.7 ± 3.4	70.6 ± 3.1
Starch	214.2 ± 8.8	226.0 ± 5.9
Other	65.9 ± 3.4	66.6 ± 3.2
Calcium, mg	766.7 ± 32.8	773.2 ± 25.2
Phosphorus, mg	1,403.2 ± 43.5	1,396.5 ± 33.2
Iron, mg	19.3 ± 0.6	18.9 ± 0.4
Potassium, mg	3,879.2 ± 116.8	3,777.8 ± 89.6
Magnesium, mg	424.1 ± 14.9	416.9 ± 10.3
Cholesterol, mg	499.2 ± 20.5	486.6 ± 15.1
Mean percent desirable weight	166.9 ± 3.62	153.9 ± 2.25

Values are expressed as mean ± SE.   [a] Components may not add to total, due to rounding.

80

cerned with the presence of diabetes. The total carbohydrate ($P < 0.05$) and sucrose ($P < 0.001$) intakes were significantly lower in the diabetic group. The percent of desirable weight of the diabetics was significantly higher, 166.9%, among diabetics than among non-diabetics, 153.9% ($P < 0.005$), but there was no significant difference in caloric intake between the groups (Table 3).

TABLE 4

Comparison of nutrient intakes of Pima women working outside the home and nonworking women

Nutrients	83 Workers	194 Non-workers	Signif-icance
Calories[a]	2,869.7 ± 91.6	3,289.5 ± 67.5	0.001
Protein, total, g	85.4 ± 2.2	91.2 ± 1.7	0.05
Animal	47.0 ± 1.5	40.2 ± 1.1	0.01
Vegetable	38.4 ± 1.5	51.0 ± 1.2	0.001
Fat, total, g	139.2 ± 4.6	161.7 ± 3.5	0.001
Saturated	49.6 ± 1.7	58.6 ± 1.3	0.001
Monounsaturated	63.2 ± 2.3	73.0 ± 1.6	0.01
Polyunsaturated	18.0 ± 0.6	20.5 ± 0.5	0.01
Carbohydrate, total, g	314.8 ± 11.7	364.9 ± 8.1	0.01
Sucrose	65.6 ± 4.6	63.7 ± 2.7	NS
Starch	175.9 ± 6.8	237.7 ± 5.5	0.001
Other	73.2 ± 4.1	63.5 ± 2.7	0.05
Calcium, mg	812.9 ± 35.0	752.5 ± 22.4	NS
Phosphorus, mg	1,360.2 ± 42.0	1,407.3 ± 30.4	NS
Iron, mg	17.4 ± 0.5	19.6 ± 0.4	0.01
Potassium, mg	3,739.6 ± 109.2	3,811.7 ± 83.8	NS
Magnesium, mg	390.3 ± 13.1	427.6 ± 9.9	0.05
Cholesterol, mg	460.6 ± 21.2	501.4 ± 13.8	NS

Values are expressed as mean ± SE. NS = not significant.   [a] Components may not add to total, due to rounding.

Thirty percent of the women interviewed were employed outside the home. Their calorie intakes were significantly lower than the uptakes for women who stayed home, but their animal protein intake was significantly higher (Table 4). Age did not prove to be a significant factor; for the selected nutrients, no significant differences were noted between the two adjacent 10-year age groups.

The gallbladder study population (3, 4) was composed of 50 males and 50 females from each of six decades. Of the 100 women in the two decades that correspond to the present diet study (25 to 34 years and 35 to 44 years), 64 were also members of the diet study population, so that there was overlapping of the two study populations (Table 5). No significant differences in dietary intakes were noted between 48 subjects with gallbladder disease and 16 subjects without disease.

Discussion

High caloric intake, in addition to relative inactivity of the subjects, accounted for the overweight of the study population (mean, 157% of desirable weight). Although the percent of calories contributed from protein, fat, and carbohydrate was comparable to the Department of Agriculture 1965 food consumption survey, it should be noted that the latter was economic rather than physiologic consumption. Protein intake of 89 g daily was above the recommended allowance; 53% of the protein, however, originated from plant sources. Hesse (6) found a protein intake of 105.2 g daily with 84% of the protein originating from plant sources. It is difficult to equate carbohydrate components in this study with the Department of Agriculture survey because we classified carbohydrate in three groups: *1)* sucrose, *2)* starch, and *3)* "other" which was predominantly fruits and vegetables. The Agriculture Department has classified carbohydrate in two groups: *1)* fruits, sugars, and sweeteners as "sugar," and *2*) vegetables and grain mainly as "starch" (15).

Few significant differences were noted in the various group comparisons. The diabetics showed a significantly lower sucrose and total carbohydrate intake, but a higher mean percent of desirable weight. Many of the diabetics had been instructed by the physician in the clinic and the public health nurse (who makes frequent home visits) to avoid high carbohydrate foods, especially cakes, pies, and sweets that are so popular. It appears that these instructions have resulted in decreased sucrose and total carbohydrate intake for this group.

TABLE 5

Comparison of nutrient intakes of Pima women with gallbladder disease and those without disease[a]

Nutrients	48 with disease	16 without disease
Calories[b]	3,054.5 ± 150.1	3,237.5 ± 176.1
Protein, total, g	87.2 ± 3.7	90.6 ± 5.2
Animal	42.2 ± 2.3	42.6 ± 5.0
Vegetable	44.9 ± 2.5	47.7 ± 2.9
Fat, total, g	148.4 ± 7.2	158.6 ± 10.1
Saturated	52.8 ± 2.6	57.8 ± 4.0
Monounsaturated	67.2 ± 3.6	71.9 ± 4.5
Polyunsaturated	19.5 ± 1.0	19.4 ± 1.3
Carbohydrate, total, g	339.8 ± 18.8	359.1 ± 20.6
Sucrose	56.1 ± 6.5	62.0 ± 8.2
Starch	210.4 ± 11.3	234.4 ± 15.9
Other	73.4 ± 5.7	62.7 ± 7.3
Calcium, mg	767.0 ± 41.8	840.1 ± 97.1
Phosphorus, mg	1,357.2 ± 64.2	1,413.8 ± 107.2
Iron, mg	18.3 ± 0.9	18.6 ± 1.0
Potassium, mg	3,772.2 ± 170.8	3,681.5 ± 210.1
Magnesium, mg	407.1 ± 19.4	400.9 ± 23.7
Cholesterol, mg	482.8 ± 31.2	511.2 ± 49.6

Values are expressed as mean ± SE.   [a] The gallbladder study was composed of 50 males and 50 females from each of six decades between 15 and 74 years of age (4). Sixty-four of these females were also included in the present diet study. [b] Components may not add to total due to rounding.

Working women showed a significantly lower caloric intake but a higher animal protein intake than women who stayed home, probably because added income provided for more meat consumption. The lower magnesium and iron intakes in the working group were the result of decreased bean consumption. The decreased bean intake was also reflected in lower vegetable protein intake. Women who work rely on quick, easy-to-prepare, convenience foods and do not routinely prepare time-consuming food items such as beans.

Although there was no significant difference in nutrient intakes in patients with or without gallbladder disease, it was frequently noted that women with gallbladder disease before surgery avoided hot, spicy foods containing chili peppers, but did not find it necessary to avoid fatty foods.

Intakes of selected nutrients in this study were not associated with prevalence of either diabetes or gallbladder disease. Prevalence of diabetes as determined by impaired glucose tolerance using standardized methods has been estimated in several other countries where diets and environmental factors are widely different. Prevalence rate in both males and females over 30 years of age was 4.6% in six Central American countries (23); 7.3% in Venezuela, 6.9% in Uruguay, 3.5% in Malaya, and 1.5% in East Pakistan (24). Thirty-four percent of those in Uruguay and 15% of those in Venezuela were obese, whereas obesity was rare in the Asian groups; obesity was more common in females. The prevalence rate of diabetes was higher in females in all countries except Malaya. The most consistent association in these studies was between obesity and prevalence of diabetes. Results of studies in the United States suggest that the prevalence rate of diabetes is roughly 15 to 17% for this age group (24–27) but the Cherokee Indians of North Carolina, who are quite obese, have a prevalence rate of roughly 25% in this age group (28). The mean percent of desirable weight in the

United States is 116% for females in this age group (29). In comparison, 97% of the Pimas studied were overweight, the mean percent of desirable weight being 157%, and the prevalence of diabetes among the women in this study population aged 25 to 44 years was 32%.

Summary

Pima Indians are a well-defined population living in close proximity to off-reservation communities. Food is procured through any of three sources: trading posts, local off-reservation grocery stores, and surplus food commodities. Although the Pimas have adopted many of the white communities' food habits, beans, chili, and tortillas are still the most prominent items in the Pima diet.

Dietary histories of 277 females, 25 to 44 years of age, showed that their diet meets or exceeds the National Research Council's recommended allowances for calories, protein, calcium, iron, and magnesium. The P/S fat ratio was lower than desirable, although it is commensurate with the intake of the general United States population. Fluoride intake from water was higher and cholesterol intake was comparable to the present dietary of this country.

The subjects were classified into various subgroups for statistical comparisons on selected nutrients. The subgroups were determined by presence of diabetes, gallbladder disease, employment status, and district of residence. There were few significant differences in the group comparisons when the two groups were compared in respect to 18 nutrients. Diabetics showed significantly lower total carbohydrate ($P < 0.05$) and sucrose ($P < 0.001$) intakes than the non-diabetics. Women working outside the home had a significantly lower caloric ($P < 0.001$) intake and a higher animal protein intake ($P < 0.01$) than the non-working women. There were no significant differences in the nutrient intakes between women with gallbladder disease and those without disease.

The chief animal protein contributors to the diet were beef, pork, variety and organ meats, eggs, and Longhorn cheese. Beans, in addition to supplying the major portion of vegetable protein, also contributed significant amounts of calcium, iron, and magnesium.

The nutrient intakes of the group interviewed and the internal comparisons do not appear to be markedly different from nutrient intakes in the general United States population.

Results of this diet survey did not indicate an association between dietary intake of selected nutrients and the prevalence of either diabetes or gallbladder disease. This study is a base line for prospective investigation in the following 10 years. This age group of women has the highest incidence of diabetes and an extraordinarily high prevalence of gallbladder disease; the incidence of diabetes is high enough so that new cases developing in a few years may demonstrate whether or not individuals with different dietary intakes develop diabetes at different rates.

We are indebted to the Tribal Council of the Gila River Indian Community for their encouragement and assistance. We also thank the women of the community for their participation in the study; without their cooperation, this study would not have been possible. Special thanks are due to Mrs. Bertha Evans and Mrs. Virginia Marrietta who served as guides and interpreters.

References

1. MILLER, M., P. H. BENNETT AND T. A. BURCH. Hyperglycemia in Pima Indians: a preliminary appraisal of its significance. In: *Biomedical Challenges Presented by the American Indian*. Washington, D.C.: Pan Am. Health *Organ. Sci. Publ.* No. 165, 1968.
2. COMESS, L. J., P. H. BENNETT, T. A. BURCH AND M. MILLER. Congenital anomalies and diabetes in the Pima Indians of Arizona. *Diabetes* 18: 471, 1969.
3. COMESS, L. J., P. H. BENNETT AND T. A. BURCH. Clinical gallbladder disease in Pima Indians. *New Engl. J. Med.* 277: 894, 1967.

4. SAMPLINER, R. E., P. H. BENNETT, L. J. COMESS, F. A. ROSE AND T. A. BURCH. Gallbladder disease in Pima Indians. *New Engl. J. Med.* 283: 1358, 1970.

5. FRIEDMAN, G. D., W. B. KANNEL AND T. R. DAWBER. The epidemiology of gallbladder disease. Observations in the Framingham study. *J. Chronic Diseases* 19: 273, 1966.

6. HESSE, F. G. A dietary study of the Pima Indian. *Am. J. Clin. Nutr.* 7: 532, 1959.

7. WORMINGTON, H. M. *Prehistoric Indians of the Southwest*. Denver: Denver Museum Natural History, 1966, p. 120.

8. CASTETTER, E. F., AND W. H. BELL. *Pima and Papago Indian Agriculture*. Albuquerque: Univ. New Mexico Press, 1942.

9. HAURY, E. H. First masters of the American Desert—The Hohokam. *J. Natl. Geographic Soc.* 1131: 670, 1967.

10. BURKE, B. S. The dietary history as a tool in research. *J. Am. Dietet. Assoc.* 23: 1041, 1947.

11. WATT, B. K., AND A. L. MERRIL. Composition of Foods—Raw, Processed, Prepared. *Agr. Handbook No. 8* (rev.). Agr. Res. Serv., U.S. Dept. Agr. Washington, D.C.: U.S. Govt. Printing Office, 1963.

12. BOWES, A. B., AND C. F. CHURCH. *Food Values of Portions Commonly Used* (10th ed.). Philadelphia: Lippincott, 1966.

13. GODDARD, V., AND L. GOODALL. Fatty Acids in Food Fats. *Home Econ. Res. Rept.* No. 7. Dept. Agr. Washington, D.C.: U.S. Govt. Printing Office, 1959.

14. Food Consumption of Households in the United States, Spring, 1965. *U.S. Dept. Agr. Rept.* No. 1. Washington, D. C.: U.S. Govt. Printing Office, 1968.

15. FRIEND, B. Nutrition in United States food supply. A review of trends, 1909–13 to 1965. *Am. J. Clin. Nutr.* 20: 907, 1967.

16. Recommended Dietary Allowances (7th rev. ed.). *Natl. Acad. Sci.–Natl. Res. Council Publ.* 1694. Washington, D.C., 1968.

17. Report of the Council on Foods and Nutrition of the American Medical Association. The regulation of dietary fat. *J. Am. Med. Assoc.* 181: 411, 1962.

18. UNDERWOOD, E. J. *Trace Elements in Human and Animal Nutrition* (2nd ed.). New York: Academic, 1962, p. 276.

19. WALDBOTT, G. L. Fluoride in food. *Am. J. Clin. Nutr.* 12: 455, 1963.

20. MAHLE, W., E. W. SCOTT AND J. TREON. Normal urinary fluoride excretion and the fluoride content of food and water. *Am. J. Hyg.* 29: 139, 1939.

21. McCLURE, F. J. Ingestion of fluoride and dental caries. *A.M.A. J. Diseases Children* 66: 362,

1943.
22. SIEVERS, M. Serum cholesterol levels in Southwestern American Indians. *J. Chronic Diseases* 21: 107, 1968.
23. WEST, K. M., AND J. M. KALBFLEISCH. Diabetes in Central America. *Diabetes* 19: 656, 1970.
24. WEST, K. M., AND J. M. KALBFLEISCH. Glucose tolerance, nutrition, and diabetes in Uruguay, Venezuela, Malaya, and East Pakistan. *Diabetes* 15: 9, 1966.
25. HAYNER, N. S., M. O. KJELSBERG, F. H. EPSTEIN AND T. FRANCIS. Carbohydrate tolerance and diabetes in a total community, Tecumseh, Michigan. *Diabetes* 14: 413, 1965.
26. GORDON, T. Glucose tolerance of adults, United States, 1960–62, diabetes prevalence and results of glucose tolerance tests by age and sex. *Vital Health Statistics, Ser.* 11, No. 2, Washington, D.C.: U. S. Govt. Printing Office, 1964.
27. UNGER, R. H. The standard two-hour oral glucose tolerance test in the diagnosis of diabetes mellitus in subjects without fasting hyperglycemia. *Ann. Internal Med.* 47: 1138, 1957.
28. STEIN, J. H., K. M. WEST, J. M. ROBEY, D. F. TIRADOR AND G. W. MCDONALD. The high prevalence of abnormal glucose tolerance in the Cherokee Indians of North Carolina. *Arch. Internal Med.* 116: 842, 1965.
29. U.S. National Center for Health Statistics. *Weight, Height and Selected Body Dimensions of Adults, United States,* 1960–62. Washington, D.C.: U.S. Dept. Health, Education and Welfare, 1965.

Diabetes

Diabetes in the Pima Indians
Evidence of Bimodality in Glucose Tolerance Distributions

Norman B. Rushforth, Ph.D., Peter H. Bennett, M.B., M.R.C.P.,
Arthur G. Steinberg, Ph.D., Thomas A. Burch, M.D., M.P.H.,
and Max Miller, M.D.

SUMMARY

Venous plasma glucose levels two hours after a 75 gm. carbohydrate load were determined on over 2,900 Pima Indians, a population known to have an extremely high prevalence of diabetes mellitus. In each sex and in each decade above twenty-five years of age, the frequency distributions of the logarithms of the glucose levels were clearly bimodal, but below this age a single symmetrical unimodal distribution was found. A maximum likelihood procedure was used to derive the best fitting theoretical gaussian distributions for each group of data, together with the parameters of each distribution.

The observed bimodal distributions were found to be in satisfactory agreement with a model of two overlapping gaussian distributions, indicating that a logical separation between those with normal and high levels of glucose is possible, although the presence of overlap indicates that some misclassification will occur if any finite level is used to subdivide the population.

The data indicate that among the Pima: 1. The frequency distributions of two-hour glucose tolerance levels can be used to identify objectively and describe a hyperglycemic population without recourse to other criteria for diabetes. 2. There are small changes in the parameters of "normal" glucose tolerance between the ages of twenty-five and sixty-four years. 3. The increase in mean glucose level found with rising age in this population is mainly the result of an increasing proportion of subjects who are in the group characterized by marked glucose intolerance.

The bimodal distributions of plasma glucose levels among the Pima Indians contrast with those described so far in other groups. It seems likely that differences are attributable to the lower prevalence of diabetes elsewhere which would obscure the identification of bimodality.

Diabetes mellitus is regarded generally as a specific disease entity characterized by symptoms related to a failure to metabolize glucose normally. The disease is also associated with a number of specific vascular complications, such as retinopathy and nephropathy, which are related to the duration of the diabetes.

The presence of carbohydrate intolerance is often accompanied by glycosuria; for many years the detection of reducing substances (and later glucose) in the urine formed a basis for the diagnosis. With the development of chemical methods to determine glucose concentration in the blood it was found that elevated levels, especially after a carbohydrate load, were characteristic of persons with diabetes mellitus. Many subjects were found to have carbohydrate intolerance without evidence of the classical symptoms and signs of diabetes, however. More recently glucose tolerance tests have been used in attempts to define more precisely the frequency of diabetes in various populations. In such studies no clear point of separation was found between individuals with normal and abnormal carbohydrate tolerance tests. The frequency distributions of glucose levels were reported to be continuous and unimodal.[1-3]

When the characteristics of the frequency distributions were examined it was apparent that mean and variances of the glucose levels tended to become greater with increasing age. Some of this rise could be attributed to a higher prevalence of diabetes mellitus among older persons. Many investigators have postulated, however, that most of this rise was the result of a normal or "physiologic" impairment of glucose tolerance among the majority of subjects. The resolution of these problems may have been obscured by a relatively low frequency of diabetes or the frequent occurrence of other diseases associated with impaired carbohydrate intolerance in the reported studies.

These problems have been re-examined in the Pima Indians, a group known to have an extraordinarily high prevalence of diabetes when conventional diagnostic criteria for carbohydrate intolerance were applied[4] and who also have a high prevalence of the specific vascular complications of diabetes mellitus.[5]

The present analysis attempts to determine:

1. The nature of the distributions of glucose tolerance levels in a population with a high prevalence of diabetes mellitus.
2. Whether the rise in mean glucose tolerance level with increasing age is mainly the result of an increasing prevalence of diabetes mellitus or a "physiologic" deterioration of glucose tolerance among the majority of subjects.

METHODS

The data were collected as part of a continuing epidemiologic study of diabetes mellitus among the Pima Indians, who reside mainly on the Gila River Indian Reservation in Central Arizona. The sample contained those persons living in the eastern portion of this reservation, which is relatively isolated geographically from other Indian communities. Its inhabitants receive free comprehensive medical care in a central location, the United States Public Health Service Hospital at Sacaton, Arizona.

The present report considers the results of a modified glucose tolerance test carried out between 1965-69 on 2,911 (1,340 males and 1,571 females), half to full-blooded Pima Indians aged five to seventy-four years, regardless of whether or not they were known to have diabetes. These subjects constituted approximately 82 per cent of those residents on the reservation as determined by our census in 1966. Because of the small number of subjects aged seventy-five years and over living on the reservation (forty-one males and twenty-three females tested) their results have been omitted from the present analyses.

The glucose tolerance test consisted of determination of a venous plasma glucose level two hours after the ingestion of a 75 gm. carbohydrate equivalent load.* The vast majority of the subjects were ambulatory at the time of the examination and during the two-hour interval of the test a number of diabetes and arthritis related examinations were performed. Two hours after the carbohydrate load, 7 ml. venous blood was drawn

---

*Glucola, Ames Company, Elkhart, Indiana, or Dexcola, Custom Laboratories, Baltimore, Maryland.

into a Vacutainer* containing 30 mg. sodium fluoride. After mixing, the blood was allowed to stand for two to twelve hours and then centrifuged and separated. The plasma glucose level was determined on the Auto-Analyzer using the modified Hoffman method.†

The distributions of the two-hour plasma glucose values and their relationships to sex and age by decade were examined. The histograms of glucose levels were unimodal in the younger age groups and indicative of bimodality in the older age groups in both sexes. Plots of cumulative frequencies of percentage distributions of the plasma glucose levels on probability paper suggested that they might conform to a model of a single gaussian (normal) distribution in the younger age groups and two overlapping gaussian curves in the older age groups. A single gaussian distribution may be expressed mathematically by the equation for the probability function $f(x)$ as

$$f(x) = \frac{1}{\sigma\sqrt{2\pi}}\, e^{\frac{-(x-\mu)^2}{2\sigma^2}}$$

where μ is the mean and σ is the standard deviation and x is a single observation. The model of two overlapping gaussian distributions[6] may be expressed as

$$f(x) = \frac{\alpha e^{\frac{-(x-\mu_1)^2}{2\sigma_1^2}}}{\sigma_1\sqrt{2\pi}} + \frac{(1-\alpha)e^{\frac{-(x-\mu_2)^2}{2\sigma_2^2}}}{\sigma_2\sqrt{2\pi}}$$

where μ_1 and μ_2 are the means of the two distributions: σ_1 and σ_2 their respective standard deviations, α is the proportion of individuals belonging to the first curve. These parameters may be estimated using graphical methods,[7] or more precisely by using a maximum likelihood procedure.[6]

---

*Vacutainer, No. 4752, Becton Dickinson & Co., Rutherford, New Jersey.

†Technicon Instruments Corporation, Tarrytown, New York, Method File N-20.

Estimates of the parameters of the gaussian distributions were obtained by dissecting the plots of the observed glucose distributions on probability paper by the method of Harding.[7] Using these values as initial estimates, the final maximum likelihood estimates of μ_1, μ_2, σ_1, σ_2 and α* were obtained with the aid of a computer program first devised by Cicchinelli for the analysis of blood pressure measurements.[6]

Chi square goodness of fit tests were employed to compare the observed frequency distributions with those predicted by the model of the composite gaussian distribution.

RESULTS

Table 1 shows the means and standard deviations of the two-hour plasma glucose values by decade for both sexes. There was a progressive increase in mean glucose levels with age for both sexes up to the age of sixty-five, but the mean decreased in the last age group (65-74 years). In all but one age group (25-34 years), glucose values for females were higher than those for males, significantly so for the groups aged five to fourteen, forty-five to fifty-four and fifty-five to sixty-four years ($p < 0.01$).

The frequency distributions of the two-hour plasma glucose values, when plotted on an arithmetic scale for various decades in both sexes, were highly skewed and indicated bimodality for the older age groups. Examples of such plots are shown in figure 1.

In order to examine whether the frequency distributions conformed to a gaussian model the cumulative frequency distributions were plotted on normal and log normal probability paper. On log normal probability paper plots yielded essentially straight lines for the younger age groups and above age twenty-five the plots contained two straight line segments, suggesting that the distributions consisted of two gaussian curves (figure 2).

A simple hypothesis consistent with these findings and with the clinical impression that the hyperglycemia of diabetes mellitus is a specific disease was proposed.[8]

---

*Subsequently these same algebraic symbols are used to signify *estimates* of the parameters rather than the parameters themselves.

TABLE 1

Plasma glucose levels (mg./100 ml.) determined two hours after an oral 75 gm. carbohydrate load

Age group	Males			Females		
	No. examined	Mean	S.D.*	No. examined	Mean	S.D.*
5-14	550	99.9	19.6	606	104.8	24.0
15-24	245	107.4	61.8	314	112.1	50.5
25-34	139	154.4	117.4	195	151.2	96.3
35-44	146	204.8	166.7	186	226.2	165.9
45-54	96	208.7	140.5	112	256.6	165.7
55-64	83	214.9	143.2	106	293.1	161.5
65-74	81	210.0	141.1	52	229.4	130.6
Total	1,340			1,571		

*Standard deviation.

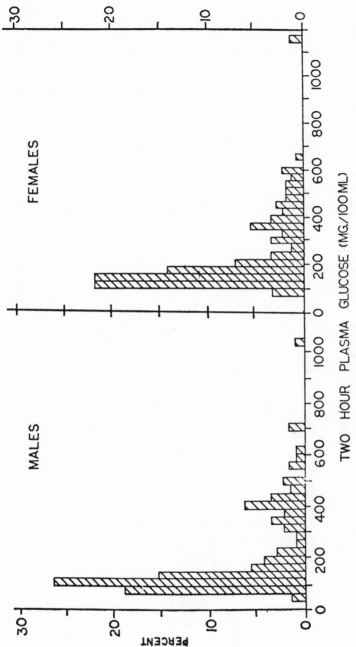

FIG. I. Histograms showing the distribution of two-hour glucose levels plotted on an arithmetic scale. Males aged thirty-five to forty-four and females aged thirty-five to forty-four.

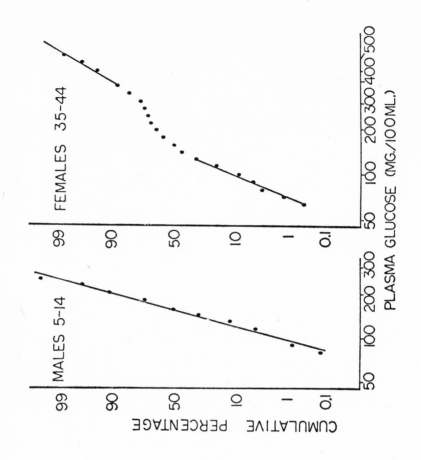

FIG. 2.

Cumulative percentage distribution of plasma glucose values plotted on a log-normal probability plot. Males aged five to fourteen and females aged thirty-five to forty-four.

The hypothesis stated that the distribution of glucose tolerance in natural populations consists of two components which are distributed to form overlapping gaussian curves.

The previously described methods were employed to estimate the parameters of the two component distributions and to examine the applicability of the hypotheses.

The parameters of the model distributions were calculated for each sex and in each decade using the arithmetic and the logarithmic values of the glucose levels. When statistical tests were applied to the parameters of mean, variance, skewness and kurtosis it was found that the distributions derived using the logarithmic values gave a closer fit to the observed distributions. For this reason only the results for the logarithmic values are presented.

When logarithms of the glucose values were plotted as histograms the frequency distributions were symmetric and unimodal in the five to fourteen age groups. Above age twenty-five there was clear evidence of bimodality in every decade. The histograms of the observed glucose distributions and predicted composite and component curves are shown in figure 3 (a and b). The predicted composite curve is represented as a continuous line and the two component curves as interrupted lines (these are only apparent in the regions where the component curves overlap). For both males and females aged five to fourteen years the frequency histograms were unimodal and only a single gaussian curve could be fitted to these distributions. For the fifteen to twenty-four year age group 2 to 3 per cent of the higher values appeared as outlying observations from the first ("normal") curve and constituted the only evidence of a second curve in this age group in each sex.

For age groups twenty-five to thirty-four years, there was more visual evidence of bimodality in each sex. Between thirty-five and sixty-four years each ten-year age group in both sexes had distributions which were clearly bimodal. Above age sixty-four in the males there was clear separation of the modes (and a close fit for the predicted curve), but in the females separation of the component distributions was less obvious.

Chi square goodness of fit tests showed satisfactory agreement between the observed frequency distributions

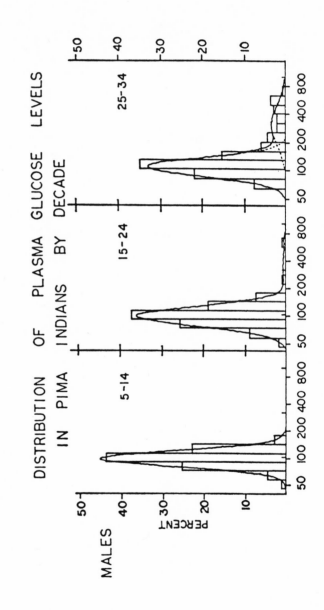

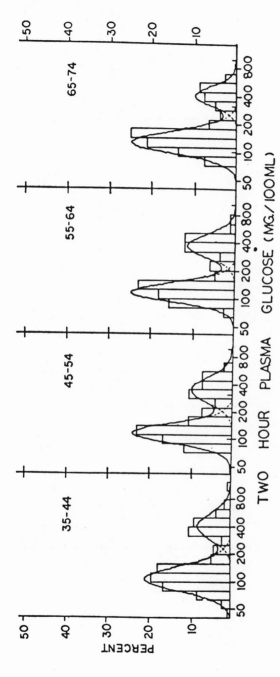

FIG. 3a. Histograms and superimposed composite curve and the component curves derived to describe the distribution of the two-hour glucose levels for males by decade. See text for further explanation.

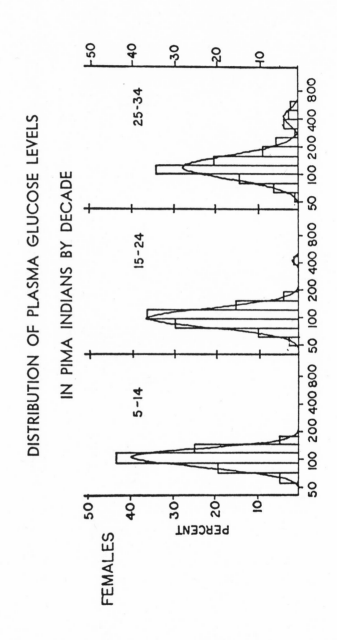

DISTRIBUTION OF PLASMA GLUCOSE LEVELS

IN PIMA INDIANS BY DECADE

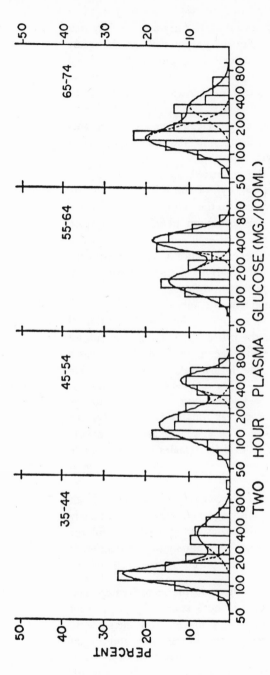

Fig. 3b. Histograms and superimposed composite curve and the component curves derived to describe the distribution of the two-hour glucose levels for females by decade. See text for further explanation.

and those predicted using the model, for all age groups ($p > 0.1$) except males aged twenty-five to thirty-four ($p < 0.05$) and males aged forty-five to fifty-four ($0.05 < p < 0.1$). For the purposes of the chi square test for each decade the data were grouped in 0.05 log glucose units (rather than in 0.1 log units shown in the histograms) in order to increase the power of the statistical test.

As the model proved satisfactory the data were analyzed to determine changes in the various estimated parameter values with age.

Table 2 shows the estimated means (μ_1, μ_2), the standard deviations (σ_1, σ_2) of the two curves and the percentage of individuals in the "normal" curves (100 x α) determined by the maximum likelihood procedure. The values of the means of each component are plotted against age for both sexes in figure 4, and the estimates of percentage of individuals in the second component (100 x ($1—\alpha$)) are shown in figure 5.

In the first component the mean levels (figure 4) were constant below age twenty-four, with a value of 98 mg./100 ml. for the males and 103 mg./100 ml. for the females. Above this age in the males there was a linear increase of the logarithmic values up to age seventy-four where the mean value was 129 mg./100 ml. In the females there was a linear increase up to age fifty-four, and the level was roughly constant over the fifty-five to seventy-four year age range at approximately 150 mg./100 ml. The level for females was significantly higher in each age group except sixty-five to seventy-four years.

The mean levels of the second component did not change significantly with age and were approximately 350 mg./100 ml. for the males and 420 mg./100 ml. for the females. These values were not significantly different from each other, but the sample sizes were small and the standard errors large.

The percentage of subjects in the second component (figure 5) rose steeply in both sexes from 0 per cent below age fifteen years, to a maximum at fifty-five to sixty-four years of 36 per cent in the males and 49 per cent in the females. There were smaller proportions in the sixty-five to seventy-four year age groups, which may have been the result of a relatively greater mor-

TABLE 2

Maximum likelihood estimates of the parameters of the frequency distributions and their standard errors* (Log plasma glucose: Arithmetic values in mg./100 ml. in parentheses)

Sex-Age	No. examined	First component				Second component		
		Mean μ_1	Standard error of mean SEμ_1	Standard deviation σ_1	Per cent of subjects ($\alpha \times 100$) $\pm$ SE $_{\alpha \times 100}$	Mean μ_2	Standard error of mean SEμ_2	Standard deviation σ_2
MALES								
5-14	550	1.992(98)	0.004	0.088	100.0	—	—	—
15-24	245	1.987(97)	0.007	0.109	97.5±1.5	2.527(337)	0.206	0.245
25-34	139	2.029(107)	0.012	0.099	81.1±5.7	2.488(307)	0.091	0.215
35-44	146	2.037(109)	0.015	0.137	71.4±4.2	2.611(408)	0.028	0.139
45-54	96	2.069(117)	0.020	0.109	65.7±6.4	2.554(358)	0.040	0.139
55-64	83	2.073(118)	0.016	0.104	64.5±5.6	2.566(368)	0.026	0.123
65-74	81	2.112(129)	0.017	0.121	74.6±5.2	2.610(408)	0.028	0.105
FEMALES								
5-14	606	2.010(102)	0.004	0.098	100.0	—	—	—
15-24	314	2.015(104)	0.006	0.107	98.4±0.7	2.645(442)	0.018	0.040
25-34	195	2.081(120)	0.010	0.130	91.6±2.1	2.628(424)	0.027	0.088
35-44	186	2.121(132)	0.012	0.103	66.0±4.9	2.571(372)	0.038	0.169
45-54	112	2.168(147)	0.024	0.159	68.5±5.5	2.660(457)	0.025	0.104
55-64	106	2.177(150)	0.022	0.134	50.7±5.4	2.623(420)	0.017	0.103
65-74	52	2.178(151)	0.049	0.130	64.5±1.7	2.538(345)	0.092	0.148

*See text for explanation of symbols.

105

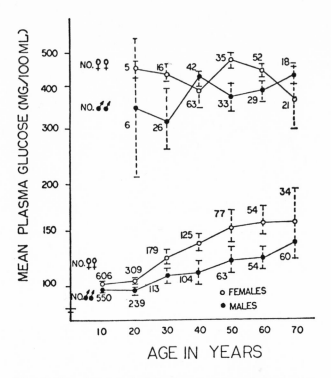

FIG. 4. Plots of the mean of the first component (μ_1) $\pm$ 2 S.E. and of the mean of the second component (μ_2) $\pm$ 1 S.E. as a function of age for males and females. The number of subjects in the component in each age-sex group is designated to the left of the respective means.

tality among the hyperglycemic subjects than among others in the older age groups.

The changes with age of the various percentile levels of glucose were also investigated to determine if the elevation of the plasma glucose levels was uniform for various segments of the distributions as age increased. In figure 6 the curves represent percentile values of plasma glucose by age. They show the plasma glucose levels for which there were 10, 30, 50, etc. per cent of the subjects with lower values in each age group (ordinate) plotted against the midpoint of the age group (abscissa).

The changes with age in the plasma glucose levels for various percentiles were not uniform. Plasma glucose

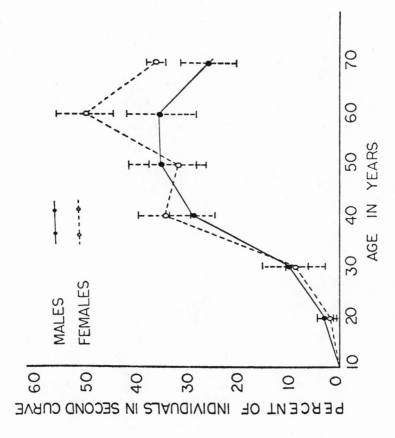

FIG. 5.

Plots of the percentage of individuals lying in the second component as a function of age for males and females. The dotted lines give the range of one standard error above and below the estimated percentage.

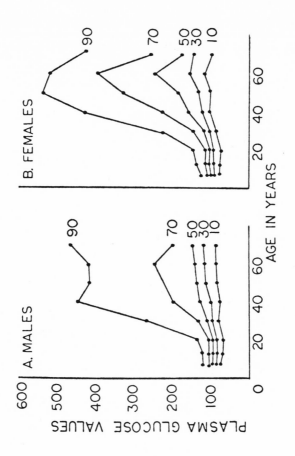

FIG. 6.

Plots of percentile values of plasma glucose levels as a function of age for males and females.

values were constant up to age twenty for both sexes. Above this age, in males below the 50th percentile and in females below the 30th percentile, glucose values rose gradually and systematically with age. In contrast, the glucose levels of the higher percentiles changed much more rapidly to peak between fifty and seventy years in the males and at age sixty years in the females. These data indicated that glucose levels did not change uniformly with age.

DISCUSSION

The observation of bimodality in the frequency distributions of the two-hour postload levels plotted on arithmetic or logarithmic scales was unequivocal in the present study. As a high proportion of the population was examined and as the subjects were distributed evenly within each age group the finding is not likely to be the result of selective sampling and, therefore, suggests that the Pima population consists of at least two subgroups. These subgroups could not be distinguished below fifteen years of age, but beyond this age there emerged a group, characterized by high postchallenge glucose levels, which increased in size progressively to age sixty and then decreased. The plasma glucose levels of this hyperglycemic group were for the most part in excess of 200 mg./100 ml. and thus by conventional standards the group contained subjects with diabetes mellitus. The second component was, therefore, assumed to represent subjects with diabetes.

The first of the two components in the frequency distributions, characterized by lower glucose levels, was assumed, as a working hypothesis, to represent the nondiabetic ("normal") population, although, in the lower age groups especially, it must have contained many individuals who would sooner, or later, develop definite evidence of glucose intolerance. The second component, characterized by high glucose levels, was incompletely separated from the upper end of the first component. This indicated that there was no specific level at which division of the two subpopulations could be made without some misclassification. With any dividing level some of the hyperglycemic population would be labeled normal and vice versa. Levels have been defined, however, which minimized the probabilities of this misclassification and have been used in genetic analyses of diabetes in this population.[9a,b]

The proportion of subjects which constituted the hyperglycemic subpopulation was determined without reference to such cutoff levels for the classification of diabetes (figure 5). This represents an important feature of the model as the parameters could then be utilized to infer changes occurring with increasing age.

The increasing proportion of subjects lying in the second ("diabetic") component presumably results from increased numbers of subjects who were initially within the first component, and who have developed glucose intolerance as they aged, thus becoming members of the hyperglycemic group.

The differences between the distributions at different ages enabled inferences to be drawn concerning the relationship of increasing age to glucose levels. Figure 4 indicates the changes in the mean glucose levels of the two individual components with age. Females in the "normal" component had higher levels than the males above the age of twenty years, the mean level increasing from 104 to 147 mg./100 ml. between twenty and fifty years, thereafter being constant. Among the males the mean level of the "normal" group rose progressively from 97 mg./100 ml. at age twenty to 129 mg./100 ml. at age seventy. The "diabetic" groups of both sexes, however, showed no consistent changes of the mean with age, but the standard errors of the means were large because of the smaller numbers of subjects falling in the second component.

The major change in the parameters with increasing age was found in the proportion of subjects falling into the second component. This proportion was assumed to represent the prevalence of "diabetes" in the sample. The proportion in the males rose rapidly from 2.5 per cent at age twenty to a maximum of 35.5 per cent at age fifty and in the females from 1.6 per cent to a maximum of 49.3 per cent in the respective age groups.

The observations that the mean glucose levels diminished in the total population beyond sixty-four years of age and that the proportion of subjects lying on the second curve diminished at age sixty and seventy are both consistent with the observed increased mortality

110

in Pima Indians with diabetes.[5] It is implicit, therefore, that in these age groups the mortality rate among diabetics exceeded the incidence (rate of development of new cases) of diabetes. Evaluation of this hypothesis will be sought in a prospective study.

In the Pima there was a relatively small age-dependent increase in the mean of the first component, but no change in the mean of the second curve (figure 4). More significantly, the proportion of individuals in the second component increased markedly with age (figure 5). Thus, the observed marked increase in the over-all mean plasma glucose level with age in the Pima (table 2) resulted primarily from an increase in the proportion of subjects who were in the category characterized by marked glucose intolerance.

These findings suggest that in populations where diabetes mellitus is unknown or very rare, a small, but definite, increase in mean glucose levels with increasing age would be observed. The relatively small (but statistically significant) increase in mean glucose levels observed in the Alaskan Eskimo and in the Athabascan Indians of Alaska, both of whom have extremely low prevalences of diabetes mellitus,[10,11] is consistent with this hypothesis. These groups showed a similar rate of change with age to the "nondiabetic" Pima subjects. A further indication that this conclusion is correct is suggested by an analysis of percentile glucose levels and age in data collected in Manitoba, Canada.[12] This study demonstrated that for 95th and 99th percentiles the glucose levels changed very rapidly with increasing age. Analysis of the Pima data (figure 6) showed similar changes above the 70th percentile. It also showed that even for the lower percentiles, e.g. 10th, there was a modest increase in glucose values with increasing age suggesting that there is some decrease in glucose tolerance with increasing age in all subjects. The hypothesis will be tested among the Pima by sequential glucose tolerance studies.

The frequency distributions of glucose levels in the Pima population appear to be the first reported to show unequivocal evidence of bimodality, and, thus, the general applicability of these findings may be questioned. We suspect, however, that the model of two overlapping distributions does indeed have general applicability. Such a model is consistent with the skewed distributions observed in several previous studies of glucose tolerance in which the prevalence of diabetes is lower than in the Pima[1-3] and has been proposed for several other biologic variables.[13-16]

While we recognize that more complex models may describe the data, the model of two overlapping gaussian distributions appeared both by visual inspection and statistical test to fit the observed glucose distributions. The reason why bimodality has not been observed for glucose distributions in other population studies of diabetes is due to the much lower prevalence of the disease. As there is overlap of the component distributions, a sizeable proportion of the population, 10 per cent or more according to our estimates, must be in the second component before clear evidence of bimodality can be seen in the frequency distributions. The model can be used, however, to test the general applicability of the hypothesis in populations with a lower prevalence of the disease, if suitable data are available. For example, among Asiatic Indians living in the Tongaat, South Africa, a population with a lower prevalence of diabetes than the Pima, a satisfactory fit to the model has been found.[9a,b]

The model appears to have general applicability and individuals in the second component have a high prevalence of the specific manifestations of diabetes. Pima Indians with hyperglycemia have a high prevalence of the pathognomonic complications of retinopathy and nephropathy, which identify the hyperglycemia specifically as diabetes mellitus.[5] Among those aged thirty-five and over diabetic retinopathy was found in 16 per cent of those who had two-hour glucose levels of 200 mg./100 ml. and over or concurrently treated diabetes, compared to 0.7 per cent in those with lower glucose levels. Proteinuria was also found more frequently among the group with glucose levels of 200 mg./100 ml. and over, and of sixty-two hyperglycemic subjects with proteinuria, twenty-two had albumin/creatinine ratios of 3.0 or more. Such levels were not encountered among subjects with lower glucose levels except in one male with a clear history of glomerulonephritis. Hence, the vast majority of individuals with the specific complications of diabetes mellitus had glucose levels which placed them in the hyperglycemic subgroup.

The identification of the bimodality in glucose tolerance distributions and of a model which describes them satisfactorily creates the opportunity to formulate many testable hypotheses related to the underlying nature of diabetes mellitus, and, in particular, enables the development of new approaches to test genetic hypotheses concerning diabetes mellitus.[9a,b]

ACKNOWLEDGMENT

This study was supported in part by Grant No. GM-12302 from the National Institutes of Health.

We wish to acknowledge with gratitude the expert programming provided by Mr. O. Morgenstern. We express our thanks also for the cooperation and help of the Tribal Council and the members of the Gila River Indian Community and the Division of Indian Health. Without their aid this study could not have been undertaken.

REFERENCES

[1] Sharp, C. L., Butterfield, W. J. H., and Keen, H.: Diabetes survey in Bedford 1962. Proc. Roy. Soc. Med. 57:193-202, 1964.

[2] Gordon, T.: Glucose tolerance of adults, United States 1960-62. U. S. Public Health Service Publication 1000, Series 11, No. 2, U. S. Government Printing Office, May 1964.

[3] Hayner, N. S., Kjelsberg, M. D., Epstein, F. H., and Francis, T.: Carbohydrate tolerance and diabetes in a total community, Tecumseh, Michigan. Diabetes 14:413-23, 1965.

[4] Bennett, P. H., Burch, T. A., and Miller, M.: Diabetes mellitus in American (Pima) Indians. Lancet II:125-28, 1971.

[5] Miller, M., Bennett, P. H., and Burch, T. A.: Hyperglycemia in Pima Indians: A preliminary appraisal of its significance. In Biomedical Challenges Presented by the American Indians, Washington, D. C.: Pan American Health Organization. Scientific Publication No. 165 (Sept.) 1968, pp. 89-102.

[6] Cicchinelli, A. L.: The composite of two gaussian distributions as a model for blood pressure distributions in man. Ph.D. thesis, Univ. of Michigan 1963, Univ. Microfilms Inc., 63-6888, Ann Arbor, Michigan.

[7] Harding, J. P.: The use of probability paper for the graphical analysis of polymodal frequency distributions. J. Marine Biol. Assn. 28:141-52, 1949.

113

[8] Bennett, P. H., Steinberg, A. G., Miller, M., and Burch, T. A.: Effect of aging on the glucose tolerance test: Evidence that the normal standards change only slightly with age. J. Lab. Clin. Med. 66:852, 1965.

[9] (a) Steinberg, A. G., Rushforth, N. B., Bennett, P. H., Burch, T. A., and Miller, M.: Preliminary Report on Genetics of Diabetes Among the Pima Indians. In Early Diabetes, Camerini-Davalos, R. A., and Cole, H. S., Eds. New York, Academic Press, 1970, pp. 11-21.

(b) Steinberg, A. G., Rushforth, N. B., Bennett, P. H., Burch, T. A., and Miller, M.: On the genetics of diabetes mellitus. Nobel Symposium 13, The Pathogenesis of Diabetes Mellitus. Cerasi, E., and Luft, R., Eds. New York, John Wiley & Sons, Inc., 1970, pp. 237-260.

[10] Mouratoff, G. J., Carroll, N. V., and Scott, E. M.: Diabetes mellitus in Eskimos. JAMA 199:961-66, 1967.

[11] Mouratoff, G. J., Carroll, N. V., and Scott, E. M.: Diabetes mellitus in Athabaskan Indians in Alaska. Diabetes 18: 29-32, 1969.

[12] Kaufman, B. J., Grant, D. R., and Moorhouse, J. A.: An analysis of blood glucose values in a population screened for diabetes mellitus. Canad. Med. Ass. J. 100:692-98, 1969.

[13] Decker, J. L., Lane, J. J., and Reynolds, W. E.: Hyperuricemia in a male Filipino population. Arthritis Rheum. 5: 144-55, 1962.

[14] Penrose, L. S.: Measurement of pheiotrophic effects in phenylketonuria. Ann. Eugen. 15:134-41, 1951.

[15] Murphy, E. A.: One cause? Many causes? The argument from the bimodal distribution. J. Chronic Dis. 17:301-24, 1964.

[16] Hopkinson, D. A., Spencer, M., and Harris, H.: Genetical studies on human red cell acid phosphatase. Amer. J. Hum. Genet. 16:141, 1964.

114

Preliminary Report on the Genetics of Diabetes among the Pima Indians*

Arthur G. Steinberg,   Norman B. Rushforth,
Peter H. Bennett,   Thomas A. Burch,   and Max Miller

There have been many reviews of the literature concerned with the genetics of diabetes (*1*), and it is not our intention to present yet another. While all acknowledge that there is an important genetic component in the determination of a predisposition to diabetes, there is considerable disagreement concerning the nature of this component.

In a review of the literature one of us (*2*) wrote "... a simple working hypothesis, not necessarily correct, but one which fits the data, is that susceptibility to diabetes is due to homozygosis for a recessive gene." This concept has been repeatedly challenged, but both this view and those in disagreement with it are based on data collected by the undesirable method of hearsay pedigrees. The information gained by interviewing the patient, by having the patient or his family complete a questionnaire, or by having a student complete a health form on entering college has not led to a universally accepted solution of the mode of inheritance of susceptibility to diabetes (see references *3* and *4* for discussions of the shortcomings of these methods). A new approach is needed.

The method of choice would be to examine all individuals in the study by some technique or techniques that could diagnose diabetes, and that could

* Supported in part by Grant No. GM-12302 from the National Institutes of Health.

detect all those liable to the disease before the appearance of clinical symptoms. No such method is recognized. In the absence of such facility, we and others have turned to an alternative procedure, i.e., the glucose tolerance test (GTT). The difficulties associated with the interpretation of the test have been well outlined by Sisk (5). In practice, an arbitrary glucose level (plasma or whole blood) obtained 1 or 2 hours after challenge with an arbitrary amount of glucose is used to determine whether the patient is or is not diabetic. The arbitrary choice of a glucose level for diagnosis is used because the plot of the data derived from tests of large numbers of individuals forms a continuous curve, skewed to the right, with, in most studies, no clear evidence of bimodality. Still other difficulties arise from the observation that multiple tests of the same individual, performed within a short time interval, may give widely different results (6), incuding variation from abnormal to normal (7). Nevertheless, in a large population, it is possible at least in theory to test various genetic hypotheses.

The uncertainties associated with the GTT make it necessary that samples include numerous diabetics. In most populations fewer than 5% have diabetes. Hence, the total sample must be almost unmanageably large to permit identification of sufficient diabetics in each of several age and sex groups to provide meaningful estimates of the parameters needed to study the genetics of the disease. The number of individuals to be studied may be reduced if relatives of diabetic probands are studied. Nevertheless, these studies also require large numbers of individuals, hence large numbers of families. Simpson (8), Thompson (9), Burkeholder et al. (7), and Sisk (5) have used this approach, but none of the studies included adequate numbers of families or patients to permit a satisfactory genetic analysis of the data.

We present a preliminary report of our continuing study of diabetes among a tribe of American Indians, the Pima of Arizona, among whom diabetes is extraordinarily frequent (among those examined thus far, more than 50% among females over 34 years and more than 35% among males over 34 years), and who compose a population of manageable size (about 3500), which is probably large enough for our purposes (10).

All individuals aged 5 and over are being given a modified GTT based on the determination of plasma glucose level 2 hours after a challenge with 75 gm of glucose. Thus far our completion rate is inadequate for most age groups (less than 70% for all except one age group for males, for example) and we have only 178 families in which both parents and at least one child were tested. Therefore this report is primarily a demonstration of a method of analysis.

Some population data based on similar tests of Asiatic Indians living in Tongaat, near Durban, South Africa are presented for comparison. These Indians were given only 50 gm of glucose, and none younger than 10 years of

116

TABLE I

Plasma Glucose Values
Determined Two Hours after Challenge with 75 gm of Glucose (Pima Indians) or with 50 gm of Glucose (Asiatic Indians)

| | Pima Indians | | | | | | | Asiatic Indians | | | | | | |
| | Males | | | Females | | | | Males | | | Females | | |
Age	No.	Mean	S.D.[a]	No.	Mean	S.D.[a]		No.	Mean	S.D.[a]	No.	Mean	S.D.[a]
5–14	236	99.6	20.0	287	105.0	23.1		66[b]	90.1	17.4	83[b]	98.0	18.6
15–24	147	98.9	24.9	228	112.5	50.5		431	86.0	15.9	443	94.6	16.9
25–34	81	154.6	124.1	152	149.0	95.6		134	84.8	17.1	248	96.2	19.1
35–44	97	180.0	155.6	147	209.5	162.0		79	83.9	18.1	158	106.8	34.8
45–54	71	194.6	128.9	96	262.3	168.4		75	113.2	67.8	116	125.3	57.8
55–64	66	223.7	155.5	88	303.3	166.7		70	106.8	44.9	49	137.6	85.5
65–74	70	206.3	130.4	55	232.6	131.3		32	146.5	114.1	18	123.4	31.3

[a] S.D. = Standard deviation
[b] Age range = 10–14

117

age were tested, otherwise the procedures used in the two studies are identical. We are grateful to Drs. W. P. U. Jackson and G. D. Campbell for permission to analyze their unpublished data.

In common with the data from other investigators, the data from these samples show that after a glucose challenge the mean plasma glucose level rises with age and is higher for females than for males (Table I). The rise with age begins earlier in the Pima Indians and reaches a much higher level.

We have assumed, as a working hypothesis, that the skewed distributions previously reported for plots of the glucose levels observed in the GTT were composed of two overlapping gaussian distributions: one to represent those individuals assumed to be normal and the other to represent those assumed to be diabetic. Because the curves overlap, a portion of the members of the sample cannot be unequivocally assigned to a given population. (Nevertheless, the relative frequencies of the populations can be estimated, and these may be used as aids in further analyses) A program written by Cicchenelli (11) to derive, by a maximum likelihood process, the means (μ), variances, (σ^2) and proportions (p) of the two curves postulated to compose the observed distribution was modified by one of us (N. B. R.) for use on the I.B.M. 1620 II. Details of this procedure will be published elsewhere. We emphasize that the only assumption made is that there are two curves, each of which represents a normal distribution.

Statistical tests showed that the derived curves fit the data better when logarithms of the observed values rather than the values themselves are used, hence these values are reported. The data for the Pima samples are shown in Table II.

Histograms of the observed data with the derived composite curve and the component curves superimposed are presented for the Pima males in Fig. 1, and for the Asiatic Indian males in Fig. 2. (Space limitations prevent us from presenting the curves for the females.) We could not derive two curves to describe the data for Pima males (or females) aged 5–14 or 15–24 years and we interpret this as indicating that there are too few individuals with high glucose values (note that the curves for age group 5–14 are not shown in Fig. 1) to permit the separation to be made. Two curves were derived for each of the five remaining age groups for each sex, and the composite curves for each of these show suggestive, if not clear evidence of bimodality.

We could demonstrate two curves for the data for only those Asiatic Indian males 45 and over (Fig. 2), and for only those females 35 and over (curves not shown). There are many fewer people with high glucose values in the Asiatic Indian sample and this accords with our surmise that the failure to observe bimodality in earlier studies of the distribution of the GTT data is due to the relatively small number of individuals with high glucose values.

118

TABLE II

Maximum Likelihood Estimates of μ_1, μ_2, σ_2, and p for $\log_{10}$ Plasma Glucose Values of a Sample of Pima Indians

Age	Males[a]						Females[a]					
	No.	μ_1	σ_1	μ_2	σ_2	p	No.	μ_1	σ_1	μ_2	σ_2	p
5–14	236	1.989	0.090				287	2.011	0.094			
15–24	147	1.978	0.106				228	2.019	0.106			
25–34	81	2.017	0.106	2.570	0.165	0.836	152	2.076	0.125	2.643	0.081	0.920
35–44	97	2.003	0.125	2.538	0.182	0.727	147	2.109	0.109	2.509	0.212	0.667
45–54	71	2.074	0.104	2.533	0.144	0.696	96	2.168	0.164	2.664	0.102	0.670
55–64	66	2.072	0.115	2.579	0.136	0.634	88	2.166	0.134	2.628	0.109	0.471
65–74	70	2.142	0.138	2.626	0.079	0.790	55	2.140	0.117	2.527	0.137	0.574

[a] μ = Mean; σ = standard deviation; p = proportion of sample included in the first curve. See text for further explanation.

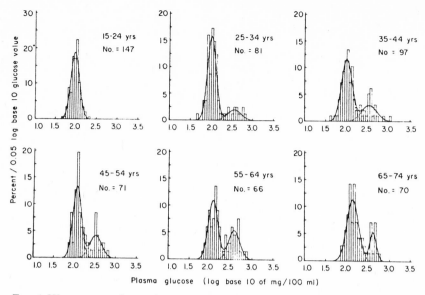

FIG. 1 Histograms and superimposed composite curve, and the component normal curves, derived to describe the distribution of the 2-hour glucose levels for Pima Indian males. See text for further explanations.

The fact that separation into two groups could be achieved among the samples for the older age groups in Asiatic Indians indicates that the separation derived for the Pima data is not unique.

The data in the column headed p in Table II indicate the weight (proportion) given to curve 1, and $1-p$ is the weight given to curve 2 when the curves are combined to estimate the observed distribution. It follows therefore, that $1-p$ represents the estimated proportion of the population assumed to be diabetic. This proportion rises in each sex, with increasing age through the 55–64 age category, and then falls. A similar pattern is apparent in the data for the Asiatic Indians. The fall is probably due to a relatively greater mortality rate among those with abnormal glucose tolerance than among those with normal tolerance (10). Except for this complication, we could in theory use $1-p$ to estimate penetrance, regardless of the genetic mechanism involved. Under the present circumstances we cannot do this, because of the fall in $1-p$ at older ages and because of perturbations introduced by the small sample sizes in some age groups. We hope to be able to do so at a later date, by using the data to be obtained from our longitudinal study of this population.

As a demonstration, we have derived values of glucose levels to classify individuals as normal or hyperglycemic. Separate cut-off points were

120

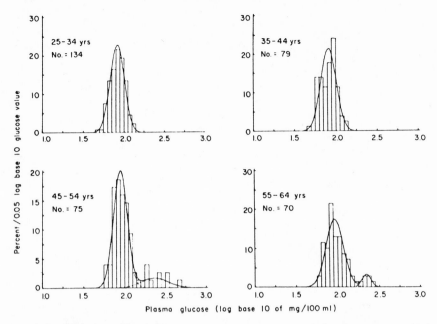

FIG. 2 Histograms and superimposed composite curve, and the component normal curves derived to describe the distribution of the 2-hour glucose levels for Asiatic Indian males. See text for further explanation.

determined for males and females between ages 25 and 74 using parameter estimates derived by methods to be described elsewhere.

Unfortunately, our family data are too few to permit satisfactory tests of hypotheses. They are presented in Tables III and IV. The parents and children were classified as normal or hyperglycemic on the basis of the commonly used glucose level of 160 mg/100 ml of plasma as the cut off point (Table III) or using 210 mg/100 ml for males and 240 mg/100 ml for females (Table IV) derived from the data for this population. The data are presented with the children grouped by age to demonstrate that most of them are younger than 25 years of age. The reader will recall that there are few hyperglycemic individuals in this age range (Table II). It is not surprising therefore that few hyperglycemic individuals were encounterd among the offspring in these 178 families. The data show the usual progression of increasing frequency of hyperglycemic children with increasing numbers of hyperglycemic parents. We call attention to the low proportion of hyperglycemic offspring when the father is affected and the mother is not (Tables III and IV). It seems likely that this observation is not of biological significance, but we shall be able to evaluate this only when the sample size has been increased.

The limited size of the sample does not justify further analysis and space

TABLE III

DISTRIBUTION OF "NORMAL" AND "DIABETIC" OFFSPRING BY SEX AND AGE, BY TYPE OF MATING[a]

	N × N[b]				Fa. D × Mo. N[b]			
	Males		Females		Males		Females	
Age	T	D	T	D	T	D	T	D
5–14	55	0	62	0	18	0	20	0
15–24	32	0	37	1	11	0	19	1
25–34	7	0	16	0	4	0	5	0
35–44	3	1	5	2	3	0	6	1
45–54	1	0	1	1	1	0	0	0
55–64	0	—	1	1	0	—	0	—

$$\% D = \frac{6}{220} \times 100 = 2.7 \qquad \% D = \frac{2}{87} \times 100 = 2.3$$

	Fa. N × Mo. D				D × D			
	Males		Females		Males		Females	
Age	T	D	T	D	T	D	D	D
5–14	21	0	19	2	4	0	14	0
15–24	17	0	29	1	13	2	14	3
25–34	10	3	11	5	10	2	16	5
35–44	3	1	7	3	4	1	11	4
45–54	2	0	0	—	0	—	0	—
55–64	0	—	0	—	1	0	1	1

$$\% D = \frac{15}{119} \times 100 = 12.6 \qquad \% D = \frac{18}{88} \times 100 = 20.5$$

[a] Cut-off for classification was 160 mg/100 ml of plasma
[b] N = "normal"; D = "diabetic"; T = total

limitations prevent us from presenting our proposed methods of procedure in detail. However, we present a summary of one approach that, to our knowledge, has not been used previously. The method estimates the gene frequency (q) and penetrance (π_{ij}) for age i, and sex j, on the assumption of a given mode of inheritance, under the following conditions: (1) recessive inheritance (other modes may be assumed); (2) essentially complete penetrance in parents;

TABLE IV

DISTRIBUTION OF "NORMAL" AND "DIABETIC" OFFSPRING BY SEX AND AGE, BY TYPE OF MATING[a]

Age	N × N[b]				Fa. D × Mo. N[b]			
	Males		Females		Males		Females	
	T	D	T	D	T	D	T	D
5–14	76	0	79	0	19	0	17	0
15–24	45	0	58	0	11	0	17	0
25–34	10	1	22	0	6	0	4	0
35–44	4	0	11	2	3	0	6	0
45–54	2	0	1	1	1	0	0	—
55–64	0	—	1	1	0	—	0	—

$$\% \text{D} = \frac{5}{309} \times 100 = 1.6 \qquad\qquad \text{D} = \frac{0}{84}$$

Age	Fa. N × Mo. D				D × D			
	Males		Females		Males		Females	
	T	D	T	D	T	D	T	D
5–14	3	0	13	0	0	—	6	0
15–24	11	0	19	0	6	0	5	1
25–34	12	3	9	1	3	0	13	1
35–44	2	0	5	0	4	1	7	2
45–54	1	0	0	—	0	—	0	—
55–64	0	—	0	—	1	0	1	1

$$\% \text{D} = \frac{4}{75} \times 100 = 5.3 \qquad\qquad \% \text{D} = \frac{6}{46} \times 100 = 13.0$$

[a] Cut-off classification was 210 mg/100 ml of plasma for males and 240 mg/100 ml for females

[b] N = "normal"; D = "diabetic"; T = total

(3) individuals examined independently of their own or their relative's phenotypes; (4) all families retained and classified into mating types of affected × normal, normal × normal, and affected × affected. With these assumptions and conditions it can be shown that the derivatives of the logarithm of the maximum likelihood equation required to solve for π_{ij} and q are:

$$(1) \quad \frac{\partial L}{\partial \pi_{ij}} = \frac{-A_{ij}q}{1 + q - \pi_{ij}q} - \frac{B_{ij}q^2}{(1 + q)^2 - \pi_{ij}q^2} - \frac{C_{ij}}{1 - \pi_{ij}} + \frac{a_{ij} + b_{ij} + c_{ij}}{\pi_{ij}}$$

$$(2) \quad \frac{\partial L}{\partial q} = - \sum \frac{A_{ij}\pi_{ij}}{(1 + q)(1 + q - q\pi_{ij})} - \sum \frac{2B_{ij}q\pi_{ij}}{(1 + q)[(1 + q)^2 - q^2\pi_{ij}]}$$
$$+ \frac{\sum_{ij}(a_{ij} + 2b_{ij})}{q} - \frac{\sum_{ij}(a_{ij} + 2b_{ij})}{1 + q}$$

Where:

A_{ij}, B_{ij}, and C_{ij} = the number of "normal" children in each of the three mating types listed above, respectively. These are estimated as $\hat{p}_{ijk} T_{ijk}$.

T_{ijk} = the total number of children of age i, sex j in mating type k, $k = 1$, 2, 3; $i = 1, n$; $j = 1, 2$.

$\hat{p}_{ijk} = \hat{p}$, the weight given to curve 1, as previously described, and is estimated by $\hat{p}$ derived from the data for offspring of age i, sex j from mating type k.

a_{ij}, b_{ij}, c_{ij} = the number of "affected" children in each of the three mating types listed above, respectively. These are estimated as $(1 - \hat{p}_{ijk}) T_{ijk}$.

Substitution of the constants appropriate for each $_{ij}$ in equation (1) yields a total of $n \times 2$ equations. Hence a total of $2n + 1$ simultaneous equations each equated to zero must be solved to estimate q and π_{ij}. The method requires large numbers of children at each $_{ijk}$ used.

The values of π_{ij} may be used to estimate the expected numbers of families of size (s) with "a" children having glucose levels above the cut-off point. These expected numbers may be compared with the observed numbers by the usual χ^2 comparison or by other standard genetic methods. The method is lengthy, hence the details cannot be present here. They will be reported elsewhere.

Summary

We have demonstrated that following a glucose challenge the 2-hour levels may be bimodally distributed if large enough numbers of hyperglycemic individuals are included in the sample, and we have derived normal distributions to describe the two populations (one normal and one "diabetic") postulated to comprise the sample. Too few families have been tested to date to permit us to test various alternative hypotheses of the inheritance of diabetes. We have presented a summary of a new approach to the analysis of family data based on the glucose tolerance test.

124

ACKNOWLEDGMENTS

We acknowledge with gratitude the expert programming provided by Mr. O. Morgenstern. We express our thanks also for the cooperation and help of the Tribal Council and the members of the Gila River Indian Community and the Division of Indian Health. Without their aid this study could not have been undertaken.

REFERENCES

1. Rimoin, D. L., *Diabetes* **16**, 346 (1967).
2. Steinberg, A. G., *Excerpta Med. Intern. Congr. Ser.* **84**, 601 (1965).
3. Steinberg, A. G., and Wilder, R. M., *Am. J. Human Genet.* **4**, 113 (1952).
4. Klimt, C. R., Meinert, C. L., Irwin, P., and Briese, F. W., *Diabetes* **16**, 40 (1967).
5. Sisk, C. W., *Lancet* **1**, 262 (1968).
6. Hayner, N. S., Waterhouse, A. M., and Gordon, T., *U.S. Public Health Serv. Publ.* **1000**, Ser. 2, No. 3 (1963).
7. Burkeholder, J. N., Pickens, J. M., and Womak, W. N., *Diabetes* **16**, 156 (1967).
8. Simpson, N. E., *Ann. Human Genet.* **26**, 1 (1962).
9. Thompson, G. S., *J. Med. Genet.* **2**, 221 (1965).
10. Miller, M., Bennett, P. H., and Burch, T. A., *Pan-Am. Health Organ. Sci. Pub.* **165**, 89 (1968).
11. Cicchinelli, A. L., Ph.D. Thesis, Univ. of Michigan, Ann Arbor, Michigan, 1963.

DIABETES MELLITUS IN
AMERICAN (PIMA) INDIANS

PETER H. BENNETT
THOMAS A. BURCH
MAX MILLER

Summary The prevalence of diabetes mellitus among the Pima Indians, who live in a hot desert environment in Arizona, U.S.A., has been determined by means of systematic glucose-tolerance tests. Using conservative conventional criteria the prevalence was 50% among those aged 35 years and over. Frequency distributions of the two-hour post-carbohydrate-load plasma-glucose levels were clearly bimodal above 35 years of age. The findings indicate that the Pima Indians have the highest prevalence of diabetes mellitus yet recorded, and that in this population normal and hyperglycæmic groups may be logically separated on the basis of the bimodality of the frequency distributions of two-hour post-load glucose levels.

Introduction

THE prevalence of diabetes mellitus has been determined carefully in several populations and, despite methodological differences which frequently vitiate comparison, it appears to vary considerably from country to country and from one ethnic group to another.

We present data which indicate that the Pima Indians of Arizona, U.S.A., have the highest prevalence of diabetes mellitus yet reported.

Methods

The Pima Indians, American Indians of the Uto-Aztecan linguistic group, reside mainly on the Gila River Reservation in south-central Arizona in the southwestern United States. This tribe and their ancestors have probably resided in this same area of the hot, dry Sonoran Desert, cultivating crops through judicious use of irrigation, for at least two thousand years.[1] The geographically well-defined eastern portion of the reservation was selected for study with the objective of examining each inhabitant, aged 5 years and over, with a glucose-tolerance test.

The glucose-tolerance test consisted of determination of the venous *plasma*-glucose level two hours after the ingestion of a 75 g. oral carbohydrate load (Glucola, Ames Company, Elkhart, Indiana; Dexcola, Custom Laboratories, Baltimore, Maryland). This was administered to all subjects regardless of age, weight, time of day, or last meal, or whether they were known previously to have

126

diabetes. The medical history of each respondent was reviewed to determine the basis for any previous diagnosis of diabetes and the nature and time of last dose of any hypoglycæmic medication. Between 1965 and 1969, 2917 half to full blooded Pima Indians were examined. This number contains 2491 of the 3035 reservation residents aged 5 years and over at the time of the census (1966), 250 of approximately 310 who became 5 years of age before completion of the study, and 176 others who returned to live on the reservation.

For the purposes of defining prevalence, those subjects with a two-hour post-load glucose level of ≥ 160 mg. per 100 ml. or unequivocal evidence of diabetes mellitus were considered to be affected.

Results

Prevalence

The glucose-tolerance results by sex and age group at the time of examination are shown in table I. Half of those with two-hour glucose levels of ≥ 160 mg. per 100 ml. had been recognised to have diabetes mellitus prior to this study, mainly as a result of presentation for medical care with the usual spectrum of classical symptoms. 11 of these 279 subjects had lower two-hour glucose levels, but had either taken hypoglycæmic medication shortly before the tolerance test or had unequivocal evidence of previous diabetes.

Fig. 1 shows the age-specific prevalence of diabetes, which rose to 47% in the 65–74-year-old males and to

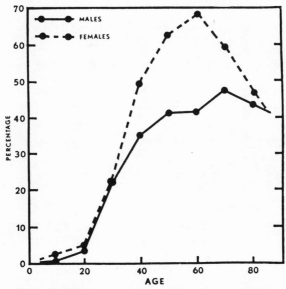

Fig. 1—Age-specific prevalence of diabetes in Pima Indian males and females.

TABLE I—TWO-HOUR POST-LOAD GLUCOSE LEVELS AND PREVALENCE OF DIABETES IN HALF TO FULL BLOODED PIMA INDIANS

Age-group (yr.)	No. examined	Two-hour venous plasma-glucose (mg./100 ml.)							With diabetes					
		0–99	100–139	140–159	160–199	200–299	300–399	400 and over	Previously recognised		Using 2-hour glucose level ≥160 mg./100 ml.*		≥200 mg./100 ml.*	
									No.	%	No.	%	No.	%
Males:														
5–14	547	280	249	16	2	:	:	:	0	0·0	2	0·4	0	0·0
15–24	239	121	95	15	3	2	1	2	1	0·4	8	3·4	5	2·1
25–34	135	39	58(1)	8	8	8	3	10	8	5·9	30	22·2	22	16·3
35–44	142	39(1)	44(1)	8	6	8	15	20	26	18·3	51	35·9	45	31·7
45–54	94	12	35	8	7	7	12	12	21	22·3	39	41·5	32	34·0
55–64	84	16	25	8(1)	4(1)	7	11	11	23	27·4	35	41·7	31	36·9
65–74	76	9(1)	20(1)	11	9	7	7	11	21	27·6	36	47·4	27	35·5
75+	41	4	13	6	5(1)	6	3	3	7	17·1	18	43·9	13	31·7
Total	1358								107	7·9	219	16·1	175	12·9
35 and over	437								98	22·4	179	41·0	148	33·9
Females:														
5–14	604	272	293	24	13	2	:	:	0	0·0	15	2·5	2	0·3
15–24	307	131	143	18	9	2	1	3	3	1·0	15	4·9	6	2·0
25–34	187	39	87	20	15	12	5	9	11	5·9	41	21·9	26	13·9
35–44	178	11	64(1)	14	26(3)	17	21	21	41	23·0	89	50·0	63	35·4
45–54	107	9	26	5(2)	12(2)	17	8	26	40	37·4	67	62·6	55	51·4
55–64	102	4	16(1)	12(1)	4(4)	15	18	27	54	52·9	70	68·6	66	64·7
65–74	59	1	15	8	6	13	9	7	21	35·6	35	59·3	29	49·2
75+	15	2	6	..	..	5	2	..	2	13·3	7	46·7	7	46·7
Total	1559								172	11·0	339	21·7	254	16·3
35 and over	461								158	34·3	268	58·1	220	47·7
Both sexes:														
Total	2917								279	9·6	558	19·1	429	14·7
35 and over	898								256	28·5	447	49·8	368	41·0

* Includes subjects, shown in main table in parentheses, who had diabetes clearly confirmed by medical record review and who were mostly taking hypoglycæmic agents, but in whom the two-hour plasma level was lower than 160 or 200 mg. per 100 ml.

69% in the 55–64-year-old females, and then fell in the older age-groups. The prevalence in females was higher than in males beyond 35 years of age ($\chi^2 = 26 \cdot 5$; $p < 0 \cdot 001$). Below this age the prevalence in the two sexes was rather similar, although the females did have a significantly higher rate in the 5–14-year age-group ($\chi^2 = 8 \cdot 6$; $p < 0 \cdot 01$).

Age at Diagnosis

The majority of the 279 subjects with an established diagnosis had been recognised to have diabetes between the ages of 25 and 64 years. When related to the population at risk the modal age at diagnosis was between 45 and 54 years (table II). Among those examined no previously known cases had been recognised below 10 years of age, but 14 (5%) had presented before the age of 25 years.

Treatment

85% of the previously recognised diabetics had received specific hypoglycæmic medication by the time of this study. 39% of the males had received insulin and 41% only oral hypoglycæmic agents. Of the females 60% had taken insulin and 27% had been treated with oral agents only.

Distributions of Glucose Levels

Among subjects aged below 25 years, less than 3% of whom had "diabetes", the two-hour plasma-glucose concentrations showed a unimodal distribution in both sexes. Above 35 years of age, where glucose intolerance was much more frequent, the distributions were clearly bimodal (fig. 2). Bimodality was found also when each decade and each sex were considered separately.

TABLE II—AGE AT DIAGNOSIS AND RELATIVE " INCIDENCE " AMONG PREVIOUSLY RECOGNISED DIABETICS

Age-group (yr.)	Age at diagnosis		Ten-year relative " incidence "†	
	Males	Females	Males	Females
0– 4	0	0	0·0	0·0
5–14	0	2	0·0	0·3
15–24	5	7	2·1	2·3
25–34	18	28	13·3	15·0
35–44	24	42	16·9	23·6
45–54	25	50	26·6	46·7
55–64	20	35	23·8	34·3
65–74	12	6	15·8	10·2
75 +	3	2	7·3	13·3
Total	107	172	..	..

† Relative " incidence " = $\dfrac{\text{no of diabetics presenting at stated age} \times 100}{\text{population of stated age}}$

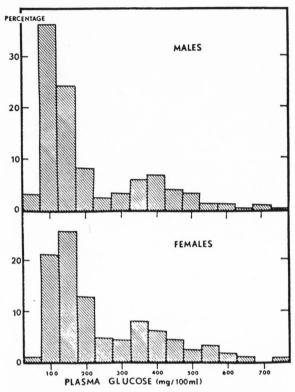

Fig. 2—Frequency distributions of two-hour post-load plasma-glucose levels in Pima Indian males and females aged 35 years and over.

Discussion

Comparisons of the prevalence of diabetes mellitus are severely hampered by the great variations in methodology. The age-groups examined, the test procedures, and diagnostic criteria vary greatly from one study to another.

Estimates of the prevalence of diabetes in western Europe and the United States generally range between 1 and 3%.[2,3] Studies employing a glucose-tolerance test yield generally higher prevalences, and in Bedford, England, and Sudbury, Massachusetts, the use of a two-hour post-load blood-sugar of 120 mg. per 100 ml. as a diagnostic criterion led to prevalence estimates of approximately 10%.[4,5] High rates have also been recorded among some other ethnic groups—for example, the urbanised East Indian population in Cape Town, South Africa (12·6% aged 35 and over),[6] the New Zealand Maori (5% aged 20 years and over),[7] and native Hawaiians (7·8% in adults).[8]

130

In contrast, among the Athabaskan Indians of Alaska [9] and the Alaskan Eskimos [10] diabetes is rare; however, some other native Americans have extremely high prevalences. The Seneca,[11] Cherokee,[12] and Cocopah Indians [13] have been reported to have diabetes-prevalence rates of 22% (aged 25 and over), 31% (35 years and over), and 34% (35 years and over), respectively.

The Pima Indians showed a prevalence of 42% among those aged 25 years and over, and 50% among those aged 35 years and over, when the criteria used in the Cocopah study were applied. These rates are significantly higher than any previously reported. They are at least ten times greater than those generally estimated for the prevalence of diabetes among the same age-groups in western Europe and the United States.

Even before systematic glucose-tolerance testing some 10% of the Pima aged 5 years and over, and 29% of those aged 35 years and over, were recognised as having diabetes mellitus.

The majority of these subjects had presented clinically as adults. Only 5% had presented before 25 years of age. This ratio is similar to that reported among clinically recognised diabetics in Great Britain and the United States.[14,15] The frequency of unrecognised glucose intolerance in the Pima children, however, was notable, suggesting that asymptomatic diabetes may be much more common in childhood than is usually suspected.

The adoption of a single venous plasma-glucose level of 160 mg. per 100 ml. and over two hours after 75 g. of glucose by mouth as the criterion for glucose tolerance abnormality is arbitrary. It corresponds to a whole-blood glucose level of approximately 140 mg. per 100 ml., and represents a conservative criterion in relation to the 120 mg. per 100 ml. post-load value used in several studies.

A more logical separation can be based on the finding that the frequency distribution of the plasma-glucose levels among those aged 35 years and over was bimodal. Further analysis showed that the frequency distributions had a similar configuration in each decade and in each sex above this age. This finding indicated a natural segregation of the population into two sub-groups, with the intersects in the distributions at plasma-glucose levels between 200 and 250 mg. per 100 ml. The biological significance of this division has been further substantiated by the observation that the specific microangiopathic lesions of diabetes—retino-pathy and nephropathy—occurred in high frequency

131

and mainly among those Pima subjects who fell in the hyperglycæmic component of the glucose distributions.[16] For these reasons, and since, because of the overlap, no single cut-off level would result in the accurate classification of all individuals, it seems likely that a cut-off point of 200 mg. per 100 ml. would result in a better estimate of prevalence than the previous criterion. By this criterion the prevalence of diabetes was still extraordinarily high—34% and 48%, respectively, in the males and females aged 35 years and over (table I).

The reasons for such a high frequency of diabetes mellitus are obscure. The Pima Indians are, in general, obese, and their diet differs somewhat from the typical American diet [17]; they have large families, they reside in a desert environment, and they are relatively inbred. We have no evidence to indicate that they suffer from " secondary " diabetes.

This natural, well-defined, and relatively homogeneous community, with such a high prevalence of diabetes mellitus, provides an opportunity to examine, by well-controlled observations, the genetics and natural history and complications of diabetes mellitus.

We thank especially all the members of the Gila River Indian Community who participated in the study, and the staff physicians, Dr. Leonard J. Comess, Dr. Robert E. Henry, and Dr. R. Gordon Senter, and other staff who conducted the examinations. We also extend our appreciation to the Tribal Council of the Gila River Indian Community, the Division of Indian Health, and staff of the United States Public Health Service Indian Hospital, Sacaton, Arizona, for permission to perform the study and for much helpful advice and assistance.

1. Haury, E. *Natn. geogr. Mag.* 1967, p. 670.
2. Jorde, R. *in* Diabetes: Proceedings of the Sixth Congress of International Diabetes Federation (edited by J. Ostman); p. 669. Amsterdam, 1969.
3. Wilkerson, H. L., Krall, C. P. *J. Am. med. Ass.* 1947, **135**, 209.
4. Butterfield, W. J. H. *Proc. R. Soc. Med.* 1964, **57**, 196.
5. O'Sullivan, J. B. *in* Diabetes: Proceedings of the Sixth Congress of International Diabetes Federation (edited by J. Ostman); p. 696. Amsterdam, 1969.
6. Marine, N., Vinik, A. I., Edelstein, I., Jackson, W. P. U. *Diabetes*, 1969, **18**, 840.
7. Prior, I. A. M., Davidson, F. *N.Z. med. J.* 1966, **65**, 375.
8. Sloan, N. R. *J. Am. med. Ass.* 1963, **183**, 419.
9. Mouratoff, G. J., Carroll, N. V., Scott, E. M. *Diabetes*, 1969, **18**, 29.
10. Mouratoff, G. J., Carroll, N. V., Scott, E. M. *J. Am. med. Ass.* 1967, **199**, 107.
11. Doeblin, T. D., Evans, K., Ingall, G., Frohman, L. A., Bannerman, R. M. *Diabetologia*, 1969, **5**, 203.

12. Stein, J. H., West, K. M., Robey, J. M., Tirador, Đ. F., McDonald, G. W. *Archs intern. Med.* 1965, **116**, 842.
13. Henry, R. E., Burch, T. A., Bennett, P. H., Miller, M. *Diabetes*, 1969, **18**, 332.
14. Fitzgerald, M. G., Malins, J. M., O'Sullivan, D. J., Wall, M. *Q. Jl Med.* 1961, **117**, 57.
15. Vital and Health Statistics, Characteristics of Persons with Diabetes, U.S. 1964-1965. National Center for Health Statistics, P.H.S. publication no. 1000, series 10, no. 40. U.S. Government Printing Office, Washington, D.C.
16. Miller, M., Bennett, P. H., Burch, T. A. *in* Biomedical Challenges Presented by the American Indian: Scientific Publication no. 165; p. 89. Pan American Health Organization, Washington, D.C., 1968.
17. Reid, J. M., Fullmer, S. D., Pettigrew, K. D., Burch, T. A., Bennett, P. H., Miller, M., Whedon, G. D. *Am. J. clin. Nutr.* (in the press).

Ethnic Variability in Glucose Tolerance and Insulin Secretion

David L. Rimoin, MD, PhD.

In an attempt to assess the ethnic variability of diabetes mellitus, a comparative study of the clinical and metabolic features of diabetes in the Navajo Indian and Pennsylvania Amish was undertaken. The Navajo have a mild form of diabetes in which the juvenile ketotic form is unknown and complications are rare, while the Amish have both juvenile and maturity-onset forms with all of the acute and chronic complications. The mean peak plasma immunoreactive insulin (IRI) concentrations attained following oral ingestion of 100 gm of glucose differed significantly in the two groups of diabetics, suggesting that they may represent distinct disorders. There was more than a threefold difference in the maximal plasma IRI response between the normal Navajo and normal Amish, indicating that there is marked ethnic variability in the normal insulin response to an orally given glucose load.

Although diabetes mellitus is a ubiquitous disorder, epidemiological surveys have revealed significant differences in the prevalence of diabetes among different populations.[1] It has become apparent that marked ethnic variability in the clinical features of diabetes also exists.[2] Although there appears to be a general correlation between overnutrition and the prevalence of diabetes[1] when the clinical form of the disease and diet are compared in different populations, no clear correlation is found (Table). For example, although the diet of the Navajo Indian is quite similar to that of the Western European in terms of relative fat and carbohydrate intake, both ketosis and vascular complications are rare in the Navajo, but common in the European.[3] On the other hand, the Japanese[4] and Ceylonese[5] consume a diet which is low in fat and carbohydrate, and yet have a form of diabetes similar to that in the Navajo. In the Pima[6] and Alabama-Coushatta Indians[7] who consume diets high in animal fat and carbohydrates, diabetic ketoacidosis

| Ethnic Group | Diet | | Ketosis | Vascular Complications |
	Fat	Carbohydrate		
European	High	High	Common	Common
Navajo Indians	High	High	Rare	Rare
Alabama-Coushatta Indians	High	High	Rare	Common
Pima Indians	High	High	Rare	Common
Lebanese	High (vegetable)	...	Rare	Common
Japanese	Low	High	Rare	Uncommon
Ceylonese	Low	High	Rare	Uncommon
South American Indians	Low	High	Rare	Very common
South African Negroes	Low	High	Common	Rare

is rare, but the vascular complications of the disease are fairly common. This same form of diabetes is found in the Lebanese who have a high vegetable but low animal fat intake.[8] The Natal Indian and Negro of South Africa have roughly similar diets, at least in terms of total fat and carbohydrate intake, but ketosis is rare in the Natal Indian and common in the South African Negro, whereas the reverse is true for vascular complications.[9] Thus the ethnic variabiliy in the clinical features of diabetes does not appear to be directly related to dietary intake.

In an attempt to define this ethnic variability, a comparative study of the clinical and metabolic characteristics of diabetes in two distinct populations, the Navajo Indian and Pennsylvania Amish, was undertaken. These two particular groups were chosen since they represent genetically homogeneous populations with clinically distinct forms of the disorder. The Navajo have a mild form of diabetes in which both ketosis and vascular complications are rare, whereas the Amish have the typical European form of the disease with all of the acute and chronic complications. Plasma insulin determinations following oral ingestion of glucose demonstrated that the clinical differences between these two groups of diabetics are paralleled by differences in the pattern of insulin secretion. Furthermore, a significant difference in the plasma insulin response to orally taken glucose was found to exist between normal members of the two populations.

The Navajo Indian

The Navajo are presently the largest Indian tribe in the United States with a population exceeding 100,000 individuals. They are an Athabascan speaking people, closely related linguistically to the Apache. The Navajo were relatively late arrivals to the American Southwest (circa 800-900 AD), arriving many centuries after the Pueblo. They are a genetically distinct group, differing from the neighboring Pueblo tribes in physical characteristics and blood group frequencies.[10]

The Navajo live in small, isolated

135

family groups scattered over a 25,000-sq mi reservation located principally in northeastern Arizona. The land is poor and their homes are without running water and electricity. The Navajo diet consists primarily of mutton stew and potatoes and bread fried in lard, and has a high content of saturated fat. Dietary surveys of the Navajo have indicated that their fat intake is similar to that of the average U. S. white.[11] In spite of this high-fat diet, the Navajo have been found to have a low prevalence of coronary heart disease, atherosclerosis, and hypertension.[12-15]

Clinical surveys have revealed that diabetes mellitus is a fairly common but extremely mild disorder among the Navajo.[3,16] In a recent retrospective analysis of 105 hospitalized Navajo diabetics, Saiki and Rimoin[3] found only three patients with a history of ketosis and seven with mild diabetic retinopathy. The juvenile form of the disease is unknown and not one case of ketoacidotic coma has been observed. Thus abnormal glucose tolerance appears to be a relatively benign chemical abnormality in the Navajo.

Pennsylvania Amish

The old-order Amish are a highly inbred religious sect widely known for their old-fashioned dress and resistance to technological advances.[17] They originated in Switzerland in 1693 as an ultraconservative wing of the Mennonite movement and migrated to eastern Pennsylvania in the 18th century. The Amish presently live in rural areas and most are farmers.

A professional dietitian visited six representative Amish households in different areas of Lancaster County and estimated their average daily intake to be approximately 2,500 calories, of which 45.9% were of carbohydrate origin, 41.5% of fat (43.3% of which was saturated) and 12.5% of protein. Thus they consume a diet which is high in carbohydrate and fat and relatively low in protein. In terms of the relative proportions of fat and carbohydrate, the diets of the Amish and Navajo are remarkably similar, although the Amish appear to have a higher total caloric intake.

Consistent with their ancestry, the Amish appear to have the typical western European form of diabetes, with both the ketotic juvenile insulin-dependent and the obese-maturity-onset varieties of the disease. Death from juvenile diabetes is well known in the community, as are the ocular and vascular complications of the disease. Since the Amish do not seek regular medical care, it was impossible to find a large group of known diabetics eliminating possibility of a survey of the clinical features of long-standing diabetes in this population. In a general health survey of the Pennsylvania Amish, Egeland[18] noted that the diagnosis of diabetes was found on the death certificates of many Amish. Six local physicians and osteopaths who were interviewed could recall 12 of their Amish patients who had diabetes. Of these 12, at least three had known coronary artery disease, 10 required insulin, 4 were known to have ketoacidosis, and 3 had significant retinopathy. A search of the medical

136

records for a two-year period in three local hospitals disclosed nine Amish patients with a diagnosis of diabetes at discharge, of whom three were admitted in diabetic coma, four had diabetic retinopathy, three had coronary artery disease, two had peripheral vascular insufficiency, and one was a 17-month old child. These individuals certainly have the more severe cases of diabetes and many undetected diabetics with mild forms of the disease exist in the Amish population as was discovered in the screening program to be discussed. Thus the type of diabetes found in the Amish is similar to the typical European form of the disease with all of the acute and chronic complications and is markedly different from the mild form of diabetes observed in the Navajo.

Plasma Insulin Responses

Methods.—Plasma glucose [19] (glucose oxidase method) and immunoreactive insulin (IRI) concentrations [20] following the ingestion of 100 gm of glucose were determined in a sample of Navajo and Amish diabetic and control subjects. All individuals were studied after they fasted overnight. Venous blood samples drawn at 0, 30, 60, 120, and 180 minutes were heparinized and the plasma was immediately separated and frozen. An individual was defined as diabetic if at least two of his plasma glucose values exceeded the following limits: fasting, 110 mg/100 ml; 30 minutes, 210 mg/100 ml; 60 minutes, 180 mg/100 ml; 120 minutes, 140 mg/100 ml; and 180 minutes, 120 mg/100 ml. If only one of the plasma glucose determinations exceeded these limits, they were classed as borderline.

As a means of ascertaining "new diabetics" in the Amish community, a screening program for diabetes mellitus was instituted. In order to obtain the highest possible yield, individuals who were known to have diabetic relatives were selected for study. Their spouses and neighbors who had no known family history of diabetes were selected as a control group.

The Navajo diabetics were selected from clinic patients of the Public Health Service Indian Hospital at Fort Defiance, Ariz, who had recently been discovered to have diabetes on the basis of routine urine or blood glucose analyses. None of these individuals had ever received insulin. The control patients were selected from Navajos living in the Fort Defiance area who had no known glucose intolerance and a negative family history of diabetes.

Results

The Navajo Indian.—The results of the Navajo's plasma glucose and insulin responses to orally given glucose have been previously published.[21] Following the ingestion of 100 gm of glucose, the Navajo controls reached a mean peak plasma insulin concentration of 141.2 ± 13.7 microunits/ml at 60 minutes (Fig 1). On the basis of the plasma glucose and insulin responses, the diabetics were separated into two distinct groups. Diabetics with marked glucose intolerance (more than 300 mg/100 ml) (group 1) had a diminished insulin response with a mean peak plasma insulin concentration of 43.9 ± 9.1 microunits/ml at two hours. There was also a group of individuals with mild glucose intolerance who had a plasma insulin response which was indistinguishable from that of the controls. These individuals were classed as group 2 diabetics, since they had abnormal glucose tolerance on the basis of criteria in whites and

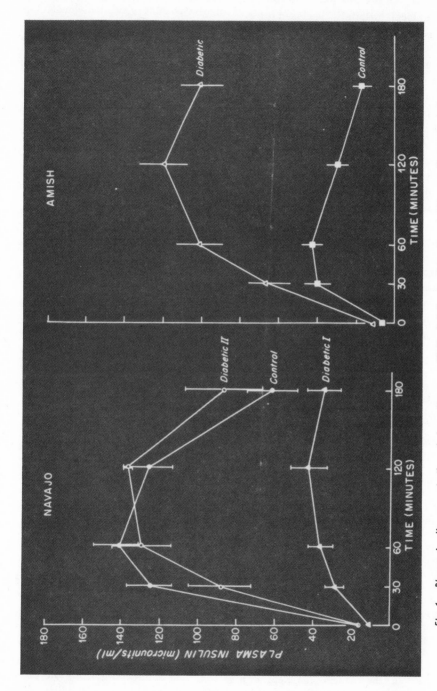

Fig 1.—Plasma insulin concentrations (microunits per milliliter) following ingestion of 100 gm glucose in diabetic and control Navajo and Amish individuals. The values are given as mean ±1 standard error.

yet had an insulin response which was normal by Navajo standards. No physical differences were apparent between these two groups, nor were there any differences in sex distribution, body weight, or blood pressure. None of the diabetics of either group had symptoms of the disease, and none had evidence of diabetic complications. Group 1 diabetics had significantly lower insulin-glucose ratios than the Navajo controls, whereas the insulin-glucose ratios of the group 2 diabetics were intermediate (Fig 2). Thus the normal Navajo has a brisk and high plasma insulin response to the ingestion of glucose and markedly diminished glucose tolerance is associated with relative insulin deficiency.

Pennsylvania Amish.—Glucose tolerance tests were performed on 83 Amish individuals, of whom 19 had definitely abnormal glucose tolerance and 7 had borderline abnormalities. Of the 57 with normal glucose tolerance, 44 had a known family history of diabetes and 13 had no known diabetic close relatives. With the standards of more than 63.5 kg (140 lb) in women and more than 81.6 kg (180 lb) in men as a definition of overweight, 77.8% of the diabetics and 30.8% of the controls were overweight. A similar distribution of obesity in the Navajo sample was also obtained, in accord with the general association of decreased glucose tolerance with excess body weight. Thus there were no significant differences in the distribution of obesity between the Navajo and Amish samples.

Following administration of glucose, the plasma insulin concentrations of the normal Amish with negative family histories rose to a mean peak concentration of 43.0± 5.43 microunits/ml at 60 minutes (Fig 1). The mean plasma insulin concentrations of the nondiabetics with positive family histories were consistently higher than in those with negative family histories, but these differences were not statistically significant. The Amish diabetics had a delayed rise in plasma insulin to a mean peak concentration of 119.7± 12.92 microunits/ml at 120 minutes. Individuals with borderline glucose tolerance attained a peak plasma insulin concentration of 90.43±15.86 microunits/ml at 60 minutes which quickly returned to basal levels, a response which was intermediate between the Amish controls and diabetics. The mean insulin-glucose ratios of the Amish diabetics and controls were also significantly different, indicating that the differences in plasma insulin concentration were not secondary to the degree of hyperglycemia achieved (Fig 2). Thus, the normal Amish secrete a modest amount of insulin in response to a glucose load, while the maturity-onset Amish diabetic appears to have a relative hypersecretion of insulin. This high-output state is comparable to that seen in other maturity-onset diabetics. The diabetics examined were too few to attempt to correlate obesity with hyperinsulinism, but at any specific body weight, the peak insulin response of the diabetics was greater than that of the nondiabetics.

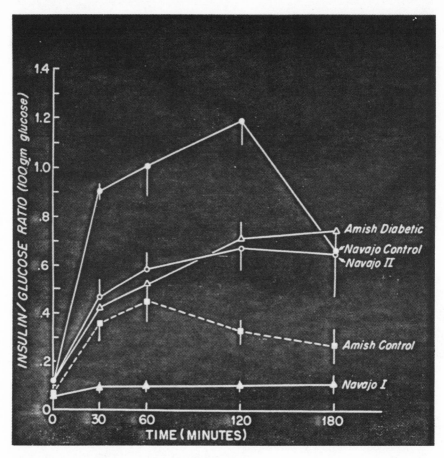

Fig 2.—Mean (±1 standard error) plasma insulin-glucose ratios achieved after ingestion of 100 gm glucose at time 0.

Comment

Epidemiologists have long used racial comparisons to detect variability in the prevalence and pattern of infectious disease. The techniques of medical ecology can also prove useful in delineating pathogenetic mechanisms in diseases of noninfectious origin.[22] Variability in the prevalence and pattern of disease among ethnic groups can be secondary to both genetic and environmental modifying factors, but it may also indicate the presence of heterogeneity, the symptom complex in question consisting of a number of distinct disorders. Marked ethnic variability in the prevalence and clinical features of diabetes mellitus has been well documented.[2] The comparative study described here demonstrates that ethnic variability in the metabolic features of diabetes as well as in the normal insulin response to glucose may also be important phenomena.

140

The Navajo Indians and Pennsylvania Amish represent two racially distinct populations. Although they inhabit markedly different environments, they both consume diets high in fat and carbohydrates. A comparison of their plasma insulin responses to a standard orally given glucose load has led to two striking observations. First, there is more than a threefold difference in the maximal plasma IRI response to orally taken glucose between the *normal* members of both populations. Plasma insulin rose to a mean peak concentration of 141.2 microunits/ml in the normal Navajo, as compared to a mean of only 43.9 microunits/ml in the normal Amish (Fig 1). This difference in insulin secretion does not appear to be related to differences in physical habitus nor is it related to differences in blood glucose concentrations achieved, as there are also significant differences in their mean insulin-glucose ratios (Fig 2). This difference in normal insulin secretion could possibly be related to environmental factors, such as the amount of prior carbohydrate ingestion, as carbohydrate deprivation has been found to be associated with decreased glucose tolerance and hyperinsulinism.[23] Although the average caloric intake of the Navajo does not appear to be as large as that of the Amish, the Navajo does consume a diet high in carbohydrates and all of the Navajo tested claimed that they had eaten well for the week proceeding the tolerance test. Furthermore, the relative hyperinsulinism observed in the normal Navajo is not associated with glucose intolerance.

Thus dietary differences alone cannot account for the marked difference in normal insulin secretion between these two populations. It is likely that other factors among which may be genetic effects are also involved. The marked similarity in insulin secretory patterns of identical twins observed by Cerasi and Luft [24] suggest that genetic factors do contribute significantly in determining the normal pattern of insulin secretion.

The clinical form of diabetes mellitus is markedly different in these two populations. The juvenile ketotic form of the disease is common in the Amish, but unknown in the Navajo. Severe ketoacidosis and coma often occur in the Amish, but even mild ketosis is rare in the Navajo. The vascular complications of diabetes seldom develop in the Navajo, whereas retinopathy, nephropathy, coronary artery disease, and peripheral vascular disease are common in Amish diabetics. Thus abnormal glucose tolerance is associated with all of the known complications of diabetes mellitus in the Amish, but it appears to be a relatively benign chemical abnormality in the Navajo.

The clinical differences observed between the Navajo and Amish diabetics are paralleled by differences in their plasma insulin response to orally given glucose. Amish diabetics secrete large amounts of insulin in comparison to the Amish controls, while Navajo diabetics have a diminished insulin response to glucose given orally in comparison to the Navajo controls. The differences in plasma insulin concentrations of the group 1 Navajo diabetics and Amish diabetics are apparently not secondary to the degree of hyperglycemia achieved, since the mean insulin-glucose ratios of these two groups of diabetics are significantly different (Fig 2). Furthermore, this difference does not appear to be related to body habitus, as approximately 80% of both groups of diabetics were overweight.

The group 2 Navajo diabetics remain an enigma. These individuals have mild abnormalities in glucose tolerance, but their plasma insulin concentrations were identical to those of the Navajo controls. Although they could represent mild diabetics in whom marked glucose intolerance and insulinopenia will develop in time, no clinical differences were apparent between them and the group 1 diabetics. On the other hand, their mild glucose intolerance may be completely unrelated to insulin secretion and secondary to some other factor. Finally, normal plasma glucose levels may be higher in the Navajo than in the European, and the group 2 individuals may, in reality, be normal and only artifically designated as diabetics on the basis of criteria in whites for normal glucose tolerance. Since these group 2 individuals had plasma insulin concentrations and insulin-glucose ratios which were similar to those of the Amish diabetics, the question arises as to whether the Amish diabetics and group 2 Navajo diabetics may with time both progress to an insulinopenic state. Only long-term follow-up of the insulin response of these two groups of diabetics can definitively answer this question. It is unlikely, however, that these two groups of diabetics are identical since their insulin responses in relationship to their own controls are markedly different. The group 2 Navajo diabetics had an insulin response similar to that of the Navajo controls, whereas the insulin response of the Amish diabetics was more than five times as great as that of the Amish controls. Furthermore, in many Amish diabetics all of the acute and chronic complications of the disease eventually develop, while the majority of the Navajo diabetics remain asymptomatic.

This evidence suggests that these two forms of diabetes mellitus may represent distinct disorders. The data presented here do not allow one to decide whether these differences are due primarily to genetic or environmental factors, and it is extremely unlikely, of course, that the necessary mating to test for genetic differences between these two groups of diabetics will ever be realized. Evidence derived from other sources, however, indicates that genetic heterogeneity may well account for the variability observed in the clinical and metabolic features of diabetes.[2] The hypothesis of genetic heterogeneity in diabetes is supported by the fact that at least 16 distinct genetic disorders, apparently secondary to mutations at different loci, are associated with abnormal glucose tolerance.[25] Most of the current studies of prediabetics are based on the premise that diabetes is a single homogeneous disorder inherited as an autosomal recessive trait. The supposition is then made that all offspring of two diabetics must have the diabetic genotype and thus be either diabetic or prediabetic. In all of these studies, however, only about 50% of such individuals are found to have the prediabetic marker in question.[26,27] If diabetes is heterogeneous genetically, this is what would be expected, since all such offspring would be prediabetic only if both parents had identical forms of a diabetic disorder which was inherited as an autosomal recessive trait. If two individuals with different genetic forms of diabetes mated, anywhere from 0 to 100% of the offspring would be affected depending on whether or not the mutant genes were allelic, were additive in their action, and on their degree of penetrance. Thus in studying the offspring of conjugal diabetics, the nature of the disorder in both parents must be established. Unless the true heterogeneity of diabetes is recognized, it will be impossible to delineate the various possible pathogenetic mechanisms involved in the production of decreased glucose tolerance. Diabetes mellitus is commonly diagnosed on the basis of hyperglycemia alone. One might speculate that hyperglycemia may be no more specific than hypertension, hypercalcemia, or anemia.

The marked difference in insulin secretion between the normal members of the Navajo and Amish populations demonstrates the variability that can exist in the normal pattern of insulin secretion. This variability can completely mask basic metabolic differences between normal and diabetic individuals if proper controls are not used. Indeed, the plasma insulin response of the Amish diabetics was indistinguishable from that of the Navajo controls, while the insulin response of the group 1 Navajo diabetics was indistinguishable from that of the Amish controls. If Amish controls were used in a study of Navajo diabetics, or vice versa, no differences between the plasma insulin responses of diabetics and controls would be found. It thus appears important to establish normal standards for insulin secretion for each population studied. Furthermore, in any study involving plasma IRI concentrations, appropriate controls from the same ethnic group and environment must be selected.

This study was supported in part by Public Health Service graduate training grant 5-TI-GM-624-04 and Research Career Development Award 1-KO3-HD 38651-01.

John Harris Saiki, MD, collaborated in the Navajo study and Victor A. McKusick, MD, and Thomas J. Merimee, MD, provided assistance. John Wachter provided technical assistance and Norma Watts assisted in the Amish study.

References

1. West, K.M., and Kalbfleish, J.M.: Glucose Tolerance, Nutrition and Diabetes in Uraguay, Venezuela, Malaya and East Pakistan, *Diabetes* 15:9-18, 1966.

2. Rimoin, D.L.: Genetics of Diabetes Mellitus, *Diabetes* 16:346-351, 1967.

3. Saiki, J.H., and Rimoin, D.L.: Diabetes Mellitus Among the Navajo: I. Clinical Features, *Arch Intern Med* 122: 1-5, 1968.

4. Rudnick, P.A., and Anderson, P.S.: Diabetes Mellitus in Hiroshima, Japan, *Diabetes* 11:533-543, 1962.

5. De Zoysa, V.P.: Clinical Variations of the Diabetic Syndrome in a Tropical Country (Ceylon), *Arch Intern Med* 88: 812-818, 1951.

6. Genuth, S.M., et al: Hyperinsulinism in Obese Diabetic Pima Indians, *Metabolism* 16:1010-1015, 1967.

7. Johnson, J.E., and McNutt, C.W.: Diabetes Mellitus in an American Indian Population Isolate, *Texas Rep Biol Med* 22:110-125, 1964.

8. Khachadurian, A.K., and Somerville, I.: Diabetes Mellitus in Lebanon: A Retrospective Clinical Study of 560 Patients, *J Chron Dis* 18:1309-1315 1965.

9. Walker, A.R.P.; Richardson, B.D.; and Mistry, S.D.: Studies on Glucose Metabolism, *Brit Med J* 2:1394, 1964.

10. Mourant, A.E.; Kopec, A.C.; and Domaniewska-Sobczak, K.: *The ABO Blood Groups*, Springfield, Ill: Charles C Thomas, Publisher, 1958.

11. Darby, W.J., et al: A Study of the Dietary Background and Nutriture of the Navajo Indian, *J Nutr* 60 (suppl 2):1-85, 1956.

12. Fulmer, H.S., and Roberts, R.W.: Coronary Heart Disease Among the Navajo Indians, *Ann Intern Med* 59:740-764, 1963.

13. Gilbert, J.: Absence of Coronary Thrombosis in Navajo Indians, *Calif Med* 82:114-115. 1955.

14. Smith, R.L.: Cardiovascular-Renal and Diabetes Deaths Among the Navajos, *Public Health Rep* 72:33-38, 1957.

15. Streeper, R.B., et al: An Electrocardiographic and Autopsy Study of Coronary Heart Disease in the Navajo, *Dis Chest* 38:305-312, 1960.

16. Prosnitz, L.R., and Mandell, G.L.: Diabetes Mellitus Among Navajo and Hopi Indians: The Lack of Vascular Complications, *Amer J Med Sci* 253:700-705, 1967.

17. McKusick, V.A., et al: The Distribution of Certain Genes in the Old Order Amish, *Cold Spring Harbor Sympos Quant Biol* 29:99-114, 1964.

18. Egeland, J.A.: Belief and Behavior as Related to Illness: A Community Care Study of the Old Order Amish, thesis, Yale University, New Haven, Conn, 1962.

19. Saifer, A., and Gerstenfeld, S.: The Photometric Microdetermination of Blood Glucose With Glucose Oxidase, *J Lab Clin Med* 51:448-460, 1958.

20. Yalow, R.S., and Berson, S.A.: Immunoassay of Endogenous Plasma Insulin in Man, *J Clin Invest* 39:1157-1175. 1960.

21. Rimoin, D.L., and Saiki, J.H.: Diabetes Mellitus Among the Navajo: II. Plasma Glucose and Insulin Responses, *Arch Intern Med* 122:6-9, 1968.

22. Lilienfeld, A.M.: "Epidemiologic Methods and Inferences Applied to the Study of Noninfectious Diseases," in B. S. Blumberg (ed.): *Proceedings of the Conference on Genetic Polymorphisms and Geographic Variations in Disease*, New York: Grune & Stratton, Inc., 1961, pp 61-72.

23. Hales, C.N., and Randle, P.J.: Effects of Low Carbohydrate Diet and Diabetes Mellitus on Plasma Concentrations of Glucose, Nonesterified Fatty Acid, and Insulin During Oral Glucose Tolerance Tests, *Lancet* 1:790-794 (April 13) 1963.

24. Cerasi, E., and Luft, R.: Insulin Response to Glucose Infusion in Diabetic and Nondiabetic Monozygotic Twin Pairs: Genetic Control of Insulin Response? *Acta Endocr* 55:330-345, 1967.

25. Rimoin, D.L.: "The Genetics of Diabetes Mellitus" in Ellenberg, M. and Rifkin, H. (eds.): *Diabetes Mellitus: Theory and Practice*, New York: McGraw-Hill Book Co., to be published.

26. Siperstein, M.D.; Unger, R.H.; and Madison, L.L.: Studies of Muscle Capillary Basement Membranes in Normal Subjects, Diabetic and Prediabetic Patients, *J Clin Invest* 47:1973-1999, 1968.

27. Taton, J., et al: Genetic Determinism to Diabetics and Tolerance to Glucose, *Lancet* 2:1360-1362, 1964.

144

Asymptomatic Parotid Enlargement in Pima Indians

Relationship to Age, Obesity, and Diabetes Mellitus

STEPHEN B. LEVINE, M.D., RICHARD E. SAMPLINER, M.D.,

PETER H. BENNETT, M.B., M.R.C.P., NORMAN B. RUSHFORTH, Ph.D.,

THOMAS A. BURCH, M.D., and MAX MILLER, M.D.

The association of diabetes and asymptomatic parotid enlargement was examined in the Pima, an American Indian tribe with a high prevalence of diabetes mellitus. The parotid gland size of 290 subjects was graded by two independent observers without knowledge of the diabetes status. Palpable parotid glands were found in 61% of subjects. Parotid gland size was associated with age, sex, obesity, and diabetes. Multiple correlation analyses demonstrated that in both sexes age and obesity were more important than plasma glucose in predicting parotid size. The relationship of asymptomatic parotid enlargement and diabetes mellitus in the Pima Indians was mainly the result of the common association of both factors to age and obesity.

ASYMPTOMATIC enlargement of the parotid glands has been reported to occur with diabetes mellitus in both hospitalized patients (1) and diabetic outpatients (2). Recently Davidson, Leibel, and Berris (3) reported 16 patients with asymptomatic parotid enlargement, 14 of whom were considered to have diabetes.

145

The Pima Indians were selected for investigation of the relationship of asymptomatic parotid enlargement to diabetes because of their extraordinary prevalence of hyperglycemia (4) and the clinical impression of a high frequency of parotid enlargement among Southwestern Indians (5). The common occurrence of characteristic diabetic renal and retinal complications (4) indicates that this hyperglycemia is diabetes mellitus. Among the Pima Indians an apparent association of parotid enlargement with diabetes resulted primarily from the common association of both factors with age and obesity.

Methods

The majority of the Pima Indians reside on the Gila River Reservation in the desert southeast of Phoenix, Ariz. Those on the eastern part of the reservation receive their medical care from a single Indian Health Service hospital. Since 1965 the National Institutes of Health have conducted prospective studies on diabetes and arthritis in the Pima Indians. An effort is made to administer a modified glucose tolerance test to each member of the population every 2 years.

Two hundred ninety Indian residents of the Gila River Reservation who were 5 years of age or older were examined over a 6-week period. They included routine respondents to the NIH study, outpatients of the general medical and obstetrical clinics of the hospital, and a few inpatients. Ninety-three percent of the subjects were at least half Pima. To avoid observer bias no subjects were obtained from the diabetes clinic. Only three persons refused to participate.

The diagnosis of diabetes was based on the results of the most recent modified glucose tolerance test done in the NIH study. Plasma glucose levels 2 hr after a 75-g glucose equivalent load* were determined on the AutoAnalyzer using the modified Hoffman method†. All the subjects had been tested within the last 4 years, 255 subjects within the last 2 years. Subjects with a glucose level of 140 mg/100 ml or less were defined as nondiabetic, 141 to 199 mg/100 ml as intermediate, and 200 mg/100 ml or greater as diabetic. This latter level is as high as any previously recommended criterion and is clearly abnormal. In addition, almost all retinopathy, elevated serum creatinine levels,

---

* Glucola®, Ames Co., Elkhart, Ind.; or Dexcola®, Custom Laboratories, Baltimore, Md.
† Technicon AutoAnalyzer Method File N-20, Technicon Instruments Corp., Chauncey, N.Y.

and heavy proteinuria occurred in Pima Indians with glucose levels over 200 mg/100 ml (4).

Percent desirable weight calculated by dividing the subject's weight by the desirable weight for the subject's age, sex, and height (6, 7) was used as an index of obesity. Subjects with a percent desirable weight of 125 or greater were defined as obese.

The size of each parotid gland was graded independently by two observers without knowledge of the subject's diabetes status. The scale used was 0 = undetectable, 1 = small, 2 = large, and 3 = readily visible and very large. Both observers' grades of each parotid gland were added to give parotid scores ranging from 0 to 12. The detectable parotid glands were discrete, nontender, firmer than adipose tissue, and generally symmetrical. The subjects were unaware of the parotid enlargement, and none had complaints referable to it at the time of examination.

Results

The prevalence of subjects with parotid scores of 4 to 12 (palpable glands) was 61.4%, 71.6% in males and 55.9% in females (Table 1). The prevalence of subjects with parotid scores of 8 to 12 (enlarged glands) was 31.4%, 45.1% in males and 23.7% in females. Both palpable and enlarged glands were more frequent in males aged 15 years and over and in females aged 25 years and over.

Fifty-six diabetics could be matched by sex and age (within 6 years) with an equal number of nondiabetics. The mean parotid score was significantly greater among diabetics than among nondiabetics ($P < 0.02$, Table 2 (*top*)). Since a significant correlation coefficient ($r = 0.28$) between parotid score and percent desirable weight was found, the data were reexamined matching for obesity using percent desirable weight within a range of five percentage points. The association between parotid size and diabetes then disappeared (Table 2 (*bottom*)).

Multiple correlation analyses (8) were performed to determine the degree of dependence of the total parotid score on the variables of age, percent desirable weight, and plasma glucose. From the significant correlation coefficients found it was estimated that 52% of the variability in parotid score in the males ($r = 0.72$) and 41% in females

147

Table 1. Distribution of Parotid Scores by Age, Sex, Obesity, and Diabetes

Age	Obesity Status	Number Examined	Parotid Score 0 to 3			4 to 7			8 to 12		
			Non-diabetic	Inter-mediate	Diabetic	Non-diabetic	Inter-mediate	Diabetic	Non-diabetic	Inter-mediate	Diabetic
Males											
5-14	Nonobese	11	9	—	—	2	—	—	—	—	—
	Obese	3	2	—	—	1	—	—	—	—	—
15-34	Nonobese	19	12	—	1	3	—	1	1	—	1
	Obese	22	3	—	—	5	1	—	4	4	5
35-54	Nonobese	5	1	—	—	—	1	1	—	1	1
	Obese	15	—	—	1	1	—	1	5	1	6
55+	Nonobese	18	—	—	—	3	—	3	7	—	5
	Obese	9	—	—	—	—	4	—	2	1	2
Subtotals		102	27	—	2	15	6	6	19	7	20
Females											
5-14	Nonobese	17	16	—	—	1	—	—	—	—	—
	Obese	4	3	1	—	—	—	—	—	—	—
15-34	Nonobese	30	24	1	1	1	2	1	—	—	—
	Obese	58	19	3	2	12	3	4	9	4	2
35-54	Nonobese	9	3	2	—	2	—	1	—	—	1
	Obese	49	4	—	—	18	—	5	12	2	8
55+	Nonobese	9	1	—	2	3	1	—	—	—	2
	Obese	12	1	—	—	4	—	2	3	—	2
Subtotals		188	71	7	5	41	6	13	24	6	15
Totals		290	98	7	7	56	12	19	43	13	35

Table 2. Matched Pair Analyses of Parotid Score and Diabetes

	Diabetic	Nondiabetic
Age-sex matched		
Number with scores 8-12	31	22
Number with scores 0-7	25	34
Mean parotid score	6.79	5.50
Significance (paired *t* test)	$P < 0.02$	
Age-sex-percent desirable weight matched		
Number with scores 8-12	18	19
Number with scores 0-7	18	17
Mean parotid scores	6.97	6.36
Significance (paired *t* test)	$P > 0.1$	

($r = 0.64$) could be explained by a linear combination of the three variables.

The simple correlation coefficients between parotid score and each of the three independent variables were positive and of decreasing magnitude for age, percent desirable weight, and plasma glucose in both sexes (Table 3).

Partial correlation coefficients were calculated to measure the association of plasma glucose with parotid score, holding age, and percent desirable weight constant. These coefficients were small, -0.06 for males and 0.19 for females, emphasizing the relatively minor importance of plasma glucose in predicting parotid score.

Discussion

Examination of the parotid gland by palpation is a subjective procedure that gives only an estimate of

Table 3. Correlation Coefficients Among Parotid Score, Age, Percent Desirable Weight, and Plasma Glucose

Parotid Score	Age	Percent Desirable Weight	Plasma Glucose
Males			
Correlation coefficient			
Simple	0.54	0.45	0.17
Partial	0.62	0.56	-0.06
Females			
Correlation coefficient			
Simple	0.50	0.47	0.28
Partial	0.41	0.44	0.19

the relative size of the gland. Nevertheless, the inter-observer agreement in scoring glands was high, the correlation coefficient being 0.77.

No attempt was made to define normal and abnormal parotid glands in this study. Only the size of the gland was graded. Some authors (9, 10) have stated that the normal parotid gland is not detectable by palpation; if so, even parotid scores of 4 to 7 represent abnormally large glands. Parotid scores of 8 to 12 undoubtedly represent enlarged parotid glands.

Enlarged parotid glands were no more frequent among diabetics than among nondiabetics matched for age, sex, and obesity (Table 2 (*bottom*)). The multiple correlation analyses showed that the plasma glucose contributed much less to parotid enlargement than did either age or percent desirable weight (Table 3). For the Pima Indians, therefore, the relationship of parotid enlargement and diabetes was mainly the result of their common association with age and obesity.

An association between asymptomatic parotid enlargement and diabetes may be masked in the Pima by the high frequency of obesity (Table 1) or by unknown environmental or genetic factors causing parotid enlargement. Methodologic differences between this and other studies were striking, however, and may account for the discrepant results. The possible effect of obesity was not considered in the report by Davidson and associates (3). Although many of their subjects were obese, the importance of this variable could not be assessed because of the lack of control data. In contrast to studies that selected patients because of large parotid glands (3, 11-13), the association of parotid enlargement and diabetes in the Pima was tested in a natural population. This provided observations on the frequency of parotid enlargement in nondiabetics as well as in diabetics.

In view of the limitations of previous reports the relationship of asymptomatic parotid enlargement and diabetes mellitus needs to be reexamined in other populations, taking into account the roles of age and obesity.

ACKNOWLEDGMENTS: The authors thank the Indian Health Service, the Tribal Council, and the members of the Gila River Indian Community for their cooperation.

References

1. KENAWY MR: Endemic enlargement of the parotid gland in Egypt. *Trans Roy Soc Trop Med Hyg* 31:339-350, 1937
2. TAKAOKA Y, YAMAGUCHI T, YAMADA N, et al: Der Hormonale Einfluss der Parotisdrüsen auf den Kohlenhydrat- und Eiweiss-Stoffwechsel. *Klin Wschr* 32:369-375, 1954
3. DAVIDSON D, LEIBEL BS, BERRIS B: Asymptomatic parotid gland enlargement in diabetes mellitus. *Ann Intern Med* 70: 31-38, 1969
4. MILLER M, BENNETT PH, BURCH TA: Hyperglycemia in Pima Indians: a preliminary appraisal of its significance, in *Biomedical Challenges Presented by the American Indian.* Washington, D.C., Pan American Health Organization, 1968, pp. 89-103
5. SANDSTEAD HR, KOEHN CJ, SESSIONS SM: Enlargement of the parotid gland in malnutrition. *Amer J Clin Nutr* 3:198-214, 1955
6. *Recommended Dietary Allowances,* Publication 1146. Report of Food and Nutrition Board. Washington, D.C., National Research Council, National Academy of Sciences, 1964
7. FALKNER F: Some physical growth standards for White North American children. *Pediatrics* 29:467-474, 1962
8. SNEDECOR GW, COCHRAN WG: *Statistical Methods,* sixth ed. Ames, Iowa, Iowa State University Press, 1967
9. WOLFE SJ, SUMMERSKILL WHG, DAVIDSON CS: Parotid swelling, alcoholism and cirrhosis. *New Eng J Med* 256:491-495, 1957
10. BORSANYI S, BLANCHARD CL: Asymptomatic enlargment of the parotid glands. *JAMA* 174:20-22, 1960
11. KATSILAMBROS L: Asymptomatic enlargement of the parotid glands. *JAMA* 178:513-514, 1961
12. FLAUM E: Parotishypertrophie, ein Symptom des Diabetes Mellitus. *Klin Wschr* 11:1704-1705, 1932
13. JOHN HJ: Mikulicz's disease and diabetes. *JAMA* 101:184-187, 1933

Hyperglycemia in Washoe and Northern Paiute Indians

Gregory W. Bartha, M.D., Thomas A. Burch, M.D., M.P.H., and Peter H. Bennett, M.B., M.R.C.P..

SUMMARY

The prevalence of hyperglycemia in two American Indian tribes, the Washoe and Northern Paiute, was evaluated by determining the number of individuals aged fifteen years and older with a history of concurrently treated diabetes or with a plasma glucose level of at least 160 mg./100 ml. (AutoAnalyzer) two hours after a 75-gm. glucose equivalent load. One hundred and twelve Washoe Indians, representing 74.2 per cent of the Washoe study population, and 131 Paiute Indians, 60.6 per cent of the Paiute study population, were examined. The prevalence of hyperglycemia was 10.7 per cent for the Washoe and 11.5 per cent for the Paiute group. These rates, when adjusted for age and sex, did not differ significantly from each other or from that reported for the Cocopah Indians. The adjusted rates for these three tribes were significantly lower than the adjusted rate for the Pima. In both the Washoe and Paiute populations, the prevalence of hyperglycemia increased with age, but was not related to parity.

In 1968, Miller and co-workers[1] reported that 23.5 per cent of 1,881 Pima Indians from the Gila River Reservation over five years of age (32.0 per cent of those aged fifteen and older) either had plasma glucose levels of at least 160 mg./100 ml. two hours following a 75-gm. glucose equivalent load or were receiving hypoglycemic medication. Using identical methods and criteria, Henry and co-workers[2] found the prevalence

152

of diabetes in the Cocopah tribe for those over five years of age to be 17.0 per cent (for those aged fifteen and older, 24.4 per cent). The difference in prevalence between the two linguistically distinct tribes* was found to be statistically significant. The same methods have been extended to two other tribes, the Washoe and Northern Paiute, and the results are presented in this report.

The Washoe and Northern Paiute formed part of the Desert Culture, which began 9,000 to 15,000 years ago in the Great Basin area of the United States. The Washoe occupied the eastern slopes of the Sierra Nevada in the region of Lake Tahoe, while the Paiute ranged over a wide area including western Nevada and southern Oregon.[3] Despite geographic proximity, they are linguistically different: The Washoe constitute a branch of the Hokan family of languages, while the Paiute, like the Pima, are part of the Uto-Aztecan family. Today each tribe lives in small, predominantly homogeneous colonies and reservations in western and central Nevada and eastern California. There is no census of this area currently available that enumerates Indians by tribe, but an unofficial estimate of its total Indian population in 1970 was 7,700, of which 60 per cent were probably Paiute.[4] The estimated number of Washoe was 600. Occupations are chiefly farming and ranching, although employment in service and manufacturing industries is increasing. The diets of neither of the tribes have been closely studied, but the impression has been that they contain much carbohydrate.

METHODS

The Washoe population selected for study included all individuals aged fifteen years and older, putatively one-half or more Washoe, and residing (in the summer of 1970) in the communities of Dresslerville, Nevada, and Woodfords, California. Those persons aged fifteen years and older and one-half or more Paiute residing on the Fort McDermitt Indian Reservation (Nevada) comprised the Paiute study population. These particular communities were chosen because of the homogeneity

*The Pima derive from the Uto-Aztecan linguistic family, while the Cocopah belong to the Yuman family.

of tribal composition and the relatively large number of available subjects. One hundred and twelve individuals, or 74.2 per cent of the Washoe group, and 131, or 60.6 per cent of the Paiute group, were evaluated either by determination of the plasma glucose level two hours ($\pm$ thirty minutes) after a 75-gm. glucose equivalent load,* or by eliciting a history of concurrently treated diabetes. The glucose load was administered irrespective of time of day or time of last meal. Twenty-nine per cent of the tests were performed in the morning, 38 per cent in the afternoon, and 33 per cent in the evening after 5 p.m. A blood sample was also collected for serum creatinine determination, and a urine specimen was obtained, tested for protein with Labstix,† and saved for quantitative determinations if a trace or more of protein was registered. For each subject examined, information on age, weight, height, and parity was recorded.

The serum, plasma, and urine samples were frozen and shipped in dry ice to the laboratory of the Southwestern Field Studies Section, National Institute of Arthritis, Metabolism, and Digestive Diseases in Phoenix, Arizona, where the analyses were performed. The plasma glucose concentration was measured with the AutoAnalyzer by the modified Hoffman method.[5] The serum and urine creatinine and the urine albumin concentration were measured, and the urine albumin/creatinine ratio‡ were calculated.

RESULTS

In the Washoe group, twelve individuals, or 10.7 per cent, were hyperglycemic by the criterion of either a two-hour post-load plasma glucose level of at least 160 mg./100 ml. or by a history of concurrently treated diabetes. Seven of these hyperglycemic individuals were previously known to have diabetes. In the Paiute group, fifteen individuals, or 11.5 per cent, were hyperglycemic,

---

*Dexcola, Custom Laboratories, Baltimore.

†Ames Company, Elkhart, Ind.

‡The albumin/creatinine (A/C) ratio is thought to give an estimate of the twenty-four-hour protein excretion.[1] A value equal to or greater than one was interpreted in this study to indicate significant proteinuria.

and eleven of these were previously known.

Tables 1 and 2 present the data on the prevalence of hyperglycemia in both populations by age and sex. Although the prevalence was higher in the females of both tribes, in neither group was there a statistically significant difference in rates between the sexes ($p > 0.2$). Comparison of the prevalence in the fifteen through thirty-four-year age group with that in persons thirty-five years of age and older revealed a significant increase in the older category in both tribes ($p < 0.05$).

No statistically significant relationship was found between parity and the frequency of hyperglycemia in the females of either population ($p > 0.2$). An accurate assessment of the association between hyperglycemia and obesity could not be made, as values for height and weight had to be estimated in a large number of cases, but approximately 20 per cent of the respondents of each tribe were obese.*

Finally, the number of abnormalities detected in serum creatinine and urine albumin/creatinine ratio was too small to permit definite conclusions: Two Washoe and four Paiute subjects† with significant proteinuria (A/C ratio $\geq$ 1) and an additional two Washoe and one Paiute subjects with elevated serum creatinine levels.‡ Three of these nine individuals with abnormal kidney function were hyperglycemic.

Direct comparisons of the observations made on the Washoe and Paiute groups with those on the Pima and Cocopah Indians were possible because variations in method were minimized.§ To correct for age and sex differences, prevalence rates were adjusted to a standard population, the sum of the individuals in the four populations. Ninety-five per cent confidence limits were

---

*Obesity is defined as $\geq$ 150 per cent of desirable weight.[6]
†Two Paiutes with proteinuria also had elevated creatinine levels.
‡$>$ 1.5 mg. per cent for males; $>$ 1.3 mg. per cent for females.
§The Pima study[1] also included half- to full-blooded Pima Indians, whereas the Cocopah study included one-quarter to full-blooded Cocopah Indians (about 70 per cent were full blood). In the present study, approximately 80 per cent of those examined were putatively full-blooded Indians of their respective tribes.

TABLE 1

Prevalence of hyperglycemia in Washoe Indians by age and sex

Age group (yr.) by sex	Number evaluated	With previously diagnosed diabetes		Plasma glucose level ≥160 mg./100 ml.*		Plasma glucose level ≥200 mg./100 ml.*†		Total hyperglycemia*‡	
		No.	%	No.	%	No.	%	No.	%
Males									
15-34	16	—	—	—	—	—	—	—	—
35-64	22	1	4.5	—	—	—	—	1	4.5
65+	12	2	16.7	—	—	—	—	2	16.7
Total male	50	3	6.0	—	—	—	—	3	6.0
Females									
15-34	30	1	3.3	—	—	—	—	1	3.3
35-64	25	2	8.0	1	4.0	1	4.0	3	12.0
65+	7	1	14.3	4	57.1	1	14.3	5	71.4
Total female	62	4	6.5	5	8.1	2	3.2	9	14.5
Total male + female	112	7	6.3	5	4.5	2	1.8	12	10.7
15-34	46	1	2.2	—	—	—	—	1	2.2
35-64	47	3	6.4	1	2.1	1	2.1	4	8.5
65+	19	3	15.8	4	21.1	1	5.3	7	36.8

* Not including previously diagnosed diabetics.
† This information included for comparison with other studies.
‡ Previously diagnosed diabetes or two-hour post-load plasma glucose level ≥ 160 mg./100 ml.

TABLE 2
Prevalence of hyperglycemia in Northern Paiute Indians by age and sex

Age group (yr.) by sex	Number evaluated	With previously diagnosed diabetes		Plasma glucose level ≥160 mg./100 ml.*		Plasma glucose level ≥200 mg./100 ml.*†		Total hyperglycemia‡	
		No.	%	No.	%	No.	%	No.	%
Males									
15-34	39	—	—	1	4.5	—	—	—	—
35-64	22	4	18.2	—	—	—	—	5	22.7
65+	5	—	—	—	—	—	—	—	—
Total male	66	4	6.1	1	1.5	—	—	5	7.6
Females									
15-34	38	1	2.6	—	—	—	—	1	2.6
35-64	24	6	25.0	3	12.5	2	8.3	9	37.5
65+	3	—	—	—	—	—	—	—	—
Total female	65	7	10.8	3	4.6	2	3.1	10	15.4
Total male + female	131	11	8.4	4	3.1	2	1.5	15	11.5
15-34	77	1	1.3	—	—	—	—	1	1.3
35-64	46	10	21.8	4	8.7	2	4.3	14	30.4
65+	8	—	—	—	—	—	—	—	—

* Not including previously diagnosed diabetics.
† This information included for comparison with other studies.
‡ Previously diagnosed diabetes or two-hour post-load plasma glucose level ≥160 mg./100 ml.

TABLE 3

Adjusted rates, with standard error* and 95 per cent confidence limits,†
for hyperglycemia‡ in four Indian populations

	Tribe			
	Pima	Cocopah	Washoe	Paiute
Hyperglycemia				
A. ≥140 mg./100 ml.§				
Adjusted prevalence rate (%)	—	25.0	14.5	18.1
Standard error of rate (%)	—	3.6	3.2	3.6
95% confidence limits of rate (%)	—	17.8-32.2	8.1-20.9	10.9-25.3
B. ≥160 mg./100 ml.				
Adjusted prevalence rate (%)	31.9	21.7	10.6	15.3
Standard error of rate (%)	1.1	3.4	2.7	3.4
95% confidence limits of rate (%)	29.7-34.1	14.9-28.5	5.2-16.0	8.5-22.0

* The adjusted prevalence rate for a group was calculated by applying age-, sex-specific rates from the original surveys to the corresponding subgroups in the standard population, the sum of individuals in the four study groups. The standard error (S.E.) of the adjusted prevalence is expressed as:

$$\sqrt{\frac{\Sigma \, N_i^2 V(P_i)}{\Sigma \, (N_j)^2}}$$

where N_i is the size of each subgroup in the standard population; $V(P_i)$ is the variance of the rate for a subgroup in a survey which in turn equals pq/n, where p is the rate, q is 1-p, and n is the size of the sample from which the rate was calculated.

† 95 per cent confidence limits equal rate ± 2 S.E.

‡ Elevation of the two-hour post-load plasma glucose level or history of concurrently treated diabetes.

§ Rates by the 140 mg./100 ml. criterion not available for the Pima.

calculated for the adjusted rates, and the criterion for a significant difference between values was taken to be no overlap of the confidence limits. Under these terms, the prevalence rate of hyperglycemia for those of both sexes aged fifteen years and older, was significantly higher in the Pima (31.9 per cent) than in the Cocopah (21.7 per cent), Washoe (10.6 per cent), and Paiute (15.3 per cent) groups. There were no statistically significant differences in the rates for the latter three populations (see table 3).

DISCUSSION

Over the past ten to fifteen years a number of papers have appeared on the subject of diabetes mellitus in American Indian populations.[7-9] A major stimulus for this work has been the question of whether the prevalence and pattern of the disease vary among tribes and whether there are general differences in its presentation in Indian and non-Indian groups. Unfortunately, the problem remains unsolved chiefly because of the wide variation in both the criteria used to define diabetes and hyperglycemia and in the methods employed to identify the condition. O'Sullivan and Williams[10] have shown that such differences alone, when applied to a survey population in Sudbury, Massachusetts, could yield prevalence rates ranging from 0.8 per cent to 13.4 per cent. Thus, for example, the rate of 1.3 per cent reported for diabetes in the Eskimo,[11] and based on an elaborate series of screening tests, cannot be directly compared with the figure of 29.0 per cent described for the Cherokee,[12] based on the results of one blood sample following a glucose load. The need for standardization of methods and definitions is obvious.

The only data from a non-Indian United States population suitable for approximate comparison with the figures from the present study were those from a study of the prevalence of diabetes in Sudbury, Massachusetts.[10] O'Sullivan and Williams reported that 13.4 per cent of a 5 per cent random sample of individuals aged fifteen and older in Sudbury had a plasma glucose level of at least 135 mg./100 ml. (AutoAnalyzer)* two

---

*The standard actually employed was a whole venous blood glucose value of 110 mg./100 ml. This value is approximately equivalent to a plasma glucose level of 135 mg./100 ml.[13]

159

hours following a 100-gm. glucose load. The 135 mg./ 100 ml. standard would yield a rate of hyperglycemia of 14.3 per cent for the Washoe and 17.6 per cent for the Paiute (including concurrently treated diabetics). If one considers the variations in method to be of minimal importance and assumes similar age distributions in the three populations, there is no significant difference among the prevalence rates.

In both the Paiute and Washoe groups, hyperglycemia was associated with increased age but was independent of sex and parity insofar as could be ascertained with available sample sizes.

While the prevalence of obesity was not accurately determined among the Washoe and Paiute, the estimated frequency (20 per cent in each group) was less than that found in the Cocopah (37 per cent), but was roughly similar to that in the Pima Indians (24 per cent).[2] Since the prevalence of diabetes was much lower in the Washoe and Paiute Indians than in the Pima, and the prevalence of obesity appeared to be similar, it seems unlikely that the differences in the prevalence of diabetes can be explained by differences in the prevalence of obesity.

The higher prevalence of hyperglycemia in the Pima Indians than among the Washoe, Paiute, or Cocopah establishes that there are variations in prevalence in different tribal groups. In addition, the present study demonstrates that the rates and patterns of hyperglycemia are very similar in three linguistically distinct tribal groups and, in fact, for the two tribes currently studied, the prevalence rates show no statistically significant difference from those for the Sudbury, Massachusetts, population.[10]

ACKNOWLEDGMENT

We would like to express our gratitude to the Washoe communities of Dresslerville, Nevada, and Woodfords, California, and to the Paiute community of Fort McDermitt, Nevada, for their cooperation; to Dr. R. M. Acheson, Dr. G. F. Sheckleton, Dr. J. R. MacBride, Mr. Elmer Lidstone, Mr. James Padbury, and Mr. Lee Truro for their assistance; to Miss P. E. Sperling for the laboratory determinations; and to Dr. R. A. Greenberg for statistical advice.

REFERENCES

[1] Miller, M., Bennett, P. H., and Burch, T. A.: Hyperglycemia in Pima Indians: A preliminary appraisal of its significance. *In* Biomedical Challenges Presented by the American Indian. Pan American Health Organization Publication No. 165, 1968, pp. 89-103.

[2] Henry, R. E., Burch, T. A., Bennett, P. H., and Miller, M.: Diabetes in the Cocopah Indians. Diabetes *18*:33-37, 1969.

[3] d'Azevedo, W. L., Davis, W. A., Fowler, D. D., and Suttles, W.: The Current Status of Anthropological Research in the Great Basin: 1964. Reno, Desert Research Institute, 1966.

[4] Schurz Service Unit Program Plan, Fiscal Year 1970. Phoenix, U. S. Department of Health, Education, and Welfare, Public Health Service, Division of Indian Health, 1969.

[5] Technicon AutoAnalyzer Method File N-2b. Tarrytown, N.Y., Technicon Instruments.

[6] Recommended Dietary Allowances. Report of Food and Nutrition Board. National Academy of Sciences, Publication 1146, 1964, p. 4.

[7] Cohen, B. M.: Diabetes mellitus among Indians of the American Southwest: Its prevalence and clinical characteristics in a hospitalized population. Ann. Intern. Med. *40*:588-99, 1954.

[8] Prosnitz, L. R., and Mandell, G. L.: Diabetes mellitus among Navajo and Hopi Indians: The lack of vascular complications. Amer. J. Med. Sci. *253*:700-05, 1967.

[9] Saiki, J. H., and Rimoin, D. L.: Diabetes mellitus among the Navajo. I. Clinical features. Arch. Intern. Med. *122*:1-5, 1968.

[10] O'Sullivan, J. B., and Williams, R. F.: Early diabetes mellitus in perspective: A population study in Sudbury, Massachusetts. JAMA *198*:579-82, 1966.

[11] Mouratoff, G. J., Carroll, N. V., and Scott, E. M.: Diabetes mellitus in Eskimos. JAMA *199*:961-66, 1967.

[12] Stein, J. H., West, K. M., Robey, J. M., Tirador, D. F., and McDonald, G. W.: The high prevalence of abnormal glucose tolerance in the Cherokee Indians of North Carolina. Arch. Intern. Med., *116*:842-45, 1965.

[13] Standardization of the oral glucose tolerance test. Report of the Committee on Statistics of the American Diabetes Association. Diabetes *18*:299-310, 1969.

161

Gallbladder Disease

Gallbladder Disease in Southwestern American Indians

Bruce D. Nelson, MD, John Porvaznik, MD,
and John R. Benfield, MD.

Southwestern American Indians suffer from gallbladder disease at a rate more than double that of the American non-Indian population. This report describes a two-year experience with 101 patients undergoing cholecystectomy at the Fort Defiance Indian hospital on the Navajo Indian Reservation in Northern Arizona. Our results show a high female-to-male sex ratio (4.6:1), a low average age in women undergoing cholecystectomy (42.4 years), a high incidence of associated common duct stones (16%), and a high rate of gallbladder malignancy (6 percent).

D uring the past decade it has been noted that Southwestern American Indians suffer from an unusually high incidence of gallbladder disease. For example, the Pima Indians of Southern Arizona were admitted to their local health facility for cholecystitis at the rate of 2.3 per hundred adult population yearly.[1] Reviews of operative experience reveal that cholecystectomy was the most common major surgical procedure performed at the Phoenix Indian Hospital, outnumbering appendectomies by a ratio of 2.7:1.[2] At the Shiprock In-

dian Hospital, serving the Navajo tribe, the incidence of common duct stones, cholecystoenteric fistula, and gallbladder cancer were considerably higher than expected from a comparative white population.[3] Autopsy reports of various Indian tribes showed a 40% incidence of gallbladder disease[4] including cholelithiasis in 24.4% to 29.9% of the adults examined.[5,6] This incidence is more than double that found in the American non-Indian population.[7] Finally, a recent epidemiological study noted a 48.6% prevalence rate for gallbladder disease in the Pima Indians.[8] It is clear that cholecystitis and its complications are frequent and serious threats to the health of the Southwestern American Indians.

This report will describe a two-year experience with gallbladder disease on the Navajo Indian Reservation in Northern Arizona. Comments about sociologic factors pertaining to this illness in the Indian population and evidence suggesting an inordinately high incidence of gallbladder ailments in young Indian women, a high rate of common duct stones, and a high incidence of gallbladder cancer will be presented.

Methods

The Fort Defiance Indian Hospital is a 100-bed general care facility located within the Navajo Indian Reservation, a 25,000-square-mile area situated mainly in Northern Arizona. The Hospital is the primary care facility for about 40,000 people. it also serves as a referral center for remote areas of the reservation. About 95% of the patients are full-blooded Navajo Indians while about 5% are Hopi Indians who live on a separate reservation now totally surrounded by Navajo lands.

Most people live scattered in desolate areas far from water and power and without ready access to transportation. The climate is dry and harsh with temperature variations from −40 F in winter to 105 F in summer. The terrain is quite variable with dessert, canyon, mountains, and woods scattered throughout. With the winter snows and spring thaws, roads are frequently impassable and access to medical facilities limited.

The records of all patients who underwent a cholecystectomy during the two-year period from July 1966, to July 1968 were reviewed. Sex, age, duration of symptoms, operative findings, operation performed, morbidity, mortality, and the results of therapy were tabulated. The obstetrical histories of the women patients were noted.

Results

Cholecystectomy, the most common major operative procedure, was performed on 101 patients (Table 1). There were 83 women and 18 men. The average age of the women at operation was 42.4 years, the men, 56.2 years, with an overall average of 44.9 years. It is noteworthy that only 28% of the women as compared to 56% of the men were over 50 years of age, and that the average woman patient was about 14 years younger than the average man (Figure).

Duration of Preoperative Symptoms.—The duration of preoperative symptoms was greater than one year in 67 patients, between one year and one month in 20 patients, and less than one month in 13 patients, while one patient was asymptomatic. Eighty patients had oral cholecystograms, 44 of which showed stones while 35 simply failed to visualize the gallbladder despite a double dose of contrast medication. Although all patients in this series had proved gallbladder disease by pathologic examination, one had a normal cholecystogram.

Obstetrical Histories.—Obstetrical histories were available for 71 of the 83 women. Forty-seven of them indicated five or more pregnancies while 20 told of ten or more. The average number of pregnancies among the women in this series was 6.3, and only one of the women was nulliparous.

Operative Findings.—At operation 95 patients had cholecystitis, including three with acalculous cholesterosis. Acute cholecystitis was found in 24 patients, including ten with empyema of the gallbladder. Seventy-one patients had chronic cholecystitis. Of the remaining six patients, all had cancer, all were over 50 years old, and five were women. One patient with gallbladder cancer had no stones. The average age of the patients with carcinoma was 66 years and in none of these cases was the correct preoperative diagnosis made.

Choledochotomy.—Choledochotomy was carried out in 56 patients whose average age was 48.8 years. Common duct stones were found in 16 patients who averaged almost six years older than the group which had no stones in the ducts. All but one of the calculous ducts measured at least 0.9 cm in diameter.

Mortality.—The mortality among the 95 patients without cancer was 1.1%. The one death was an 80-year-old patient whose gallbladder had perforated by the time of oper-

Table 1.—Gallbladder Disease in Southwestern American Indians*

	No.	Age, yr Average (Range)	Common Duct Exploration	Common Duct Stones	Cancer
Men	18	56.2 (30-90)	11	2	1
Women	83	42.4 (15-95)	45	14	5
Total	101	44.9 (15-95)	56	16	6

* Fort Defiance Hospital, 1966-1968.

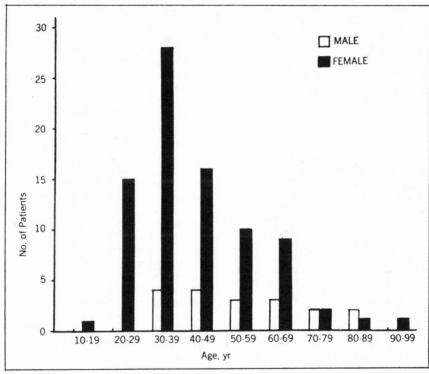

Comparison of incidence of cholecystectomy in men and women at various age levels. Total patients: 101.

Table 2.—Average Age at Cholecystectomy

Indian Series	Female	Male	Total	No. Patients
Kravetz (mixed)	39.1	48.6	41.4	105
Brown & Christensen (Navajo)	39.9	56.8	43.0	104
Sampliner & O'Connell (Major Navajo)	30.0	65.5	38.8	237
Present study	42.4	56.2	44.9	101
Non-Indian Series Colcock & Perry	53.4	53.7	53.5	1,756

ation. Only one other patient suffered a major complication—subphrenic abscess which required drainage. There were nine minor complications, including three spontaneous abortions, two pneumonias, two urinary tract infections, one polyarthritis, and one wound infection.

Late follow-up information was available for 87 patients. Excluding those with cancer, all but four were asymptomatic. Those with symptoms described them as mild, only slightly resembling their preoperative symptoms.

Comment

Modern medical care is a relatively new benefit for Navajo Indians, dating essentially to 1955 when the US Public Health Service took over the responsibility for administering and delivering their health care. Prior to that time, it was largely the task of medical missionaries and a few physicians employed by the Bureau of Indian Affairs. The Navajo has been somewhat reluctant to accept "white man's medicine," for cultural and religious reasons, and still today he may prefer to seek medical care from the native medicine man who is able to offer spiritual as well as certain therapeutic aids for various illnesses.[9] When the Public Health Service began caring for the Indians, it recognized the seriousness of these cultural conflicts and initiated a continuing campaign for a program of cooperation and improved understanding. As a result, it is now not infrequent to see Navajo medicine men within the hospital performing certain rituals prior to operations. The effect has been a steady increase in the Indians' trust in modern medicine, as a result of which an increasingly accurate picture of disease patterns of the Indian population is being obtained.

The preponderance of women suffering from gallbladder ailments is remarkable. Our female-male sex ratio of 4.5:1 is similar to that of other reports about Southwestern Indians in which the ratio varies from 3:1 to 7:1.[1-4,10] By way of contrast, women generally outnumber men only by a factor of 2:1 to 3:1 in the non-Indian population.[7,11] As most Indian men on the reservation are unemployed, they are not lacking in time to seek medical help for their ailments. The women, however, are more in demand to remain at home caring for the children and tending their sheep. If anything, these factors tend to delay the women's seeking aid while leaving the men free to do so, and it is therefore likely that the sex ratio which we have pointed out is real.

It appears that Southwestern American Indians suffer from gallbladder disease earlier in life than other Americans. For example, the average age of our patients was almost nine years younger than that of 1,756 non-Indian patients reviewed by Colcock and Perry.[12] This difference is totally accounted for, however, by the lower average age in the Indian women. In our series it was 42.4 years, or about 11 years less than that noted for non-Indian women. Comparison of age incidence between Indian and non-Indian men does not reveal a similar difference, and the data we have presented relative to Indian women have been corroborated by the observations of others which are summarized in Table 2.[2,3,10]

It is apparent that Indians seek medical attention for biliary tract ailments late in the course of the disease. For example, 67% of our patients had symptoms greater

167

than one year in duration, and 24% of the group treated required operation for acute cholecystitis. Most likely these facts are the result of the Indian's relative willingness to accept symptoms of gallbladder disease as a natural part of life and of his reluctance to seek help except under dire circumstances.

The high incidence of choledocholithiasis is another feature of biliary tract disease in Indians. While the non-Indian population has approximately a 6% to 8% incidence of common duct stones associated with cholecystectomy,[13,14] 16% of our patients had choledocholithiasis and similar results have been reported from other Indian hospitals.[3,10]

For this reason, the standard indications for choledochotomy were liberally used (56%) and the justification for this approach is apparent in that 29% of the explorations were positive for stones. This is similar to the 27.6% rate reported in over 500 duct explorations by Colcock and Perry in non-Indians.[13]

Of most significance in this study was that six patients (6%) had cancer of the gallbladder discovered at laparotomy. Rates from other reports of various Southwestern Indian tribes range from 3% to 3.8%.[2,3,10] These figures are all somewhat higher than the generally accepted 1% to 2% incidence for the non-Indian population.[15-17] Richenbach, at the Phoenix Indian Hospital reviewing autopsies, noted that the rate of gallbladder and biliary tract cancer in Indians was six times that of the non-Indian population.[6] An important observation in our study was the high likelihood of cancer being present in the elderly female with five of the 23 women (21.7%) over 50 years of age having cancer at laparotomy.

The relationship between cholelithiasis, cholecystitis, and pregnancy has been controversial for years.[11,18] Despite the fact that only one woman in our series was nulliparous and that all the women we operated upon had an average of 6.3 pregnancies, whether or not this is related to their gall bladder disease is still questionable.[2,8] However, it would appear that the Indian population is fruitful for clinical research directed at resolving this perennial question.

The differential diagnosis of cholecystitis in Southwestern Indians deserves comment because it is definitely less difficult than in the non-Indian population. Indians appear to be almost immune from duodenal ulcer disease. During the two-year period of this study, no patient with duodenal ulcer disease was encountered, and during an eight-year period at the Phoenix Indian Hospital there were only three patients with documented duodenal ulcer disease, and they came from tribes outside the Southwest.[19] Thus, signs and symptoms of right upper quadrant peritonitis are almost uniformly due to cholecystitis in Indians.

We have presented evidence that gallbladder disease is a frequent, virulent public health problem in Southwestern American Indians. It appears particularly to affect young women and includes a high incidence of common duct stones and cancer. The fact that this population is easily identified, relatively uniform in its dietary habits, and centrally located on reservations suggests that Southwestern American Indians should be intensively studied to answer important questions relative to the etiology and pathogenesis of cholecystitis and cholelithiasis.

References

1. Hesse F: Incidence of cholecystitis and other diseases in the Pima Indians of southern Arizona. *JAMA* 170:1789-1790, 1959.
2. Kravetz R: Etiology of biliary tract disease in the southwestern American Indians. *Gastroenterology* 46:392-398, 1964.
3. Brown JE, Christensen C: Biliary tract disease among the Navajos. *JAMA* 202:1050-1052, 1967.
4. Sievers M, Marquis J: The southwestern American Indian's burden: Biliary disease. *JAMA* 182:570-572, 1962.
5. Hesse F: Incidence of disease in the Navajo Indian. *Arch Path* 77:553-557, 1964.
6. Richenbach D: Autopsy incidence of disease among southwestern American Indians. *Arch Path* 84:81-86, 1967.
7. Lieber M: The incidence of gall stones and their correlation with other diseases. *Ann Surg* 135:394-405, 1952.
8. Sampliner RE, Bennett PH, Comess LJ, et al: Gallbladder disease in Pima Indians: Demonstration of high prevalence and early onset by cholecystography. *New Eng J Med* 283:1358-1364, 1970.
9. Porvaznik J: Traditional Navajo medicine. *GP* 36:179-182, 1967.
10. Sampliner JE, O'Connell DJ: Biliary surgery in the southwestern American Indian. *Arch Surg* 96:1-3, 1968.
11. Robertson H, Dochat G: Pregnancy and gall stones. *Surg Gynec Obstet* 78:193-204, 1944.
12. Colcock B, Perry B: The treatment of cholelithiasis. *Surg Gynec Obstet* 117:529-534, 1963.
13. Colcock B, Perry B: Exploration of the common bile duct. *Surg Gynec Obstet* 118:20-24, 1964.
14. Glenn F: Common duct exploration for stones. *Surg Gynec Obstet* 95:431-438, 1952.
15. Briele H, Long W, Parks L: Gallbladder disease and cholecystectomy: Experience with 1,500 patients managed 'in a community hospital. *Amer Surg* 35:218-222, 1969.
16. Derman H, Gerbarg D, Kelly J, et al: Are gall stones and gallbladder cancer related. *JAMA* 176:450-452, 1961.
17. Newman H, Nortrup J: Gallbladder carcinoma in cholelithiasis. *Geriatrics* 19:453-455, 1964.
18. Large A, Lofstrom JE, Stevenson CS: Gallstones and pregnancy. *Arch Surg* 78:966-968, 1959.
19. Sievers M, Marquis J: Duodenal ulcer among southwestern American Indians. *Gastroenterology* 42:566-569, 1962.

169

LITHOGENIC BILE AMONG YOUNG INDIAN WOMEN*

Lithogenic Potential Decreased with Chenodeoxycholic Acid

JOHNSON L. THISTLE, M.D., AND LESLIE J. SCHOENFIELD, M.D.

Abstract Chippewa Indian women have a high prevalence of symptomatic gallstones. Lithogenic bile is characterized by a low ratio of bile acids plus lecithin to cholesterol. The ratios of bile acid plus lecithin to cholesterol in duodenal bile among 12 young Indian women without gallstones were significantly lower, 9.4 ± 0.82 (mean ± S.E.), than among white controls, 16.4 ± 1.0 (p less than 0.001), and Indian men, 14.8 ± 2.2 (p less than 0.02), and not different from those previously reported among white women with gallstones: 11.3 ± 1.3. Administration of chenodeoxycholic acid resulted in a bile acid composition of 96 per cent chenodeoxycholic acid and significantly increased the ratio of bile acid plus lecithin to cholesterol to 14.2 ± 1.9, without adverse reactions. These observations suggest that lithogenic bile precedes gallstone formation in Chippewa women and that administration of chenodeoxycholic acid decreases this lithogenic potential.

HUMAN gallstones in the United States are composed predominantly of cholesterol; bile acids and lecithin are the primary solubilizing agents for cholesterol in bile.[1] Lithogenic bile exists when the physicochemical state of the bile is such that the concentrations of either or both of these solubilizing agents are sufficiently decreased in relation to cholesterol to result in crystallization, liquid crystallization or supersaturation of cholesterol.[2] We have previously reported that the administration of the primary human bile acid, chenodeoxycholic acid, to white persons with lithogenic bile and gallstones increases the ratio of bile acid plus lecithin to cholesterol to normal.[3]

An appropriate group for further investigation of this effect of chenodeoxycholic acid was initially suggested by the report of a high prevalence of gallstones among American Indians of the Southwest. Comess and his co-workers[4] reported a 30 to 40 per cent prevalence of symptomatic gallbladder disease

*Supported in part by a research grant (AM-6908) from the National Institutes of Health, U. S. Public Health Service.

among Pima Indian women 30 to 62 years of age, and more recently Burch et al.[5] have observed prospectively a total prevalence of 60 to 70 per cent among these women. A similar prevalence of symptomatic gallstones has been found among Chippewa women of northern Minnesota.[6] Having identified a high-risk group for cholelithiasis, we proposed to determine if lithogenic bile is present among young Indian women without gallstones and, if so, whether this lithogenic potential can be decreased by the administration of chenodeoxycholic acid.

MATERIALS AND METHODS

Duodenal bile was obtained from subjects 18 to 25 years of age of comparable body weight and having normal cholecystograms. Twelve nulliparous Indian women, six nulliparous white women, six Indian men and six white men were studied. Ten of the 12 Indian women were then randomly allocated to receive either chenodeoxycholic acid,* 0.75 to 1 g per day, or placebo for two months and to have repeat duodenal drainage after treatment.

Duodenal bile (pH 6 to 7) was obtained under fasting conditions by means of fluoroscopically positioned double-lumen (Dreiling) tube after the duodenum had been flushed with 50 ml of physiologic saline solution at 37°C. Cholecystokinin-pancreozymin,† 40 Ivy U, was administered intravenously during a period of 20 minutes to stimulate gallbladder contraction. During this period, dark, concentrated bile, with bile acids of 55.4 ± 5.9 mM (mean ± S.E.), of pH 6 to 7, was immediately aspirated. The sample was maintained at 37°C during passage through a 60-ml coarse, fritted-glass filter funnel (with a pore size of 40 to 60 μ) and a Millipore filter (with a pore size of 0.22 μ) to remove cholesterol crystals. The residue retained by the Millipore filter was immediately transferred to a slide and examined by light and polarized-light microscopy for crystals.

Aliquots of 0.5 or 1 ml were added immediately to 19 ml of Folch's solution (chloroform: methanol [3:1]) and to 20 ml of 95 per cent ethanol. Duplicate determinations were performed on the Folch solution for lecithin by the method of Fiske and Subba-

*Obtained from Weddel Pharmaceuticals, London, England.
†Obtained from Professor Erik Jorpes, Stockholm, Sweden.

row,[7] on a petroleum-ether extraction of the ethanol solution for cholesterol by the method of Leiberman-Burchard[8] and on the ethanol solution after cholesterol extraction for total bile acids by the steroid dehydrogenase method.[9] The ethanol and petroleum-ether fractions were taken to dryness in an atmosphere of nitrogen and stored in methanol until analysis. The reproducibility of each analytical method was established, the coefficient of variation being 2 per cent. Individual bile acids were determined from the ethanol fraction by gas-liquid chromatography. Enzymatic cleavage of the carbon-nitrogen bond of the conjugates was performed as described by Nair et al.[10] The free bile acids were dissolved in methanol and methylated with freshly distilled diazomethane in ether prepared as described by Schlenk and Gellerman.[11] Bile-acid methyl esters were converted to trifluoroacetates for gas chromatography, which was carried out as previously described[12] in an F and M Gas Chromatograph, Model 402, in which 4-foot glass columns are packed with acid-washed silanized gas-chrom P‡ (100 to 120 mesh) coated with 3 per cent QF-1. The column was operated at about 240°C, with a helium-carrier flow rate of 60 to 70 ml per minute and the flame-ionization detector at 260 to 270°C. The number of theoretical plates under these conditions was about 3000 for methyl deoxycholate, with a retention time of about 18 minutes. Quantification was made with a Digital Readout System, Model CRS-104,§ with the use of standard curves determined from pure bile acids.¶

Recoveries of total bile acids, lecithin and cholesterol added to duodenal drainage in increments of 10 to 100 per cent were 90 to 100 per cent in six experiments with each compound. Recovery of taurine and glycine conjugated cholic, chenodeoxycholic, deoxycholic and lithocholic acid (10 to 100 per cent added to bile) was 89.2 ± 1.3 per cent (mean ± S.E.) in 30 experiments. Lecithin could have been hydrolyzed to lysolecithin by pancreatic phospholipase; however, no lysolecithin was detected by thin-layer chromatography in the Folch solutions.

‡Obtained from Applied Sciences Laboratories, Inc., State College, Pa.

§Manufactured by Infotronic Corporation, Houston, Tex.

¶Supplied by Dr. A. F. Hofmann, Mayo Clinic, Rochester, Minn.

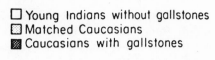

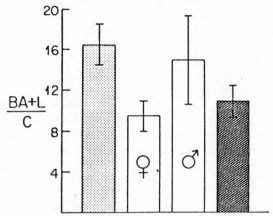

Figure 1. Ratios (Mean ± 2 S.E.) of Bile Acid (BA) plus Lecithin (L) to Cholesterol (C) Designated on the Ordinate. These ratios were significantly lower among young Indian women without gallstones than among white controls and Indian men.

Also, when lysolecithin‖ was added to the Folch solution, virtually all remained in the lower phase after washing and thus was included in the determination of total lipid phosphorus. The ratio of bile acid plus lecithin to cholesterol did not differ significantly among sequential samples or between duodenal bile and gallbladder bile obtained at subsequent cholecystectomy.

Serum glutamic oxalacetic transaminase (SGOT) and alkaline phosphatase levels were obtained after administration of chenodeoxycholic acid.

Dietary histories were available for six of the Indian women and four of the Indian men studied, as well as from 10 white women matched for age and weight. **RESULTS**

The ratios of the cholesterol-solubilizing agents, bile acids and lecithin, to cholesterol in bile from normal white men and women were similar and are combined in Figure 1. Among young Indian women without gallstones, these ratios were significantly lower than those among white controls (p less than

‖Obtained from Mann Research Laboratories, Inc., New York, N.Y.

0.001) and Indian men (p less than 0.02) and not different from those previously reported among white women with gallstones.[3] The ratios among young Indian men were not significantly different from those among either white controls or white women with gallstones. The ratios of bile acid to cholesterol and lecithin to cholesterol demonstrated the same significant differences as those of bile acids plus lecithin to cholesterol.

These differences in bile composition can be more fully appreciated when plotted on triangular co-ordinates (Fig. 2), in which any point within the triangle represents a combination of the three components, bile acids, lecithin and cholesterol, expressed as millimoles totaling 100 per cent. For scrutiny of detail, only the lower left corner of the triangle is shown. Admirand and Small[2] established, on the basis of in vitro and in vivo observations, that bile containing more than 4 per cent solids, represented by any point below a line of cholesterol saturation, has a sufficient concentration of bile acids and lecithin in relation to cholesterol to keep cholesterol in a micellar solution. Total solids in the duodenal drainage analyzed comprised more than 4

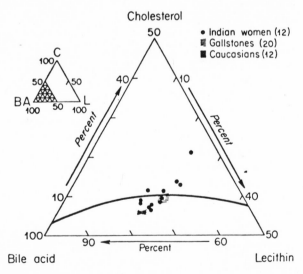

Figure 2. Relative Proportions of Bile Acids (BA), Lecithin (L) and Cholesterol (C) among White Controls, White Women with Gallstones and Young Indian Women without Gallstones Plotted on Triangular Co-ordinates (the Hatched and Stippled Areas Encompass Mean ± 2 S.E.).

per cent. Points along this line represent bile saturated with cholesterol; above the line insufficient bile acids and lecithin are present so that cholesterol will be in a crystalline, liquid crystalline or supersaturated state. When plotted on triangular coordinates, bile from the white controls fell within the micellar zone. Bile from white women with gallstones, after Millipore removal of cholesterol crystals, fell along the line of cholesterol saturation. Bile from young Indian women having normal cholecystograms was more saturated with cholesterol than that of the normal white controls and in five subjects fell above the line of cholesterol saturation. No crystalline or liquid-crystalline cholesterol was observed on microscopy immediately after aspiration of the duodenal bile of any of the Indian women, and the samples were then Millipore-filtered before analysis. This suggests that biliary cholesterol in these five subjects was in a supersaturated state. Subsequent freezing and thawing of duodenal bile resulted in the precipitation of cholesterol, but extrabiliary factors in duodenal drainage may have influenced its physical state. Cholesterol crystals were identified by thin-layer and gas-liquid chromatography.

Table 1. Percentages of Three Bile Acids in Duodenal Biliary Drainage.

SUBJECTS	NUMBER	PERCENTAGE OF DESIGNATED BILE ACIDS*		
		CHENODE-OXYCHOLIC	CHOLIC	DEOXY-CHOLIC
White men & women (untreated)	9†	53 ± 7.0	31 ± 5.0	16 ± 9.0
Indians (before treatment or untreated)	18	49 ± 5.0	33 ± 4.0	18 ± 3.0
Indians (after receiving chenodeoxycholic acid)‡	4	96 ± 2.0§	2 ± 0.5§	2 ± 0.2§
White women with gallstones¶	20	38 ± 5.0§	38 ± 4.0	24 ± 5.0

*Mean ± 2 SE.

†Percentages of individual bile acids not determined in 3 of 6 whites studied.

‡4 additional Indian women receiving placebo & 2 having no treatment showed no change in values after same period (2 mo).

§p <0.05.

¶Data from Thistle and Schoenfield.[3]

175

Among the 10 young Indian women who underwent repeat duodenal drainage, four had received chenodeoxycholic acid, four placebo, and two no medication. Bile acid composition was strikingly altered (p less than 0.001) in the women receiving chenodeoxycholic acid, the biliary bile acids becoming 96 per cent chenodeoxycholic acid (Table 1). This effect is the same as that observed among white women with gallstones who received chenodeoxycholic acid.[3] Untreated white women with gallstones have a significantly lower percentage of chenodeoxycholic acid than Indian women or normal whites. Bile-acid composition among the control Indians did not change after two months and was not different from that of Caucasian controls. The bile of the four Indian women receiving chenodeoxycholic acid underwent a significant increase in the ratio of bile acids plus lecithin to cholesterol, decreasing the lithogenic potential so that the bile composition moved well into the micellar zone in three of the four subjects (Fig. 3). No significant changes in this ratio were detected among the six Indians receiving placebo or no treatment as determined by the t-test for paired data.

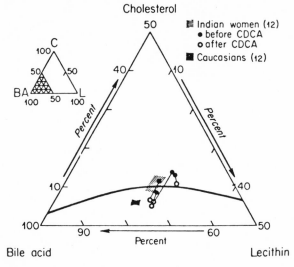

Figure 3. Relative Proportions of Bile Acids (BA), Lecithin (L) and Cholesterol (C) among White Controls and Young Indian Women without Gallstones before and after Administration of Chenodeoxycholic Acid (CDCA), Plotted on Triangular Co-ordinates (the Hatched and Stippled Areas Encompass Mean ± 2 S.E.).

Lithocholic acid, the bacterial degradation product of chenodeoxycholic acid, is hepatotoxic in the laboratory animal[13]; however, among the subjects receiving chenodeoxycholic acid, no increase in the trace amounts (less than 2 per cent) of lithocholic acid in duodenal bile was observed, and determinations of SGOT and serum alkaline phosphatase gave normal results.

Dietary histories of 10 of the young Indians studied did not reveal significant differences in the daily total calories per kilogram, in the percentages of carbohydrate, fat and protein, in the ratio of polyunsaturated to saturated fat, or in the total cholesterol intake from that of the 10 young white women interviewed in the same manner and did not differ from such histories reported by the National Research Council.[14]

DISCUSSION

The concept of lithogenic bile was fostered by the observations that both bile acids and lecithin are necessary for cholesterol solubilization in bile and that an insufficient amount of these solubilizing agents in relation to cholesterol will result in cholesterol crystallization, liquid crystallization or supersaturation.[2] In the hamster receiving a cholesterol-gallstone-inducing diet, lithogenic bile has been observed to precede the development of gallstones.[15] Lithogenic bile has been documented among human beings with gallstones in duodenal bile[3] and in gallbladder bile[2] and hepatic bile obtained during cholecystectomy.[16] Abnormal bile from persons without gallstones has not previously been reported. Lithogenic bile preceding the development of gallstones in a high-risk group for cholelithiasis supports the concept that this physicochemical change is important as a precursor to gallstone formation rather than as a secondary phenomenon. No differences in diets of Indian men and women and white women were elicited, although their bile composition was different, militating against etiologic importance of diet in gallstone formation. Past dietary histories, however, were not determined, and Sarles et al.[17] have related an increased intake of calories to cholelithiasis.

Administration of chenodeoxycholic acid suppressed hepatic bile-acid synthesis, replacing en-

177

dogenous biliary bile acids with chenodeoxycholic acid. The mechanism of the effect of chenodeoxycholic acid on the ratio of bile acids plus lecithin to cholesterol is less clear. Chenodeoxycholic acid may be more effective than cholic acid in inhibiting cholesterol synthesis or stimulating lecithin synthesis. Glycochenodeoxycholic acid, in contrast to conjugated cholic acid, has a substantial passive absorption in the jejunum as well as active ileal transport[18] and, therefore, may be more effective in increasing a diminished bile-acid pool.[19] Finally, chenodeoxycholic acid may influence the bile secretory apparatus, altering the proportions of bile acids, lecithin and cholesterol secreted.

Side effects were minimal and confined to an occasional slight increase in ' stool frequency. No change in appetite was noted. Serum cholesterol among white women with gallstones did not change significantly after four months of treatment with chenodeoxycholic acid.

The decrease in lithogenic potential induced by administration of chenodeoxycholic acid has important prophylactic implications.

We are indebted to Miss Esperanza Briones, Clinical Research Center and Department of Nutrition of the Mayo Clinic, who obtained the dietary histories, and to Miss Linda L. Livingston and Mr. Richard Tucker for technical assistance.

REFERENCES

1. Isaksson B: On the lipids and bile acids in normal and pathological bladder bile: a study of the main cholesterol dissolving components of human bile. Thesis, University of Gothenburg, 1954
2. Admirand WH, Small DM: Physicochemical basis of cholesterol gallstone formation in man. J Clin Invest 47:1043-1052, 1968
3. Thistle JL, Schoenfield LJ: Induced alteration of bile composition in humans with cholelithiasis. J Lab Clin Med 74:1020-1021, 1969
4. Comess LJ, Bennett PH, Burch TA: Clinical gallbladder disease in Pima Indians: its high prevalence in contrast to Framingham, Massachusetts. New Eng J Med 277:894-898, 1967
5. Burch TA, Comess LJ, Bennett PH: The problem of gallbladder disease among Pima Indians. Biomedical Challenges Presented by the American Indian. Washington DC, Pan American Health Organization, 1968 (PAHO Scientific Publication No 165), pp 82-88
6. Thistle JL, Schoenfield LJ: Lithogenic bile among young Indian women, a high risk group for cholelithiasis. Gastroenterology 58: 1000, 1970
7. Fiske CH, Subbarow Y: The colorimetric determination of phosphorus. J Biol Chem 66:375-400, 1925
8. Abell LL, Levy BB, Brodie BB, et al: A simplified method for

the estimation of total cholesterol in serum and demonstration of its specificity. J Biol Chem 195:357-366, 1952

9. Talalay P: Enzymatic analysis of steroid hormones. Meth Biochem Anal 8:119-143, 1960

10. Nair PP, Gordon M, Reback J: The enzymatic cleavage of the carbon-nitrogen bond in 3α, 7α, 12α-trihydroxy-5β-cholan-24-oylglycine. J Biol Chem 242:7-11, 1967

11. Schlenk H, Gellerman JL: Esterification of fatty acids with diazomethane on a small scale. Anal Chem 32:1412-1414, 1960

12. Schoenfield LJ, Sjövall J, Sjövall K: Bile acid composition of gallstones from man. J Lab Clin Med 68:186-194, 1966

13. Carey JB Jr, Wilson ID, Zaki FG, et al: The metabolism of bile acids with special reference to liver injury. Medicine (Balt) 45: 461-470, 1966

14. National Research Council, Food and Nutrition Board: Recommended Dietary Allowances. Seventh revised edition. Washington DC, National Academy of Sciences, 1968 (Publication No 1694)

15. Prange I, Christensen F, Dam H: Alimentary production of gallstones in hamsters. 11. Relation between diet and composition of the bladder bile 1. Z Ernaehrungswiss 3:59-78, 1962

16. Small DM, Rapo S: Source of abnormal bile in patients with cholesterol gallstones. New Eng J Med 283:53-57, 1970

17. Sarles H, Hauton J, Planche NE, et al: Diet, cholesterol gallstones, and composition of the bile. Amer J Dig Dis 15:251-260, 1970

18. Hislop IG, Hofmann AF, Schoenfield LJ: Determinants of the rate and site of bile acid absorption in man. J Clin Invest 46: 1070-1071, 1967

19. Vlahcevic ZR, Bell CC Jr, Buhac I, et al: Diminished bile acid pool size in patients with gallstones. Gastroenterology 59:165-173, 1970

179

Health of Children

The Health of American Indian Children

Helen M. Wallace, MD, MPH.

A summary of the present health status of major health problems in American Indian infants, children, and youth is presented. It is evident that, although considerable progress is being made, they represent a high-risk group of children from disadvantaged families. High priority in the delivery of health and related services is needed for American Indian children and their families.

There is little question that progress has been made since 1955, the year the US Public Health Service (USPHS) was assigned the responsibility of providing Indians and Alaskan Natives with health care. Nevertheless, in spite of the progress, much more is needed to narrow the gap between the health of Indian children and children belonging to other American families.

Demographic Information Relevant to Health

The American Indian population is relatively small (561,100 in 1968); it represented only 0.3% of the total population within the United States in both 1940 and 1969.[1] The rate of population increase from 1955 to 1968 was similar for Indians (20.9%) to that of the United States as a whole (21.6%), but only half as great as that

of the Alaska Native population (39.4%).[2]

The rate of migration of the American Indian from rural to urban areas has been higher than for any other ethnic group from 1930 to 1970. In this period the percentage of Indians in urban areas more than tripled from 10% to 35%[1] compared with a 1¼ increase for whites and 1¾ for Negroes.

The American Indian population is a relatively young one: in 1960 the median age of the Indian was 17.3 years and of the Alaskan Native, 16.3 years. This is in comparison to 29.5 years for the United States as a whole.[3] Furthermore, there is a much higher percentage of children and youth under the age of 20 among the Alaskan Natives (57.7%) and the Indians (55.2%) compared with the United States as a whole (38.7%). The significance of these statistics is that the Indian population has more children and youth and, therefore, a more dependent population. It has a greater need for all types of community services for children and youth—hospitals, health centers, clinics, schools, school health services, recreation programs, preschool programs such as day care, Head Start, and special health programs for youth, etc. Also, this population will be having a proportionately higher number of girls entering the childbearing age and needing maternal health services in this present decade.

Although many preschool children of Indian and Alaskan Native families come from the disadvantaged group, they nevertheless represent only a small percent of those enrolled in Head Start in 1968 and 1969—about 3.0% for the American Indian and about 0.2% for the Alaskan Native,[1] compared with about 50% for American blacks.

Births.—The birth rate among the American Indian and Alaskan Native populations (39.2 and 31.5/1,000 population) is approximately twice that of the US population as a whole (17.5) in 1969.

A high birth rate is of vital concern for health reasons. In general, maternal mortality is higher in women with a larger number of children. Infant and perinatal mortality is also higher in women who have a larger number of children. Early weaning because of an early next pregnancy is one aspect: the fact that a mother has to take care of a large number of children at any one time means less maternal time and attention per child. This is also a factor in less than optimal physical and emotional growth and development and of illness in the individual children. Frequent pregnancies also produce the "maternal depletion" picture: that of the worn-out mother, prematurely aged, with insufficient energy to take care of home and all her children adequately.

Furthermore, there is a well-known relationship between the interval separating pregnancies and the birth weight of the baby; babies of low birth weight (under 2.5 kg) have a higher mortality and higher incidence of residual neurological and brain damage (cerebral palsy, mental retardation, and epilepsy). There are many specific health reasons for concern about the birth rate, about the number and spacing of children, about family size, and about the need to make family planning services and education available to all girls and women of the childbearing age (Table 1).[1]

Another consideration is place of delivery. In a developed country such as the United States, it is considered safer for the mother to deliver the baby in the hospital. For the US population as a whole, 98.5% of the babies are born in hospitals. Some questions need to be raised about this. Is there a lack of hospital beds? Or are there enough hospital beds, but are they not easily accessible geographically to all the population? Or is it that some mothers are unwilling or afraid to deliver in a hospital (Table 2)?[2]

Annual income is an important factor in the health picture. The most recent information indicates that in the United States the American Indian is economically disadvantaged compared with other ethnic groups:

Ethnic Group	Annual Family Income for 1970
All groups	$ 9,870
Whites	10,240
Spanish-American	7,330
Blacks	6,280
American Indian	1,900

Mortality

Infant Mortality.—The infant mortality rate is a sensitive index of the socioeconomic status, stage of development of a country, and availability and utilization of health services. While the infant mortality rate has been declining for both the American Indian and the Alaskan Native popu-

Table 1.—Birth Rates*				
Year	United States	Indians & Alaskan Natives	American Indians	Alaskan Natives
1955	24.6	37.1	36.1	49.3
1960	23.7	42.5	42.2	45.6
1965	19.4	41.7	41.5	43.4
1968	17.5	38.5	39.2	31.5

* Per 1,000 population.
Source: White House Conference on Children.[1]

Table 2.—Percentage of Live Births in Hospitals				
Year	Indians & Alaskan Natives	American Indians	Alaskan Natives	United States
1955	88.2	90.8	65.1	94.4
1960	92.9	95.1	70.9	96.6
1965	95.5	96.7	84.0	97.4
1968	98.0	98.5	91.8	98.5
1971	99.0	99.3	95.0	NA

Source: Indian Health Service.[2]

Table 3.—Infant Death Rates*				
Year	Indians & Alaskan Natives	American Indians	Alaskan Natives	United States
1955	62.5	61.2	74.8	26.4
1960	50.3	47.6	76.3	26.0
1965	39.0	36.4	65.4	24.7
1967	32.2	30.1	55.6	22.4
1968	30.9	30.2	40.4	21.8
1971	28.8	23.5	27.4	19.2†

* Per 1,000 live births.
† Provisional, monthly Vital Statistics Report, NCHS, vol 20, No. 13.
Source: Indian Health Service.[2]

Table 4.—Neonatal and Postneonatal Mortality Rates*						
Population	1955	1960	1965	1967	1968	1971
Indians and Alaskan Natives						
Neonatal	22.7	19.1	15.8	15.3	14.4	12.5
Postneonatal	39.8	31.2	23.2	16.9	16.5	11.4
American Indians						
Neonatal	22.2	20.4	15.2	14.2	13.7	12.1
Postneonatal	39.0	26.4	21.1	15.9	16.5	11.4
Alaskan Natives						
Neonatal	27.8	28.5	21.8	27.5	24.1	16.9
Postneonatal	47.0	47.8	43.6	28.1	16.3	10.5
United States						
Neonatal	19.1	18.7	17.7	16.5	16.1	14.3†
Postneonatal	7.3	7.3	6.9	5.9	5.7	4.9†

* Per 1,000 live births.
† Provisional, monthly Vital Statistics Report, NCHS, vol 20, No. 13.
Source: Indian Health Service.[2]

lations, the rates are still much higher than for the United States as a whole. For example, in 1967 the rate for American Indians (30.1/1,000 live births) was 34.5% higher than that of the United States as a whole (22.4), while the rate for Alaskan Natives (55.6) was 148% higher (Table 3).[2]

Neonatal mortality (within the first 27 days of life) is an index of maternity care. The neonatal mortality rate of the American Indian is similar to that of the United States as a whole; that of the Alaskan Native is 67% higher than that of the United States, pointing up the need for improvement in maternity care.

Postneonatal mortality (the 28th day to the first birthday) is an index of the care of the baby in environmental conditions at home. Here the picture is very unfavorable: the postneonatal mortality rate in American Indians is almost three times greater than that of the United States as a whole, while that of Alaskan Natives is almost five times greater (Table 4).[2]

Table 5, showing the causes of neonatal and postneonatal mortality,

demonstrates the differences more specifically. During the neonatal period, obstetric causes play the significant role and there is a similarity to the United States as a whole. During the postneonatal period, respiratory, digestive, and other infectious and parasitic diseases have much higher mortality rates among the American Indian and Alaskan Native populations. Accidental causes also show higher mortality rates (Table 5).[2]

Mortality in Childhood.—The mortality rate in children age 1 to 14 years is almost three times greater in the American Indian and Alaskan Native population than among the United States as a whole[1] (Table 6); this is largely due to infectious diseases and accidents. Within the infectious disease group, respiratory infections, gastrointestinal infections, tuberculosis, and meningitis play prominent roles. Within the accident group all kinds of accidents are involved including motor vehicle accidents. Furthermore, homicide and suicide begin to appear, reflecting mental health problems.

Table 5.—Neonatal and Postneonatal Death Rates by Cause*

Cause of Death	Indians & Alaskan Natives, 1965 to 1967 Av	United States, 1966
Neonatal		
Immaturity	3.1	3.6
Ill-defined diseases	3.1	2.7
Postnatal asphyxia & atelectasis	2.5	3.8
Congenital malformations	1.7	2.3
Birth injuries	1.6	2.0
Postneonatal		
Respiratory diseases	7.1	2.5
Digestive diseases	3.6	0.5
Accidents	1.9	0.8
Infectious & parasitic diseases	1.6	0.3
Congenital malformations	1.3	1.1

* Per 1,000 live births.
Source: Indian Health Service.[2]

Table 6.—Causes of Death in Children 1 to 14 Years*

Cause of Death	Indians & Alaskan Natives, 1965 to 1967	United States, 1966
All deaths	144.2	57.1
Tuberculosis	2.1	0.2
Dysentery	1.5	0.1
Whooping cough	0.1	0.0
Meningococcal infections	1.3	0.7
Other infectious & parasitic diseases	3.8	1.4
Meningitis, except meningococcal & tuberculous	2.8	0.8
Diseases of heart	2.1	1.0
Influenza	0.4	0.2
Pneumonia	13.9	4.4
Bronchitis	0.7	0.4
Hernia & intestinal obstruction	0.6	0.2
Gastroenteritis	5.3	0.7
Cirrhosis of liver	0.4	0.1
Congenital malformations	6.0	4.8
Motor vehicle accidents	22.6	10.1
Other accidents	45.9	13.6
Suicide	0.6	0.2
Homicide	1.9	0.8

* Per 100,000 population.
Source: White House Conference on Children.[1]

Table 7.—Percent of Deaths by Age Group				
	Indians & Alaskan Natives		United States	
Age	1967	1969	1967	1969
Under 1	13.9	11.2	4.3	3.9
1 to 4	(20.7) 4.3	(16.9) 3.0	(5.9) 0.7	(5.4) 0.6
5 to 14	2.5	2.7	0.9	0.9
15 to 24	7.5	8.3	2.0	2.3
25 to 34	8.2	9.0	1.9	2.0
35 to 44	9.0	10.5	4.0	3.9
45 to 54	9.7	10.9	8.9	8.8
55 to 64	11.6	13.4	15.9	15.9
65 to 74	15.0	13.3	23.7	23.3
75 & over	18.2	17.6	37.7	38.4

Source: Indian Health Service.[2]

Over one fifth of all deaths occur in infants and children among the American Indian and Alaskan Native populations, in contrast to only 5.9% among the US population as a whole (Table 7).[2]

The large role played by gastroenteritis as a cause of death in infants and children among the American Indian and Alaskan Native population is shown in Table 8.[2]

Illness Among Children

Table 9 shows the major causes of illness among the Indian population; most of these are illnesses of childhood (Table 10). It is of some interest that the rank of the various diseases has changed very little since 1965. The diseases where progress has been made are measles (where the new vaccine has been available) and trachoma (Table 11).[3]

In children, most of these illnesses are preventable through better living conditions at home; more adequate housing; safer water supply and sewage disposal systems; breast-feeding of infants, safer weaning practices, and safer methods of preparation of infant feeding (including refrigeration of foods); immunization against common communicable diseases of childhood; providing easily accessible

Table 8.—Gastroenteritis Age-Specific Death Rates*					
	Indians & Alaskan Natives		United States		Ratio: Indians to United States
Age	1965 to 1967	1967 to 1969	1966	1968	
All ages	18.2	13.4	3.9	4.1	4.7
Under 1	309.6	297.5	36.9	31.7	8.4
1 to 4	16.2	13.7	2.1	1.7	7.7
5 to 14	. . .	0.7	0.2	0.2	. . .
15 to 64	2.6	2.4	1.6	1.7	1.6
65 & up	43.4	31.9	20.9	23.7	2.1

* Per 100,000 population.
Source: Indian Health Service.[2]

Table 9.—Rank of Notifiable Diseases—Indians & Alaskan Natives, 1965 to 1969					
Disease	1969	1968	1967	1966	1965
Otitis media	1	1	1	1	1
Gastroenteritis	2	2	2	2	2
Strep throat, scarlet fever	3	3	4	5	4
Pneumonia	4	4	3	3	3
Influenza	5	5	5	4	6
Gonorrhea	6	6	7	7	7
Trachoma	7	7	6	6	5
Chickenpox	8	8	9	9	10
Dysentery	9	10	8	10	9
Mumps	10	9	11	11	11
Measles	11	12	10	8	8

Source: Indian Health Service.[3]

medical and health care for well and sick infants and children; early identification of illness and prompt treatment; and health education of parents and children.

The relationship between the method of feeding infants and young children and diarrhea is illustrated by a study among Navajo children during the first two years of life.[4] In this, there was a higher incidence of diarrhea in bottle-fed babies than in breast-fed babies at all ages. There was also found a higher incidence of all illnesses in bottle-fed babies, but the difference was not statistically significant.

A study of 631 children on the Cherokee North Carolina Indian Reservation (96% of the 655 students enrolled in the elementary school) showed infection with one or more parasites in 92%.[5] The need to improve sanitation and to intensify health education is evident.

Otitis media with resultant hearing impairment is recognized as one of the most serious health problems among Indian and Alaskan Natives. As with other infectious diseases, there is a close relationship between otitis media and crowded living conditions. Those at greatest risk are children under 2 years of age. If otitis media occurs before the child reaches his first birthday, the risk of repeated attacks is increased; if hearing loss occurs, medical and surgical treatment is usually indicated, and special educational measures and vocational assistance may be required.

Unless these special services are available, speech and language development may be impaired, the child's progress in school may be poor, and his future vocational opportunities and social development may be restricted. There is every reason to try to improve general living conditions, provide continuous health supervision of well children, and provide prompt treatment of children with early respiratory infections. There is also need of prompt treatment of otitis media

Table 10.—Indian and Alaskan Native Cases by Age Group, 1969					
Disease	Total Cases	14 yr & Under		15 yr & Over	
		No.	%	No.	%
Otitis media	39,351	33,139	84	6,212	16
Gastroenteritis	29,811	20,224	68	9,587	32
Strep throat, scarlet fever	20,022	12,185	61	7,837	39
Pneumonia	13,423	10,478	78	2,945	22
Influenza	8,666	4,145	48	4,521	52

Source: Indian Health Service.[3]

Table 11.—Change in Leading Notifiable Diseases—Indians and Alaskan Natives, 1969 and 1965

Disease	Reported Cases 1969	Reported Cases 1965	% Change, 1969 to 1965
Otitis media	39,351	22,614	+74.0
Gastro-enteritis	29,811	20,000	+49.1
Strep throat, scarlet fever	20,022	7,433	+169.4
Pneumonia	13,423	13,525	+0.8
Influenza	8,666	3,652	+137.3
Gonorrhea	4,543	7,849	+59.5
Trachoma	3,388	4,731	−28.4
Chickenpox	1,735	1,867	−7.1
Dysentery	1,130	1,901	−40.6
Mumps	1,083	1,131	−4.2
Measles	774	2,508	−69.1

Source: Indian Health Service.[3]

and special medical, surgical, and educational measures for those children with chronic otitis media.

Dental problems are frequent in all children. Oral hygiene, the use of fluoride in the water supply or applied locally to children's teeth, dental care, cleaning, and treatment programs, and orthodontia programs are considered essential. There is a great shortage of dental health personnel of all types—dentists, dental hygienists, assistants, etc. Considerable progress has been made in meeting dental health needs of Indians: for example, more teeth are being filled and fewer teeth are decayed or missing. Never-

theless, only 54% of the population under 20 years of age is receiving dental service (Tables 12 and 13).[2]

Although progress is being made in control of tuberculosis, this is still an important cause of illness and mortality among children and youth in the Indian population (Tables 14 and 15).[2] Key measures in a tuberculosis prevention and control program are the use of bacille Calmette Guérin vaccine in infants and children; screening through tuberculin testing, follow-up and diagnostic work-up of positive reactors; the use of isoniazid in recent converters from negative to positive tuberculin tests; and the treatment and supervision of those in close contact with a patient with active tuberculosis.

Table 13.—Av No. of Permanent Teeth Decayed, Missing, and Filled per Child, 6 to 17 Years*

Year	1957 to 1972 Total Decayed, Missing, and Filled Teeth	De-cayed	Miss-ing	Filled
1957	4.00	2.49	0.40	1.11
1969	5.88	2.42	0.32	3.13
1972	5.92	2.43	0.32	3.17

* Average number of permanent teeth decayed, missing, and filled per child 5 to 19 years of age.
Source: Indian Health Service.[2]

Table 12.—Percent of Population Receiving Dental Treatment by Age Group, 1957 to 1972

Year	All Ages No.	All Ages %	Under 20 No.	Under 20 %	20 & Over No.	20 & Over %
1957	72,479	19.1	56,079	29.5	16,400	8.6
1969	151,310	37.5	120,120	53.5	31,190	17.4
1972	183,689	39.1	137,809	54.6	45,880	21.0

Source: Indian Health Service.[2]

Table 14.—Tuberculosis Age-Specific Death Rates*

Age	Indians and Alaskan Natives		United States		Ratio: Indians to United States
	1965-1967	1967-1969	1966	1968	
All ages	17.4	12.8	3.9	3.1	4.5
Under 15	2.0	1.0	0.2	0.1	10.0
15 to 24	1.1	0.8	0.2	0.2	5.5
25 to 34	11.3	7.7	1.0	0.8	11.3
35 to 44	34.1	18.4	3.0	2.2	11.4
45 to 54	31.2	31.3	5.5	4.3	5.7
55 to 64	43.3	40.4	10.1	8.1	4.3
65 & over	155.7	91.2	19.2	15.7	8.1

* Per 100,000 population.
Source: Indian Health Service.[2]

Table 15.—No. of Cases and Incidence Rates for Tuberculosis, 1955 to 1969

Year	No. of Cases			Rate/100,000 Population			
	Indians & Alaskan Natives	American Indians	Alaskan Natives	Indians & Alaskan Natives	American Indians	Alaskan Natives	United States
1955	2,400	1,586	814	758.1	563.2	2,325.7	60.1
1960	1,096	877	219	322.4	292.3	547.5	39.4
1965	801	563	238	218.6	175.9	511.8	25.3
1969	623	556	67	153.2	155.7	135.6	19.1

Source: Indian Health Service.[3]

Table 16.—Venereal Diseases—Rates/100,000 Population, 1963 to 1969

Year	Gonorrhea			Syphilis		
	American Indians	Alaskan Natives	United States	American Indians	Alaskan Natives	United States
1963	833.9	541.9	147.5	119.0	Not available	65.8
1965	768.1	840.9	167.7	113.5	15.1	58.2
1967	770.1	121.8	204.6	123.4	14.5	51.8
1969	1.019.0	1,827.9	264.9	200.4	Not available	45.6

Source: Indian Health Service.[3]

Both gonorrhea and syphilis show an increase in reported incidence among the Indian and Alaskan Native population (Table 16).[2] Syphilis is of special importance because if it occurs in pregnant women, untreated, it will cause congenital syphilis in infants.

Nutrition in Indian Children.—There is evidence that the nutritional status of a significant number of Indian children is substandard. For example, the records of children born in 1964 and living on the Pine Ridge Reservation were reviewed: of 190 children who had hemoglobin determinations recorded in their health records, 40.5% of them were below 10 gm and 15.8% were below 8 gm at some time in the first two years of life.[6]

A survey of six Kodiak Island villages by Brown showed that 82 children 0 to 3 years old had an average hemoglobin level of 10.3 gm.[6]

Among 676 discharges of children age 0 to 4 years from the Tuba City Hospital, Arizona, from July 1, 1967 to April 30, 1968, there were 44 cases of malnutrition, 38 of iron deficiency anemia, 13 of marasmus (all under 1 year of age), and eight of kwashiorkor. Among 1,591 discharges of children 5 years of age and older, there were 44 with iron deficiency anemia and two with malnutrition.

Preliminary data from a study of Alaskan Natives in Kodiak Island villages disclosed a very high incidence of iron deficiency (nutritional) anemia among infants and young children. Similar iron deficiencies have been noted in other parts of the state among Alaskan Native infants and children as well as pregnant women.[6]

In the Window Rock area, in fiscal year 1966, 20% of pediatric admissions to the PHS Indian Hospitals revealed evidence of malnutrition. Of patients discharged from these hospitals in fiscal year 1966, 10% of 4,167 children age 0 to 4 years and 10% of the pregnant women had iron deficiency anemia.[6]

In a five-year period (1963 to 1967) there were 4,355 admissions to the pediatric service of the PHS Indian Hospital in Tuba City, Ariz, of children under 5 years of age. Of the total number, 616 had diagnoses of malnutrition; 44 of these had kwashiorkor or marasmus. The other 572 children were children whose weights or heights were below the norms for their ages.[7]

From this study it appeared that artificially fed Navajo infants are most apt to have malnutrition. It also appeared that infants with marasmus and kwashiorkor were weaned early in life and were not provided with a suitable, safe infant formula or weaning supplement afterwards. Kwashiorkor in an older child was frequently associated with displacement from the breast by a younger child due to too rapid successive pregnancies. Diarrhea was a frequent occurrence in the children with marasmus and kwashiorkor.

Mental Health.—At the Third National Conference on American Indian Health, it was reported that mental health was emerging as one of the major health problems among American Indians.[8] It was estimated that possibly 20% to 25% of the American Indian population may be affected by some type of mental health problem, ranging from major psychoses to personality disorders. Factors cited include disintegration of the American Indian culture, the transition in the way of life from the previous predominant Indian culture to the present social order of American society, the generally poor level of

191

education, poverty, and disturbing childhood experiences. Furthermore, removal of Indian children from their families to government boarding schools for their education may be a contributing factor.

Recommendations included pilot studies to determine the most acute needs of those with psychiatric problems; provision of consultative services to young couples on the health care of their children, to the staff of boarding schools, and to children with problems in boarding schools; development of mental health services; steps to strengthen family life and child rearing among Indian families; making it possible for Indian children to attend school while living with their families or a substitute family at home; and psychiatric services for these children and families in need of it. It is generally agreed that the parent-child relationship, especially in the first five years of life, plays an important role in fostering optimal emotional and social development of the child.

More Recent Health Problems of Youth.—School dropouts, juvenile delinquency, out-of-wedlock pregnancy, drug abuse, as well as venereal disease, are some of the more recent Indian youth problems. These are complex emotional problems related to a number of possible factors—the weakening of the family and of family life; increased sexual freedom in general in Western culture; increased movement of young people and families to the large cities with inability of the cities to provide sufficient preventive and remedial health, social, educational, recreational, housing, and employment services for them; increasing emphasis on technology and technical education and training in American society, with difficulty of adaptation among young people not so trained; lack of education and services in the field of family planning; and the need for programs of education, information, counseling, and treatment in regard to drugs and drug abuse.

References

1. White House Conference on Children-1970: *Profiles of Children.* Government Printing Office, 1970.
2. Indian Health Service: *Indian Health Trends and Services,* 1970 edition. Government Printing Office, 1971.
3. Indian Health Service: *Illness Among Indians.* Government Printing Office, July 1971.
4. French JG: Relationship of morbidity to the feeding patterns of Navajo children from birth through 24 months. *Am J Clin Nutr* 20:375-385, 1967.
5. Healy GR, et al: Prevalence of ascariasis and amebiasis in Cherokee Indian school children. *Public Health Rep* 84:907-914, 1969.
6. USDA, HEW OEO: *Hearings Before the Select Committee on Nutrition and Human Needs of the US Senate: Nutrition and Human Needs,* part 2. Government Printing Office, 1969, pp 441-444.
7. Van Duzen J, et al: Protein and calorie malnutrition among preschool Navajo Indian children. *Am J Clin Nutr* 22:1362-1370, 1969.
8. Fahy A. Muschenheim C: Third national conference on American Indian health. *JAMA* 194:1093-1096, 1965.

The Health of American Indian Children

A Survey of Current Problems and Needs

HELEN M. WALLACE, M.D., M.P.H.

TREMENDOUS progress has been made since 1955, the year the United States Public Health Service was assigned responsibility for providing Indians and Alaskan natives with health care. The evidence is widespread[1]—improvement in the health of Indian family members, as illustrated by increased clinic visits, hospital admissions and deliveries, and dental services; program expansion, shown by greater numbers of health personnel and increased training and employment of Indian personnel in the health field; and efforts to improve such environmental health facilities as water supply, waste disposal, etc. Nevertheless, despite this progress, the gap between the health of Indian children and children belonging to other American families is still much too wide. This paper will review where we stand today.

Demographic Information Relevant to Health

The American Indian population is relatively small—561,000 in 1968. Both in 1940 and in 1969, it represented only 0.3 per cent of the total U. S. population.[2] From 1955 to 1968, the rate of population increase among Indians (20.9%) was similar to that of the country as a whole (21.6%), whereas it was almost double[3] (39.4%) among the Alaskan native population.

193

The rate of migration of the American Indian from rural to urban areas from 1930 to 1970 has been higher than for any other ethnic group. In that time span, the percentage of Indians living in urban areas rose three and one half times,[3] from 10 to 35 per cent.[2]

These populations are relatively young. In 1960, the median age of the American Indian was 17.3 years, and of the Alaskan native 16.3 years, compared with 29.5 years for the U. S. as a whole.[4] The percentage of children and youth under the age of 20 years is much higher among the Alaskan natives (57.7%) and the Indians (55.2%), than for the nation (38.7%).

Having fewer adults makes these Indian populations more dependent and makes the need for all types of community health services, especially those directed toward the young, greater. Hospitals, health centers, clinics, schools, school health services, recreation programs, and such preschool programs as day care, Head Start, special health projects for youth, etc. are all needed. Later in this decade, a proportionately higher number will be entering the childbearing age.

Although many preschool children of Indian and Alaskan native families are disadvantaged, only a very small fraction were enrolled in Head Start during 1968 and 1969—only about 3.5 per cent of the enrollees were Indians, and about 0.2 per cent were Alaskan natives.[2]

Of the 177,464 American Indian children in school in 1968, about one-third were attending federal schools for Indians; the other two-third were attending regular community schools.[2]

Births

The birth rates for the American Indian and Alaskan native populations (39.2 and

31.5 per 1,000 population) were more than twice and slightly less than twice that of the U.S. population as a whole (17.5) in 1969.

A high birth rate is of vital concern for health reasons. In general, maternal mortality rates are higher in women having a greater number of children, as are also infant and perinatal mortality rates. Too many babies too rapidly produces a well-known pattern of illness—the young infant is weaned too early from the breast because of a too early next pregnancy, thereby becoming more prone to diarrhea and malnutrition. When a mother has to take care of a large number of children at any one time, she can give less time and attention to the individual child. Too frequent pregnancies produce the "maternal depletion" picture—that of the worn-out mother, aged prematurely, with insufficient energy to take care of home and all her children adequately. Shorter pregnancy intervals mean lower birth weights, and newborns (under 5-1/2 pounds) with a higher mortality and more neurologic and brain damage—cerebral palsy, mental retardation, and epilepsy. Thus, there are many specific health reasons for concern about the birth rate, about the number and spacing of children, about family size, and about the need to make family planning services and education available to all girls and women of the childbearing age.[2]

Economic Status

Annual income is an important factor in the health picture. The most recent information indicates that in the U. S. the American Indian is economically disadvantaged compared with other ethnic groups:

195

Ethnic Group	Annual Family Income for 1970 in U. S.
All groups	$ 9,870
White	10,240
Spanish-American	7,330
Black	6,280
American Indian	1,900

Infant Mortality

The infant mortality rate is a sensitive index of the socioeconomic status, the stage of development of a people, and the availability and utilization of health services. While the infant mortality rates have been declining for both the American Indian and the Alaskan native populations, they are still much higher than for the country as a whole. For example, in 1967, the rate for American Indians (30.1 per 1,000 live births) was 34.5 per cent higher than that of the country as a whole (22.4), while that for Alaskan natives (55.6) was 148 per cent higher.[4]

Neonatal mortality (within the first 27 days of life) is more an index of maternity care. The neonatal mortality rate of the American Indian is similar to that of the country as a whole; that of the Alaskan native, is 67 per cent higher.

Postneonatal mortality (the 28th day to the first birthday) is mainly an index of the care of the baby in environmental conditions at home. Here the picture is very unfavorable. The postneonatal mortality rate in American Indians is almost three times that of the country as a whole; that of Alaskan natives, almost five times.[5]

Table 1 demonstrates these differences more specifically. During the neonatal period, when obstetric causes play the significant role, there is similarity with the U. S. as a whole. During the postneonatal period, respiratory, digestive, and other infective and parasitic diseases and accidents have much higher mortality rates among the American Indian and Alaskan native populations.[3]

Mortality During Childhood

The mortality rate in children aged 1–14 years is almost three times greater among the American Indian and Alaskan native populations than in the U. S. as a whole (Table 2). The difference is largely due to the infectious diseases and accidents. Respiratory infections, gastroenteritis, tuberculosis, and meningitis play a major role. Furthermore, homicide and suicide begin to appear, pointing to mental health problems.

Over one-fifth of all deaths among the American Indian and Alaskan native populations occur in infants and children, in contrast to only 5.9 per cent among the nation's population as a whole.[3]

TABLE 1. *Neonatal and Postneonatal Death Rates by Cause*

Cause of Death	Indian & Alaskan Native 1965–67 Average	U. S.— 1966
Neonatal		
Immaturity	3.1	3.6
Ill-defined diseases	3.1	2.7
Postnatal asphyxia & atelectasis	2.5	3.8
Congenital malformations	1.7	2.3
Birth injuries	1.6	2.0
Postneonatal		
Respiratory diseases	7.1	7.5
Digestive diseases	3.6	0.5
Accidents	1.9	0.8
Infective & parasitic diseases	1.6	0.3
Congenital malformations	1.3	1.1

Source: U. S. Indian Health Service. Indian Health Trends and Services. 1970 Edition. January, 1971. 94 pp.

	Indian & Alaskan Native 1965–67	U. S.— 1966
All Deaths 1–14 years	144.2	57.1
Tuberculosis	2.1	0.2
Dysentery	1.5	0.1
Whooping cough	0.1	0.0
Meningococcal infections	1.3	0.7
Other infective & parasitic diseases	3.8	1.4
Meningitis, exc. meningococcal & Tuberculous	2.8	0.8
Diseases of heart	2.1	1.0
Influenza	0.4	0.2
Pneumonia	13.9	4.4
Bronchitis	0.7	0.4
Hernia & intestinal obstructions	0.6	0.2
Gastroenteritis	5.3	0.7
Cirrhosis of liver	0.4	0.1
Congenital malformations	6.0	4.8
Motor vehicle accidents	22.6	10.1
Other accidents	45.9	13.6
Suicide	0.6	0.2
Homicide	1.9	0.8

Source: White House Conference on Children. 1970 Profiles of Children.

Illness Among Children

Most of the infections seen in these children are preventable through better living conditions such as more adequate housing; safer water supply and sewage disposal systems; breast feeding of infants, safer weaning practices, and safer methods of preparation of infant feeding, including refrigeration of foods; immunizations against the common communicable diseases of childhood; more easily accessible medical and health care for well and sick infants and children; earlier identification of illness and prompt treatment; and health education of parents and children.

A study done by French among Navajo children under two years of age showed more diarrhea in bottle-fed than in breast-fed babies.[5] Another recent study, of 631 children on the Cherokee North Carolina Indian Reservation, representing 96 per cent of the 655 students enrolled in the elementary school there, showed that 92 per cent were infested with one or more parasites.[6] The need to improve sanitation and to intensify health education is evident.

Otitis media is one of the most serious health problems among Indian and Alaskan natives. As with the other infectious diseases, this is closely related to poor and crowded living conditions. At greatest risk are those children under two years of age. Furthermore, otitis media beginning before the first birthday carries a greater risk of repeated attacks. One unhappy consequence is permanent impairment of hearing. This in turn calls for medical and surgical treatment, and often special educational measures and vocational assistance. Without these special services, speech and language development may be restricted.

Considerable progress has been made in meeting dental health needs of Indians. More teeth are being filled, and fewer teeth are decayed or missing, but there still is a great shortage of dental health personnel of all types—dentists, dental hygienists, assistants, etc. Only 54 per cent of the population under 20 years of age is receiving dental service.[3]

TABLE 3. *Per Cent of Population Receiving Dental Treatment by Age Group, 1957 and 1969*

Year	All Ages		Under 20		20 and Over	
	Number	%	Number	%	Number	%
1957	72,479	19.1	56,079	29.5	16,400	8.6
1969	151,310	37.5	120,120	53.5	31,190	17.4

Source: U. S. Indian Health Service. Indian Health Trends and Services. 1970 Edition. January 1971. 94 pp.

Tuberculosis, gonorrhea, and syphilis are important diseases also, and the latter are rising among teen-agers and young adults.[8] Syphilis is of special importance because in an untreated pregnant woman it may lead to congenital syphilis in the infant.

Malnutrition

There is considerable evidence that the nutritional status of a significant number of Indian children is substandard. For example, a review of the records of children born in 1964 and living on the Pine Ridge Reservation showed that, of 190 who had had hemoglobin determinations, 40.5 per cent had levels below 10 gm, and 15.8 per cent had levels below 8 gm at some time during their first two years of life.[7]

A survey of six Kodiak Island Villagers by Brown showed that 82 children from birth to three years of age had an average hemoglobin of 10.3 gm.[8]

A report of discharges from the Tuba City Hospital, Arizona from July 1, 1967–April 30, 1968 revealed the following indicators of malnutrition.[7]

Children Aged 0–4 years (676 discharges)

Malnutrition	44
Iron deficiency anemia	38
Marasmus (under 1 year of age)	13
Kwashiorkor	8

Children 5 years of age and older (1,591 discharges)

Iron deficiency anemia	44
Malnutrition	2

Preliminary data from Alaskan natives in Kodiak Island villages and elsewhere revealed a very high prevalence of iron deficiency (nutritional) anemia among infants, young children, and pregnant women.[7]

In the Window Rock area in the Southwest, during fiscal year 1966, 20 per cent of the children admitted to the P.H.S. Indian

Hospitals had evidence of malnutrition. Of the patients discharged from these hospitals during fiscal year 1966, 10 per cent of 4,167 children aged 0–4 years and 10 per cent of all pregnant women had iron deficiency anemia.[7]

In the five-year period 1963 to 1967, there were 4,355 admissions to the pediatric service of the P.H.S. Indian Hospital in Tuba City, Arizona of children under five years of age. Of this total, 616 had diagnoses related to malnutrition: 44 had kwashiorkor or marasmus, and the other 572 had weights or heights below the norms for their ages.[8] Those infants with marasmus and kwashiorkor had been weaned early in life and were not provided with a suitable feeding regimen afterwards.

Mental Health

The Third National Conference on American Indian Health brought out that mental health was emerging as one of the major health problems.[9] As an estimate, possibly 20 to 25 per cent of the American Indian population seem to have some type of mental health problem, ranging from personality disorders to major psychoses. Influences cited as bearing on the development of mental illness included the disintegration of the American Indian culture, the transition in the way of life from the previous predominant Indian culture to the present social order of American society, poverty, the generally poor level of education, and disturbing childhood experiences. The removal of Indian children from their families to government boarding schools for education may be a contributing factor.

More Recent Health Problems of Youth

Among the more recent health problems may be included school dropout, juvenile delinquency, out-of-wedlock pregnancy, and

201

drug abuse, as well as venereal disease, which was mentioned earlier. These complex emotional problems are related to a number of possible factors—the weakening of the family and of family life; increased sexual freedom in general in Western culture; increased movement of young people and families to the large cities with inability of the cities to provide sufficient preventive and remedial services (health, social, educational, recreational, housing, and employment) for them; increasing emphasis on technology and technical education and training in American society, with difficulty of young people not so trained to fit in; lack of education and services in the field of family planning; the need for programs of education, information, counseling, and treatment in regard to drug abuse.

Health Is a Team Affair

Health care in the United States is changing to delivery by a health team instead of delivery by one person. On the health team are various kinds of people—the physician, dentist, nurse, nutritionist, social worker, and various supportive and educational personnel. A new trend is to use local representatives of the people to be served, in order that they may be reached more effectively. The community health representative is an example of the process of extending health services to reach people more extensively in their own homes, in order to interpret the need for health care and to explain the services available to be used.[10-12]

References

1. U. S. Indian Health Service to the First Americans. The Fourth Report on the Indian Health Program of the U. S. Public Health Service. Public Health Service Publication No. 1580. Revised 1970.
2. White House Conference on Children—1970. Profiles of Children. Washington, D. C., U. S. Government Printing Office, 1970.

3. U. S. Indian Health Service. Indian Health Trends and Services. 1970 Edition. January, 1971. 94 pp.

4. U. S. Indian Health Service. Illness Among Indians. Washington, D. C., U. S. Government Printing Office, July, 1971. 42 pp.

5. French, J. G.: Relationship of morbidity to the feeding patterns of Navajo children from birth through twenty-four months. Clin. Nutr. 20: 375, 1967.

6. Healy, G. R., Gleason, N. N., Bokat, R., Pond, H. and Roper, M.: Prevalence of ascariasis and amebiasis in Cherokee Indian school children. Public Health Reports 84: 907, 1969.

7. Hearings Before the Select Committee on Nutrition and Human Needs of the U. S. Senate. Nutrition and Human Needs. Part 2—U.S.D.A., H.E.W., and O.E.O. officials. Washington, D. C., U. S. Government Printing Office, 1969. pp. 441–44.

8. Van Duzen, J., Carter, J. P., Secondi, J., and Federspiel, C.: Protein and calorie malnutrition among preschool Navajo Indian children. Nutrition 22: 1362, 1969.

9. Faly, A. and Muschenheim, C.: JAMA 194: 1093, 1965.

10. Uhrich, R. B.: Tribal community health representatives of the Indian Health Service. Public Health Reports 84: 965, 1969.

11. U. S. Indian Health Service. Indian Community Health Representative Program. Washington, D. C., U. S. Government Printing Office, July, 1968.

12. U. S. Indian Health Service. Tribal Community Health Representative Program. Training Protocol. August. 1968. 9 pp. plus attachments.

THE WORKING MOTHER AND CHILD NEGLECT
ON THE NAVAJO RESERVATION

Lynne Oakland, B.A., and Robert L. Kane, M.D.

ABSTRACT. In this small retrospective study, child neglect was not found to be closely related to the mother's age, education, nor employment, but the significant factors appeared to be marital status and size of family. The clinical impression of physicians that child neglect was related to the phenomenon of working mothers was not substantiated by our findings. *Pediatrics*, 51:849, 1973, NAVAJO, NEGLECT, WORKING MOTHERS, INDIAN, CROSS-CULTURAL.

For many developing nations, industrialization holds the key to the 20th century. In many ways, Indian reservations within the United States resemble developing countries abroad. On the Navajo reservation, growing industrialization has dictated social changes. In this paper, we deal with one aspect of change—the emergence of the working mother and its possible relationship to child neglect.

The study was prompted by the suggestion that the incidence of child neglect was increasing in one Service Unit on the Navajo reservation where industry had recently been introduced. The clinicians hypothesized that the industry was imposing a new pattern of surrogate mothers and thus indirectly producing an epidemic of child neglect. The clinical impression of the pediatricians was even cited in a *Business Week* article:[1] "Industrialization has also brought some sociological changes on the reservation. The Public Health Service in Shiprock reports some increase in child neglect."

In order to test the validity of this observation, the authors initiated a retrospective case history study.

MATERIALS AND METHODS

A. Setting

The Shiprock Service Unit of the Indian Health Service encompasses about 5,000 square miles in the Four Corners area of New Mexico, Arizona, and Utah. The health needs of the approximately 25,000 Navajos within its boundaries are met primarily by the Public Health Service Indian Hospital at Shiprock. This facility provides both inpatient and outpatient care as well as dental, optometric, pharmacy, school health, public health, and environmental health services. For patients who require treatment not available at IHS hospitals, limited funds are available to pay for care at other hospitals.

At the time of this study the inpatient services included pediatric, medical-surgical, and obstetrical-nursery care. The hospital had 91 beds, including 16 nursery beds and 32 pediatric beds. The average daily inpatient load was 66. There were 12 physicians, including two pediatricians. Nursing coverage was provided by a staff of eight RNs, ten LPNs, and seven nursing aides. The outpatient clinics received approximately 5,000 visits each month. Field clinics were held in five outlying areas in the Service Unit at weekly or bimonthly intervals. The hospital field health program was carried out by four public health nurses and a public health nurse supervisor. These nurses provided tuberculosis case-finding and follow-up, home visits, well-baby care, and immunization conferences. Three

This study was supported in part by Traineeship Grant for Apprenticeship Training 5A07AH00178–03.

TABLE I
Mother's Employment Among Neglected and Non-neglected Children

	Neglect		Control	
	Cases	%	Cases	%
Mother's Employment				
Mother working	10	30	14	29
Mother not working	23	70	35	71
	33	100	49	100

p > .5
x^2 = .03

---

school nurses were assigned to five neighboring boarding schools.[2]

Shiprock is a community of about 5,000. It is not incorporated as a town and does not provide the usual municipal services of a community of that size, such as street lighting and paving, fire protection, police protection, or organized recreation. The three largest organizations in the town, namely the Bureau of Indian Affairs, the

TABLE II
Significant Factors

	Neglect		Control	
	Cases	%	Cases	%
A. MARITAL STATUS				
Married	16	49	38	78
Not Married	17	51	11	22
Single	(12)	(36)	(7)	(14)
Widowed	(3)	(9)	(1)	(2)
Divorced	(2)	(6)	(3)	(6)
	33	100	49	100

p < .01 (married versus not married)
x^2 = 7.4

B. NUMBER OF SIBLINGS				
0	2	6	6	14
1–4	20	65	15	35
5 or more	9	29	22	51
	31	100	43	100

p < .05
x^2 = 6.37

Public Health Service, and the Navajo Tribe, each provide some services in these categories but there has been no central planning for the community. The town has no governing body and no authority to raise funds.

A unique feature of the Shiprock area is the presence of the Fairchild Corporation, an electronics company which employs about 1,000 Navajos, most of them women. This plant began operations in 1965 and is one of the first examples of industrialization on the reservation. Fairchild Corporation has introduced a new pattern of life in the region. Previously, most Navajos lived in isolated rural settings with only a few homes in each encampment. Sheep herding had been the major method of earning a living; women contributed to this effort, often weaving rugs at home in their spare time. The average annual family income on the reservation was about $1,200.

Fairchild employees are employed under the usual industrial hourly wage pattern—an eight-hour shift, five days a week, cash salary. Many find it convenient to move into town rather than remain in remote hogans. Some stay in town during the week and return home on weekends. Because Fairchild Corporation finds that women perform better than men at the painstaking assembly work, most of the jobs are filled by women. Since other job opportunities are scarce in the Shiprock region, the husbands of the Fairchild employees are not always able to find work.

B. Methods

Cases of child neglect were selected by a review of the hospital records from the pediatric inpatient service of the Shiprock Indian Hospital for the period June 1968 to June 1970. For the purposes of this study, the working definition of neglect was established as a disturbance in the parent-child relationship which prevented the child from receiving adequate physician and/or emotional care, thereby harming his physical, intellectual, or emotional development. The physicians' diagnoses of abuse, poor

205

home situation, family problems, maternal deprivation, desertion, failure to thrive, malnutrition, and kwashiorkor were used in compiling a preliminary list of neglected children treated at the facility. The medical records of each child on the list were reviewed and several cases eliminated because an underlying cause had been found for stunted growth or malnutrition. The Public Health Service social service records and the records of the field health nurses were used to confirm or, in a few cases, overrule the physician's diagnosis.

A control group was selected by taking the name of the child (of comparable age) admitted to the hospital immediately after each of the children in the neglected group. Those children who did not fall into the age range of the neglected group (2 months to 3 years) were eliminated, as well as those with a previous history of neglect in the family. In these cases, the second child admitted after the neglected case was selected as a control.

If sufficient information was not available or if neglect could not be proved with certainty, the case was discarded. The preliminary sample of neglect cases was reduced from 49 to 33. The control group consisted of 49 subjects.

The medical records of the mothers of the children in the sample were also analyzed. The demographic data collected included mother's age and marital status at the time of the child's birth, occupation, educational level, and the extent of prenatal care. The size of the family and ages of all the children were recorded. The Fairchild Corporation employment records and the Shiprock tribal census records were used to supplement this information.

The chi-square test was used to determine the statistical significance of the data obtained.

RESULTS

The neglect among the 33 cases could be classified into seven major categories. Several children suffered from more than one form of neglect.

TABLE III

NONSIGNIFICANT FACTORS

	Neglect		Control	
	Cases	%	Cases	%
A. PRENATAL CARE VISITS				
No visits	10	40	8	26
Less than 5 visits	8	32	13	42
5 or more visits	7	28	10	32
	25	100	31	100
$p > .5$				
$x^2 = 1.31$				
B. AGE OF MOTHER (at time of child's birth)				
18	2	7	3	7
19–30	18	62	22	50
31 and older	9	31	19	43
	29	100	44	100
$p > .5$				
$x^2 = 1.13$				
C. EDUCATION OF MOTHER				
None or elementary	6	36	7	30
High school or higher	11	64	16	70
	17	100	23	100
$p > .5$				
$x^2 = 0.105$				

Poor home situation	14
Malnutrition	9
Failure to thrive	8
Unwanted child or desertion	7
Maternal deprivation	7
Kwashiorkor	2
Battered child	2
	49

Under the category of "poor home situation" are cases in which either a court decision was reached that the home was an inadequate place for care of the child, or a field health or social service nurse visited the home and identified specific problems which were considered detrimental to the child's development.

In addition to the principal hypothesis, several other factors were studied in an effort to explain the neglect found. Unfortunately all the information sought was not available in some cases; therefore, the size of each group is indicated on each of the tables shown.

If employment of mothers does increase child neglect among the population studied, then the percentage of working mothers among the neglected children should be greater than among the control group. As is shown in Table I, there is no difference in the percent of working mothers in the neglected and control groups. Most of the working mothers in this study were employees of the Fairchild Corporation.

There were two significant differences between the neglected and control children in the conditions of family life (Table II). A significantly larger percentage of the mothers of the neglected children were not married (single, widowed, or divorced) as compared to the percentage in the control group, as is shown in Table IIA. The neglected children also came from smaller families (Table IIB). Perhaps related to this, more of the neglected children had birth weights of less than 5.2 lb (chi-square $= 5.92$; $p < .025$). Seven of the neglected children were small for dates as compared with two of the control group. Table III presents other factors which were examined and found not to be significantly different between the neglect and control groups.

DISCUSSION

The results of this study would suggest that there was no relationship between neglected children and working mothers. To explore further this potential repercussion of industrialization on child-rearing practices, one of the authors (L. O.) interviewed a random sample of women working on the day shift at the Fairchild plant who had children of school age or younger. Of the 139 women asked about the care for their children while they worked, 90% left their children in the care of relatives. In only 10% of the cases were children left in the care of a sitter or the local nursery. This suggests that the close and extended family ties remained intact even when mothers became employed in industrial jobs. In a comparison of a primarily rural community and a more industrialized community near Tuba City, Arizona, Levy[3] also concluded that industrialization was not resulting in the breakdown of clan ties among the Navajo.

In this study marital instability did appear to play a significant role in distinguishing between the child neglect group and the control group. This factor has been confirmed by other studies as correlating with inadequate nurturing of the child.[4-9]

However, for the other significant factor in this study, number of siblings, conflicting evidence exists. Simons et al.[8] found a higher percentage of abuse in larger families, whereas the present research found that the neglected child came from a smaller family than did the child in the control group.

A possible explanation for these differences may lie in the type of neglect isolated. The Simons study dealt with physically abused children. In this study, the major neglect problems found were poor home situations and maternal deprivation. These types of neglect have their most critical effects during the first two or three years of life. After that, a child may be described as small for his age, of low intelligence, or socially maladapted, but not as neglected. Similarly, in larger families this type of inadequate nurturing of the very young child may be less of a problem. Older siblings may be able to assist in the mothering role. Also, when ignorance and inexperience are factors in poor nurturing, the effects are most likely to be felt in families with a young mother without an extended family.

Admittedly the definition of neglect used in this study is a broad one. Our sample contains only two battered children—the rest of the children did not receive adequate nurturing for one or another of the reasons previously mentioned. Neglect has been defined as "the outcome of what ranged from a lack of protection or inability to nurture the child to a physical assault upon the young, helpless child."[10] In this study, we considered neglect to be some disturbance in the parent-child relationship which prevented the child from receiving adequate physical and/or emotional care, thereby harming his physical, intellectual, or emotional development.

Cultural unfamiliarity can also enter the picture at the point of the determination of neglect by the examining physician. The preliminary identification of potentially neglected children depended on the impressions of physicians who come to the reservation from university medical centers. These physicians have for the most part contact with the Navajo in the hospital environment, far-removed from the main pulse of this people's way of life. For this reason, confirmatory evidence from social service and field health records was considered essential in selecting the group of neglected children. These records generally reflected the judgment of people (two of whom were Navajo) who had worked on the reservation for many years, who visited the families in their homes, and who talked directly with relatives and neighbors.

Several limitations of the present study must be acknowledged. The sample represents only that segment of the Navajo population which uses the hospital facilities and only that group of children who have been brought to the hospital. This tends to exclude those who live far from Shiprock, who have no means of transportation, and who do not accept the white man's medicine. Moreover, follow-up by social workers and field health nurses to establish evidence of neglect is more difficult for those families in remote parts of the Service Unit area.

A peripheral, but important, idea illustrated by this study was that clinical impressions can be relatively easily checked. The project came about because of the strong, admittedly often subjective, feeling among physicians, nurses, and social workers at the hospital that the problem of neglect was correlated with the changes that Fairchild Corporation had brought into the community. The decision to use a retrospective design represented a deliberate choice to sacrifice the more definitive results of a prospective approach in favor of the simpler use of available data. Had the results suggested a relationship between working mothers and child neglect, a definitive prospective study would have been carried out. As it developed, the results of the retrospective study were sufficient to cause the hospital staff to re-examine their initial assumption.

REFERENCES

1. Industry invades the reservation. Business Week, 2118:72, 1970.
2. Kane, R., and Kane, R.: Federal Health Care (With Reservations!) New York: Springer Publishing Company, 1972.
3. Levy, J. E.: Some trends in Navajo health behavior. Tuba City, Arizona, PHS Indian Hospital, 1962 (mimeo).
4. Powell, G. F., Brasel, J. A., and Blizzard, R. M.: Emotional deprivation and growth retardation simulating idiopathic hypopituitarism. N. Eng. J. Med., 276:1271, 1967
5. McHenry, T., Girdany, B. R., and Elmer, E.: Unsuspected trauma with multiple skeletal injuries during infancy and childhood. PEDIATRICS, 31:903, 1963.
6. Patton, R. G., and Gardner, L.: Growth Failure in Maternal Deprivation. Springfield, Illinois: Charles C Thomas, 1963.
7. Silver, H. K., and Finkelstein, M.: Deprivation dwarfism. J. Pediat., 70:317, 1967.
8. Simons, B., Downs, E. F., Hurster, M. M., and Archer, M.: Child abuse: Epidemiologic study of medically reported cases. New York J. Med., 66:2783, 1966.
9. Leonard, M., Rhymes, J., and Solnit, A. J.: Failure to thrive in infants: A family problem. Amer. J. Dis. Child, 111:600, 1966.
10. Solnit, A. J.: In the best interests of the child and his parents. Paper presented at annual meeting of the American Orthopsychiatric Association, San Francisco, California, 1966.

Acknowledgment

We would like to acknowledge the support of Dr. Chase P. Kimball, Director of the Yale Navajo Student Project, in facilitating the program and reviewing the manuscript. Dr. Donna Olsen provided much helpful consultation.

Health of Papago Indian Children

MORTON S. ADAMS, M.D., KENNETH S. BROWN, M.D.,

BARBARA Y. IBA, R.N., B.S., and JERRY D. NISWANDER, D.D.S.

THE HEALTH of the American Indian is a matter of increasing concern. Considerable evidence supports the impression that health-related problems are contributing significantly to the Indians' prolonged dependency upon government services. Knowledge of developmental and disease patterns of American Indian children is basic to the understanding of their medical needs. Several studies based on a review of the birth records of all American Indian infants born in Public Health Service facilities have documented various aspects of the disease and development patterns of the newborn (1–5).

This study was designed to follow up the results of examinations of newborns and obtain information on genetic and environmental factors which may be important contributors to the mortality and morbidity experienced by Indian children. In view of the approximately

Miss Lillian Watson, public health nurse supervisor, Indian Health Service, Sells, Ariz., and her staff, including the translator assistants—Mrs. Philipa Lewis, Mrs. Blanche Hendricks, and Mrs. Catherine Norris—aided in conducting the family interviews. Mrs. Aline Pournelle, health records librarian at the Sells hospital, assisted in the compilation of data from the hospital records.

10,000 Indian births each year and the wide dispersion of the various hospitals, only a selected group could be examined in the detail desired.

The Papago tribe was chosen for several reasons. Their uniform socioeconomic conditions, preservation of traditional culture patterns, and a relative absence of the confounding influence of miscegenation were each important considerations. Moreover, the availability of extensive records of lineage made possible additional genetic studies which would have been impossible in any other group (6-8).

Three major concerns influenced the collection of data on the Papago: (a) the health status of infants from birth to 1 year of age, (b) the health status of school children, and (c) the health consequences of their culture and family structure.

The Papago

The main Papago reservation occupies 2,774,000 acres of semiarid desert in southwestern Arizona along the Mexican border. This region represents the ancestral homeland of the Papago and attained official reservation status in 1916. The reservation is divided into nine political districts (fig. 1). The San Xavier Reservation which occupies 29,700 acres (with one major village) comprises district 10. Geologic formations, which traditionally limited intermarriage to some extent, define these districts (7). Thus, the members of each district are bound by biological as well as cultural ties. Approximately 40 villages (10 of them with more than 100 residents each) established along family lines are distributed throughout the main reservation (9).

The infants and children examined in this study are among the 5,000 to 7,000 Papago who live on the two reservations (table 1). The total population of the Papago tribe approaches 12,000. There is considerable mobility between the reservations and between on-reservation and

Figure 1. Political districts on the Papago reservations and principal villages with schools and medical facilities

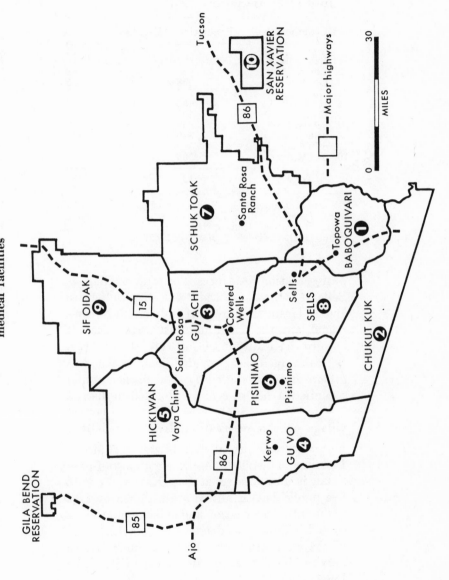

Table 1. Papago Reservation districts with approximate population in December 1967 and number of births of full-blooded Papago at Sells and Sacaton hospitals, July 1965—December 1967

District and No.	Population	Families	Births
1. Baboquivari____	627	136	17
2. Chukut Kuk____	126	27	8
3. Gu Achi_____	538	128	15
4. Gu Vo_____	287	64	6
5. Hickiwan_____	355	77	9
6. Pisinimo_____	401	94	2
7. Schuk Toak____	293	64	12
8. Sells_____	1, 349	266	46
9. Sif Oidak_____	598	116	15
10. San Xavier_____	560	115	4
Total_____	5, 134	1, 087	134

SOURCE: Demographic and socio cultural characteristics: Papago Indian Reservations, Arizona. Health Program Systems Center, Division of Indian Health, Public Health Service, September 1968.

off-reservation residences. The largest village is Sells. It is the site of the Public Health Service Indian Hospital, Bureau of Indian Affairs compound, and the tribal administrative offices. It has grown steadily in the last three decades (7).

Health facilities provided include a 50-bed general hospital staffed by four physicians and a dentist. A health center is located in district 3 (Gu Achi) at Santa Rosa, the second largest village on the reservation. It is staffed by a physician who also attends biweekly clinics at Pisinimo in district 6. A clinic with a staff physician is also located at San Xavier. Four to five public health nurses are assigned by area to the entire reservation and make regular visits to each village. Residents of the northern part of the reservation also use the Public Health Service Hospital at Sacaton on the Gila River Reservation.

Birth to 1 Year of Age

One hundred and twenty-seven full-blooded

Papago infants living on the two reservations were born in the Sells hospital from July 1965 through December 1967 and seven were born at the Sacaton hospital from May 1966 through December 1967 (table 2). During visits to 134 families, 124 examinations of infants (57 boys, 67 girls) were completed. Not examined were two stillborn infants (one boy and one girl), four boys who died in the neonatal period, and three boys and one girl who had been adopted or whose families had moved. There was one set of twins in the group of 134 children. The girl was examined; her twin brother had died 12 hours after birth.

Examinations of the infants at about 1 year of age were made during four field trips in 1967 and 1968. The examinations were done in the infant's home and consisted of the "One-Year Neurological Examination" used by the collaborative research study of the Perinatal Research Branch, National Institute of Neurological Disease and Blindness. This protocol includes a full general physical examination. Findings on the 1-year examination indicated that most of the major congenital malformations as defined by Neel (10), with the exception of some heart defects, were detected at birth and reported on the infants' records.

At the same home visit, a blood sample was drawn from the mother 1 hour following ingestion of 75 grams of glucose. The height and weight of the mother was also measured.

Records of all of the 128 living infants were examined at the Sells hospital. Records of the infants who had outpatient care at the Santa Rosa clinic were also examined. Of the 128, four who were living on the San Xavier Reservation and one whose adoptive residence was unknown had no outpatient records available. These charts were reviewed for data on well-baby care, episodes of diarrhea, respiratory disease, and other illness, and for measurements of growth.

Table 2.   Ascertainment of families selected for visits in 1967–68

Place and period of birth	All births in hospital	Fullblooded Papago infants					
		Total	When examined	Number examined	Still-birth	Neonatal death	Not living with mother
Sells hospital							
July 1965–March 1966	98	45	January–February 1967.	42	1	0	2
April–June 1966	41	13	May–June 1967	12	0	1	0
July–December 1966	88	45	November 1967	41	1	2	1
January–December 1967	172	24	May 1968	23	0	1	0
Sacaton hospital							
May 1966–December 1967	392	7	May 1968	6	0	0	1
Total	[1]791	134		124	2	5	4

[1] Includes births of 263 non-Papago infants, 197 non-fullblooded Papago infants, and 197 fullblooded Papago infants whose parents lived off the reservation. None of these infants was examined.

Birth weight. The mean birth weight of the 133 infants whose families were visited (excluding the twins) was 116.94 ounces. After eliminating the two stillbirths and six infants with malformations, the mean birth weight for 125 infants was 118.03 ounces (65 females—117.52 ounces, 60 males—118.58 ounces). The birth weight of Papago infants was examined for heterogeneity among reservation districts and none was found.

The mean birth weights for the Papago and other southwestern tribes shown in table 3 are for single, liveborn, nonmalformed infants taken from all Public Health Service Indian hospital birth records from July 1964 through June 1968. These data include non-fullblooded Papago living off the Papago and San Xavier Indian Reservations so that they compare with the information on the other tribes. The mean birth weight of the Papago is similar to that of the Pima but averages about 2 ounces lighter for both sexes. These two tribes appear to have heavier birth weights for both sexes than most other southwestern Indians except the Mohave.

The birth weight of the liveborn Papago infant is significantly affected by the status of the mother in regard to diabetes (table 4). Among mothers with plasma glucose below 150 mg. per 100 ml. 1 hour following a 75-gram glucose load, the average weight of the offspring was 117.6 ounces, while the offspring of mothers with plasma glucose of 150 mg. per 100 ml. or more had an average weight of 128.0 ounces.

Growth. The growth in weight of Papago infants during their first year of life is presented in figure 2. This study is longitudinal and, although a weight is not available for each infant every month, three-fifths of the infants were weighed in any given month. No infant had less than six recorded weights and most had between 8 and 10.

There is an indication that for the first 6 to 8 months these infants follow substantially the

Table 3. Birth weights of single, live, nonmalformed infants of eight southwestern Indian tribes, July 1964–June 1968

Tribe	Males		Females		Total	
	Mean weight (ounces)	Number	Mean weight (ounces)	Number	Mean weight (ounces)	Number
Apache	113.04	906	111.26	845	112.18	1,751
Hopi	113.26	277	110.66	280	111.97	557
Mohave	129.40	50	119.43	45	124.59	95
Navajo	114.80	5,416	111.82	5,316	113.33	10,732
Papago	120.78	388	115.15	404	117.88	792
Pima	122.08	280	118.23	264	120.13	544
Pueblo	115.27	252	110.67	273	112.90	525
Zuni	114.10	376	109.83	325	112.15	701

Table 4. Distribution of birth weights of 94 Papago infants, by maternal blood glucose levels

Birth weights of infant (ounces)	Mothers with glucose levels—	
	Less than 150 mg. per 100 ml.	150 mg. per 100 ml. or higher
Less than 88_____	5	2
88–103_____	10	1
104–119_____	35	3
120–135_____	22	5
136–151_____	7	3
152–167_____	0	1
Total_____	79	15
Average glucose level mg. per 100 ml_____	111	192
Average birth weight (ounces) [1]_____	117. 6	[2] 128. 0

[1] Excludes stillbirths and premature births.
[2] Significantly different at 5 percent confidence level.

same growth curve as white infants. Papago boys are perhaps somewhat larger. However, this advantage is lost before the end of the first year and infant girls actually fall substantially behind the white children. This dip in the growth curve may represent the burden of greater infectious disease among the Papago. To study this possibility, children who had been hospitalized were separated from those who had escaped hospitalization prior to each monthly interval. Following hospitalization the child was not returned to the "healthy" group even though he fully recovered. When these data were plotted, no change in the pattern of growth was observed, although the hospitalized children were consistently lighter than their healthy peers.

Figure 2. Growth of Papago infants during the first year of life compared to normal white infants

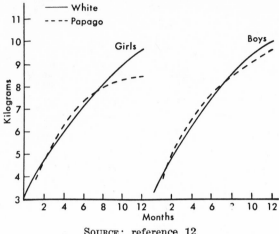

SOURCE: reference 12

Mortality. Mortality in this group of infants was 5 percent. There were two stillborn children. One was the child of a 38-year-old, diabetic, gravida 8 mother. The other infant was born at term weighing 5 lbs., 4 oz. and had severe phocomelia of all extremities. The five neonatal deaths included one premature boy (birth weight 2 lbs., 10 oz.) who was normal except for a supernumerary digit. Death was apparently due to immaturity. A second child who died 1 hour after birth had multiple malformations including congenital heart disease, low-set ears, and clubfeet. The pregnancy was complicated by polyhydramnios. The third neonatal death occurred in a 2-week-old boy. Prior to delivery his mother was febrile and there was evidence of fetal distress. He was treated with antibiotics but his illness followed a septic course. Autopsy revealed no malformations. The fourth neonatal death was due to pneumonia following prolonged rupture of membranes. He died during transfer to the hospital in Phoenix, Ariz., at 11 hours of age. The final neonatal death was that

218

Table 5. Hospitalizations in the first year of 67 Papago infants

Type of illness	Total days	Number of children	Average stay (days)
Gastrointestinal_____	669	40	16. 7
Respiratory_____	748	49	15. 3
Other_____	222	14	15. 9
Total_____	1, 639	67	24. 5

of a 3 lb., 4 oz. boy. He was the smaller of twins and died at 12 hours of age with respiratory distress. No autopsy was performed.

Morbidity. More than half the infants were hospitalized during their first year. There were two frequent causes of hospitalization—gastrointestinal illness, mostly bacterial diarrhea, and respiratory illness such as tracheobronchitis and pneumonia. These account for most of the hospitalizations and the bulk of hospital days (table 5). The average duration of hospitalization for each category of illness was about 16 days, but some children had hospitalizations for several types of illness; the average total inpatient time for this group of patients is 24.5 days. Included in the other category of diagnoses were two children with failure to thrive as a result of malnutrition and neglect who had prolonged hospital stays. Cases of meningitis, measles, suspected tuberculosis, dilation of postoperative anal atresia, kerosene ingestion, omphalitis, otitis media, and milk allergy were also in the other category.

The pattern of outpatient visits was similar (table 6). These infants averaged 3.2 outpatient visits for upper respiratory infections, 1.4 visits for diarrhea, and 1.1 visits for other complaints including otitis media, conjunctivitis, dermatitis, and chickenpox. No child with pneumonia was treated on an outpatient basis.

Any assessment of morbidity among this

population must be coupled with a consideration of hospital use and population distribution. From table 6 it is clear that the distribution of infants using health facilities is far from uniform over the reservation. More than half the children live within the three districts (1, 7, 8) closest to the Sells hospital. These children make more use of its facilities than those living in more remote areas. The average rate of use falls off proportionally and significantly as the travel time from the hospital increases.

The correlations of average travel time to the hospital and the rate of outpatient use are all significantly negative (table 6). This finding suggests that a major factor in use of hospital services is difficulty in getting to the clinic. The same factor does not appear to apply to hospital admissions for which there was no significant correlation between admission and district.

School Children

School children were examined at all nine schools on the reservation (fig. 1). There is a public school in Sells with classes through the ninth grade. The Federal Government maintains elementary day schools in three smaller villages (Santa Rosa Ranch, Vaya Chin, Kerwo) and a boarding school in Santa Rosa. Franciscan Fathers administer mission grade schools in four other villages (Topowa, San Xavier, Covered Wells, Pisinimo). High school education is not available on the reservation but may be obtained in Government boarding schools.

More than 900 children were weighed and measured. Visual acuity and color vision ability were tested using a vision screener equipped with Landolt ring charts for acuity testing and reproductions of Ishihara plates for color vision testing. Glucose tolerance of 292 unselected children who were 10 years of age or older was tested. Blood was drawn 1 hour after a 75-gram oral glucose load. Dr. Thomas L. Burch

Table 6. Use of outpatient clinic in the first year of 123 Papago infants, by district

District	Average travel time (minutes)	Number of children	Average outpatient visits per child for—					Average hospital admissions per child
			Well baby care	Gastrointestinal illness	Upper respiratory illness	Other complaints	Total	
1	27	17	4.0	2.0	4.0	1.2	11.2	1.2
2	37	8	2.9	1.6	3.4	1.2	7.9	.6
3	36	14	2.7	1.6	2.6	.7	4.5	2.0
4	107	6	.2	.5	1.3	.0	2.0	1.7
5	77	9	.1	.2	1.0	.3	1.7	1.1
6	61	2	4.5	1.0	5.5	1.5	12.5	2.0
7	33	10	2.3	2.0	2.2	.8	7.3	1.4
8	21	43	3.6	1.6	4.4	1.5	11.1	1.3
9	75	14	1.7	.8	1.3	.6	4.4	.4
Total		123	2.8	1.4	3.2	1.1	8.5	
Correlation of usage rate and travel time			-.73	-.89	-.58	-.75	-.67	+.03

made the glucose determinations at the field laboratory of the National Institute of Arthritis and Metabolic Diseases in Phoenix. One hundred and ninety-three older children received dental examinations, and a random sample of 140 had impressions made for the fabrication of dental casts.

Growth. The values of the mean heights and weights observed for Papago school children by age are presented in table 7 and plotted with the comparable data for white children in figures 3 and 4. Their stature is typical of similar age white children and they are somewhat taller than Navajo or Japanese children (*11–13*). Weight, however, shows a rather dramatic increase beginning at about 8 years among the girls and approximately a year later among the boys. Some measure of ponderosity was therefore necessary to document this growth pattern.

The mean ponderal index

$$\left(PI = 3\sqrt{\frac{ht.(cm.)}{wt.(kg.)}} \right)$$

of the Papago children and comparative data on white children are presented in figure 5. The mean PI of Papago boys remained stable between 41 and 43 from age 6 to 15 years. Papago girls show a decreasing PI after age 9, falling from 42.1 to 38.1 by age 15. These PI patterns are very different from those of white children who show a steady increase in PI of a similar type for both sexes from age 5 to 12. White children of both sexes have higher ponderal indexes than do Papago at all ages, and the difference between the two populations increases with age up to 14 years. These differences in PI are almost entirely a reflection of increased weight among the Papago rather than lack of growth in stature, since until age 14 the Papago children match the stature of white children of the same age. The ponderal index continues to drop in the Papago children to adult values of 38.9 for men and 37.1 for women. The adult Papago values are from a sample of 33

222

Table 7. Anthropometric measurements of 929 Papago school children

Age (years)	Stature (cm.)			Weight (kg.)		
	Number	Mean	Standard deviation	Number	Mean	Standard deviation
Males						
5	18	100.33	4.82	18	19.20	2.11
6	40	115.13	11.55	40	22.53	3.64
7	58	122.93	6.14	57	26.19	7.15
8	73	130.05	5.93	73	29.58	7.24
9	50	134.05	6.26	49	32.67	7.61
10	55	138.49	6.09	55	37.04	9.87
11	57	147.12	7.79	57	42.61	12.98
12	47	153.32	7.19	47	48.44	12.09
13	41	159.38	6.29	41	58.42	14.68
14	21	164.77	7.68	21	60.66	17.70
15	9	165.10	6.62	9	64.30	15.02
Females						
5	17	109.56	4.14	17	18.85	2.08
6	50	117.15	5.01	52	22.09	3.03
7	70	121.26	5.71	71	24.75	4.31
8	47	126.23	5.35	47	27.12	5.94
9	58	136.05	8.17	58	34.89	9.12
10	50	141.45	8.43	50	39.16	9.12
11	44	146.96	5.56	43	46.04	12.11
12	38	153.56	3.74	37	53.54	21.33
13	52	152.77	7.41	52	56.02	13.69
14	24	155.12	4.19	24	52.94	10.94
15	10	158.10	4.39	10	71.42	10.24

Figure 3. Growth in weight of Papago school children compared to normal white children

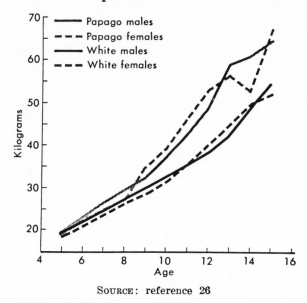

SOURCE: reference 26

Figure 4. Growth in height of Papago school children compared to normal white children

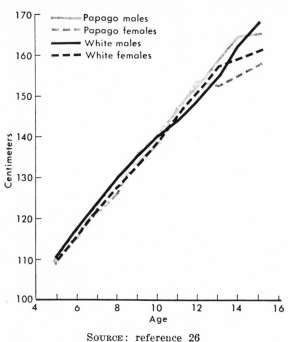

SOURCE: reference 26

men from ages 24 to 77 and 107 women from ages 18 to 68.

Health. Table 8 shows the results of the glucose tolerance tests for 137 boys and 155 girls. There was no appreciable difference in glucose tolerance between boys and girls and no trend with age. There were two boys with blood sugars above 210 mg. per 100 ml., a 13-year-old with a blood sugar of 406 mg. per 100 ml. and a 15-year-old with a blood sugar of 214 mg. per 100 ml. This number is a frequency of 0.68 percent (approximately 1 in 150). The overall frequency of blood sugar levels of 150 mg. or more was 2.4 percent.

Table 9 summarizes the data on visual acuity obtained using a Landolt ring test for far vision in a sample of 323 Papago children and adults. The distribution of visual acuity differed between the old and the young and between the sexes at younger ages. Among those more than 45 years old the sex difference was not present. More than half of the older group had visual acuity of 20/40 or less, and only three of 42 had acuity of 20/17 or better. In the age range 30 to 44 years more than half had acuity of 20/22 or better. Among those under age 30 a difference between the sexes was apparent. Males had better acuity than females. Females were much more prone to have acuity of 20/40 or less while males were more likely to have acuity of 20/17 or better. Sixty-three percent of boys under 15 had acuity of 20/22 or better while only 45 percent of girls were in the same range. More than 37 percent of girls age 10 to 15 had acuity of 20/40 or less while only 12 percent of the boys are in this range.

The significance of these results of acuity tests is not clear. Several factors are involved in the interpretation of the records. Myopia does occur and was observed in 12 of the persons scoring 20/40 or less. Endemic trachoma is a major medical problem of the Papago and accounts for much of the reduced visual acuity

Table 8. Blood sugar levels of 292 Papago school children following a 1-hour glucose tolerance test

Age (years)	Number	Mean level (mg. per 100 ml.)	Standard deviation
Boys_____	137	_____	
10_____	13	103. 7	15. 61
11_____	36	102. 4	17. 10
12_____	30	93. 4	21. 64
13_____	35	99. 4	16. 67
14_____	17	95. 6	12. 21
15_____	6	93. 0	22. 61
Girls_____	155	_____	
10_____	12	108. 6	18. 40
11_____	29	96. 1	29. 95
12_____	41	99. 1	20. 07
13_____	46	101. 7	20. 03
14_____	20	96. 9	15. 15
15_____	7	112. 5	20. 41

Table 9. Visual acuity of 323 Papagos, by age and sex

Visual acuity and sex	10–15 years	16–29 years	30–44 years	45 years or older	Total
20/40 or less:					
Male_____	8	7	9	12	36
Female____	30	13	11	13	67
20/35 to 20/25:					
Male_____	17	5	4	4	30
Female____	14	10	5	4	33
20/22 to 20/18:					
Male_____	24	5	4	2	35
Female____	23	9	7	4	43
20/17 or better:					
Male_____	19	13	10	2	44
Female____	13	10	11	1	35
All males____	68	30	27	20	145
All females___	80	42	34	22	178

Figure 5. Ponderal index of school-age Papago and white children

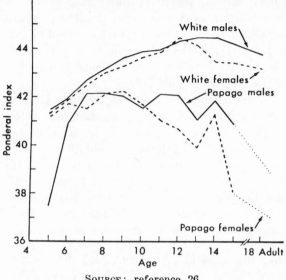

SOURCE: reference 26

among the adults. Active programs of prevention and therapy may account for much of the difference between younger and older groups.

The primary concern of the dental studies was the evaluation of tooth alignment and other morphological variations of dentition. An almost constant finding in the dentition of the 193 children examined was the presence of shovel-shaped incisors, a trait characteristic of Mongoloid populations. These teeth have thickened marginal ridges on their lingual surface, giving the incisor crowns a definite shovel-like appearance. It was observed in a moderate to marked degree in 94 percent of the group. This trait is of little clinical significance except that in some persons it appears to contribute to malalignment of the upper incisors.

A relatively common variation in upper lateral incisor morphology found among many Indian groups, a barrel-shaped incisor, was encountered in 7 percent of the children. This variation may represent an extreme form of the shovel-shape trait and is of significance in that a deep lingual pit particularly susceptible to the initiation of dental caries is often present. Caries forming in such a pit may extend to the pulp of the tooth and result in a periapical abscess with practically no evidence of a lesion on the surface of the tooth.

Malocclusion was assessed using Angle's classification of anterior-posterior jaw relationship (14). Frequencies of the four major categories were as follows: no significant malocclusion, 33 percent; class I malocclusion, 48 percent; class II malocclusion, 14 percent; and class III malocculsion, 5 percent. Comparable figures in an earlier study of Japanese children using similar criteria were normal occlusion, 41 percent; class I, 44 percent; class II, 12 percent; and class III, 3 percent (15). For white school children residing in Utah the frequencies were normal occlusion, 36 percent; class I, 30 percent; class II, 24 percent; and class III, 10 percent (Niswander, unpublished data).

In general, the dental status of the Papago children is characterized by low caries rates, moderate to severe fluorosis, moderate abrasion, and relatively poor oral hygiene with an accompanying high prevalence of gingivitis. One 12-year-old girl with multiple papules of the oral mucosa was observed. The lesions were similar in appearance to those of focal epithelial hyperplasia previously described (16, 17). Focal epithelial hyperplasia of the oral mucosa is unusual because it is apparently restricted to Indians. More than 40 cases have been observed in young Indians of North, Central, and South America, but none have been reported in whites or Negroes. The clinical and histological characteristics of the lesions suggest a viral etiology. The papules and nodules can be extensive throughout the buccal and lingual mucosa and may present a rather dramatic picture if traumatized or seen with superimposed herpetic ulcerations.

Congenital defects. Congenital malformations among American Indians have been reported from a review of records of newborns (4). American Indians as a whole have a total frequency of major congenital defects similar to other major racial groups, although they differ in the frequency of specific defects. From our study it became evident that the distribution of specific major malformations in subsets of the population is not uniform. Certain malformations did not occur at all in the Papago in the period studied, whereas myelodysplasia and microphthalmia occurred with extremely high frequency.

The diagnosis of myelodysplasia, including both spina bifida and anencephaly, is easily and accurately made. Review of the records of the Sells Indian Hospital and the Phoenix Area Indian Hospital, which is the center for medical care for the entire area, led to the ascertainment of seven cases of myelodysplasia in Papagos. Extended pedigrees were drawn for each case and juxtaposed with sections of a map of the reservation to reveal the mating patterns of families which produced affected persons. Two main clusters and one sporadic case were identified (fig. 6).

One cluster had its origin in the village of Choulic in Chukut Kuk District (district 2). This family group had three affected children, all descended from three brothers who married women from nearby villages. Two of the affected siblings were the product of a consanguineous mating between first cousins once removed ($F=1/32$).

The second cluster originated in the village of Sikal Hamatk in Gu Achi District (district 3) and resulted in two propositi and a third affected person from the same district who can be tentatively linked with this cluster. The isolated case occurred in Nestor's in the Pisinimo District (district 6), and all blood relatives except the

Figure 6. Areas of residence and pedigrees of Papagos with myelodysplasia

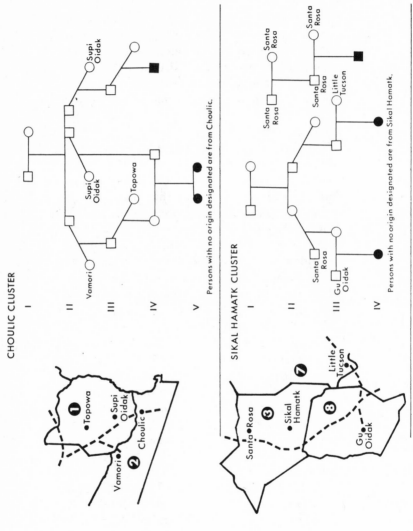

CHOULIC CLUSTER

Persons with no origin designated are from Choulic.

SIKAL HAMATK CLUSTER

Persons with no origin designated are from Sikal Hamatk.

230

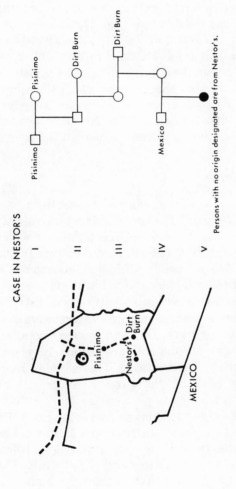

CASE IN NESTOR'S

I

II

III

IV

V

Persons with no origin designated are from Nestor's.

■ Myelodysplasia

MAP SECTIONS HAVE THE SAME SCALE AS FIGURE 1

Pisinimo

Dirt Burn

Dirt Burn

Pisinimo

Mexico

Pisinimo

Nestor's Dirt Burn

MEXICO

father were from this district. There is no evidence for the last five generations that the Choulic and Sikal Hamatk groups have shared genetic material, and they probably have been isolated for much longer.

A rare malformation, microphthalmia, occurred in a cluster in Sif Oidak District (district 9). Four cases were diagnosed by ophthalmologists at the Phoenix Indian hospital. Anecdotal reports of two affected antecedents are available. An extensive pedigree of this group was constructed (fig. 7), and the four affected persons (V, 7; VI, 1–3) almost certainly all descended from brothers (II, 2, 3) both of whom lived in the village of Cockleburr. All relatives of the four persons with microphthalmia come from Cockleburr or the neighboring village of Chui Chu. No other cases of microphthalmia are known among the Papago.

Discussion

Evaluation of the health of American Indians (in this paper, Papago children) necessarily leads to comparison with populations which differ genetically (racially) and culturally and which live in vastly different environments. Each of these factors affects health parameters. There are well-recognized differences between races for the anthropometric measurements used to evaluate growth. Diet and disease also affect normal growth, and both are intimately related to culture and environment. This complex interplay is part of the process recognized as adaptation.

The Papago and Pima newborns are generally heavier than other southwestern Indians. The differences in birth weight may reflect differences in body structure and metabolism. The Pima and Papago have relatively high frequencies of diabetes, which is associated with increased birth weight. However, the relation to diabetes is probably not a major factor in these

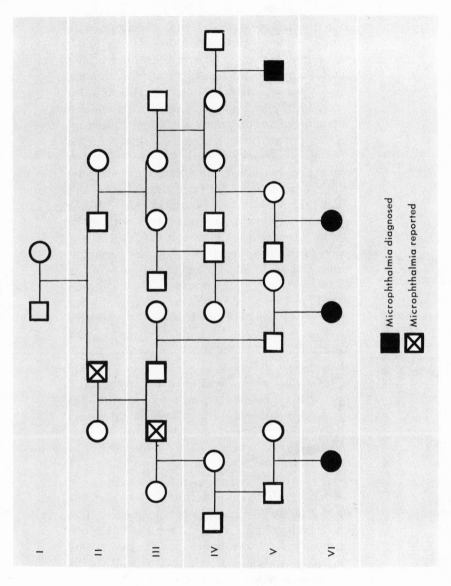

Figure 7. Pedigree of Papagos diagnosed or reported to have microphthalmia

Microphthalmia diagnosed
Microphthalmia reported

tribal differences because the Hopi and Zuni also have high frequencies of diabetes but low mean birth weights (*18*).

The growth pattern of Papago children during the first year of life was consistent with many other reports of children living under substandard nutritional and health conditions. This pattern characteristically shows children of all races and conditions paralleling each other for the first 6 months. Thereafter the disadvantaged infant shows a marked falling off of his growth rate. Salber (*19*) has reported this phenomenon for South African infants, as have Parsons (*20*) for Australian aborigines and Su and Liang (*21*) for Chinese. Meredith's (*22*) review of the first postnatal year of North American Negro infants compared with white babies revealed that although the Negro baby was somewhat lighter throughout the period, he did not show the decreased rate of gain during the second half of the first year if he was well cared for. Comparable data are not available for American Indian infants. However, it is possible that the growth pattern we observed in the first year reflects malnutrition to a greater degree than genetic differences.

Infectious diseases, especially diarrhea and pneumonia, present the greatest health problem of Papago children during the neonatal period and through the first year. It is unlikely that these children have a peculiar susceptibility to these disorders (*23*).

However, the impact of infectious disease is certainly affected by cultural and environmental factors. During the hot summer months, diarrhea becomes a serious problem as the opportunity for transmission of infective agents increases. Because the Papago frequently do not have refrigerators it is impossible to keep artificial formulas sterile. Water is hauled considerable distances in unsanitary containers and is stored in open vats and pots.

The infant is the one most seriously affected

234

by diarrhea and, too often, the parents do not get him to the hospital until the infection is considerably advanced. Although treatment with intravenous fluids is usually successful, it has been suggested that such febrile illnesses associated with extreme dehydration may cause irreversible changes in perceptual and mental abilities. Hospitalization for diarrhea is usually prolonged (an average of 16.7 days), since staff physicians have learned that recurrences are frequent if the child is returned to the home environment before he has completely recovered and shown a significant weight gain.

Breast feeding and closer medical supervision would greatly reduce the morbidity from diarrhea. Unfortunately, breast feeding frequently is not possible with Papago mothers. Children are often placed in the care of babysitters or grandparents while the mother is working or otherwise occupied. The long distances which separate most villages make intensified medical supervision difficult. The possibility remains that an intensive program especially aimed at reducing mortality and morbidity resulting from diarrhea might well be an entering wedge toward controlling the health problems of the Papago.

Pneumonia in the Papago children is also seasonal and is apparently due to secondary bacterial invasion in infants predisposed by viral infections of the upper respiratory tract. These infections are extremely common during the colder months when the family is confined to close quarters and viral infections are common. Physical or X-ray evidence of pneumonia uniformly warrants hospitalization since treatment and diet can be more closely supervised.

Hospital use varies due to transportation problems. Families from outlying districts in particular find it difficult to travel to the Sells hospital. For example, two children have died from neonatal tetanus since this study was completed. Neither was born in the hospital, although the mothers had tried to obtain transportation. These deaths have led to a policy of immunizing mothers during the prenatal period. However, the basic difficulty of delivery of health services on the reservation remains unsolved.

The differences in correlation of the various types of outpatient visits to distance of residence from the hospital show that cultural factors as well as simple distance are involved. Well-baby visits, which are prearranged, and visits for respiratory illness, which is recognized as serious by the mother, have lower correlations to distance than do visits for diarrhea, which is considered an Indian disease. This lower correlation may reflect the mother's recognition of the seriousness of different types of illness or her acceptance of hospital services for certain types of illness.

The lack of correlation between inpatient admissions and distance of residence from the hospital may reflect several factors. There is actually a positive correlation of inpatient admission to distance of residence from the hospital once the child appears at the outpatient department. This situation reflects the reluctance of physicians to send a potentially ill child home if home is a long distance from the hospital, as well as the increased severity of illnesses of children who have been brought by their parents over longer distances. Both factors reflect the major effect transportation has on the medical care of Papago infants. Also, acceptance of medical care may be low among those living in the areas of the reservation most remote from the hospital, contributing to delay in seeking transportation to the hospital.

The growth of school-age Papago children is remarkable in the early onset of obesity. This phenomenon has been repeatedly observed by the medical personnel working on the reservation and is recognized by the Indians themselves as the typical growth pattern. Doubtless the Papago's high carbohydrate diet contributes to this obesity. Unfortunately, dietary manipulation is difficult for both cultural and financial reasons. The frequency of diabetes mellitus in the adult Papago is high. Among the children we tested, at least two had blood sugars, 1 hour after a glucose load, which were unequivocally in the diabetic range. Neither child experienced polyphagia nor considered himself ill. Both were obese.

Niswander has recently commented on the apparently greater prevalence of malocclusion among modern industrialized populations compared with ancient man and modern primitive groups (24). The reasons for this prevalence are not clear, although there is a suggestion that environmental factors play an important role, perhaps through the disruption of highly adapted oral-facial growth pattern relationships. It would be of considerable interest to know if the high prevalence of malocclusion among the present Papago children is of recent origin or characteristic of Papagos living prior to disruption of aborginal culture patterns by the white man.

To obtain information on this point we attempted to locate skeletal remains of ancestors of the present-day Papago Indians. Although a moderate amount of such skeletal material exists, most of it is not well enough preserved to allow reliable assessment of dental alignment. Dr. Charles Di Peso made available skeletal material at the Amerind Foundation, Dragoon, Ariz., and Dr. Walter Birkby assisted us in examining the skulls in the collection of the University of Arizona, Tucson.

To date only 10 skulls sufficiently intact for comparative purposes have been found. These date roughly from the period between 1300 and 1700 A.D. All showed nearly perfect occlusion. Although the sample is extremely small and there can be no absolute certainty that these persons are, in fact, direct antecedents of the present-day Papago, it suggests a striking increase in the prevalence of malocclusion among the Papago occurring sometime in the last 600 years. Such a wide timespan allows for either genetic or environmental factors to be responsible for this temporal change.

Pedigree analysis suggests that, in this population, the frequency of several congenital defects is principally consequent to the cultural factors dictating the mating pattern. Thus, nearly all cases of microphthalmia and myelodysplasia are accounted for by several small endogamous mating groups. A conservative estimate of the frequency of myelodyplasia among the Papago can be obtained for the last 5 years for which we have reasonably complete records of the number of births. During these years, births averaged approximately 200 per year, occurring almost exclusively in the Sells (64 percent) and Sacaton (33 percent) hospitals. During this period, there were five cases of myelodysplasia, a frequency of 1 in 200 births. This exceedingly high frequency, attributable to small clusters of cases, may well account for the high frequency of this malformation in much larger Indian populations (*3*).

Microphthalmia is a heterogenous entity, and various modes of inheritance have been observed in clinically undistinguishable cases. The cluster of cases occurring in the Sif Oidak District most likely represents simple autosomal recessive inheritance. If so, the large number of cases reflects a high level of endogamy present in this group of adjacent villages.

The etiology of myelodysplasia is not as simple. It would appear that an interaction between a specific polygenic predisposition and environmental factors is important. The high frequency of diabetes mellitus (*18*) present in adult members of the tribe may be significant. It has been suggested that this disease is related to "anti-insulin" activity in the synalbumin fraction of human plasma. Elevated levels of anti-insulin have also been reported in the mothers of myelodysplastic children (*25*).

238

Summary

The Papago Indians reflect their genetic potential in birth weight, growth and development, and metabolic patterns. These have all been shaped by their prolonged residence in the arid southwest which has become more desert-like during the past 1,000 years. These traits seem to be shared with their linguistic and historic relatives, the Pima. The high frequency of certain malformations can be attributed to cultural patterns which were also adaptive in this environment.

The pattern of disease seen in Papago infants and children is associated with a harsh environment. Lack of water and sanitation are major components in the etiology of diarrhea, and the cold desert winter, which results in crowding into largely unheated houses, contributes to the burden of pneumonia and respiratory disease. A major limitation on the use of hospital services appears to be isolation by distance. These conditions are preventable.

REFERENCES

(*1*) Niswander, J. D., and Adams, M. S.: American Indian congenital malformation study. National Institutes of Health, Bethesda, Md., 1966–67.

(*2*) Niswander, J. D., and Adams, M. S.: Oral clefts in the American Indian. Public Health Rep 82: 807–812, September 1967.

(*3*) Adams, M. S., and Niswander, J. D.: Birth weight of North American Indians. Hum Biol 40: 226–234, May 1968.

(*4*) Adams, M. S., and Niswander, J. D.: Health of the American Indian: congenital defects. Eugen Quart 15: 227–234, December 1968.

(*5*) Adams, M. S., MacLean, C. J., and Niswander, J. D.: Discrimination between deviant and ordinary low birth weight: American Indian infants. Growth 32: 153–161, June 1968.

(*6*) Hackenberg, R. A.: The Papago population register. National Cancer Institute, Bethesda, Md., 1965.

(*7*) Niswander, J. D., et al.: Population studies on southwestern Indian tribes. I. History, culture and genetics of the Papago. Amer J Hum Genet 22: 7–23, January 1970.

(8) Workman, P. L., and Niswander, J. D.: Population studies on southwestern Indian tribes. II. Local genetic differentiation in the Papago. Amer J Hum Genet 22: 24–49, January 1970.

(9) Hoover, J. W.: Generic descent of the Papago villages. Amer Anthrop 37: 257–264, April–June 1935.

(10) Neel, J. V.: A study of major congenital defects in Japanese infants. Amer J Hum Genet 10: 398–445, December 1958.

(11) Steggerda, M., and Densen, P.: Height, weight and age tables for homogeneous groups. Child Develop 7: 115–120, June 1936.

(12) Stuart, H. C.: With particular reference to Navajo Indians and Dutch whites. *In* Preventive pediatrics, by P. A. Harper. Appleton-Century-Crofts, New York City, 1962, pp. 81–94.

(13) Greulich, W. W.: A comparison of the physical growth and development of American-born and native Japanese children. Amer J Phys Anthrop 15: 489–515 (1957).

(14) Anderson, G. M.: Practical orthodontist. Ed. 9. C. V. Mosby Co., St. Louis, 1960.

(15) Schull, W. J., and Neel, J. V.: The effects of inbreeding on Japanese children. Harper & Row, Publishers, Inc., 1965.

(16) Archard, H. O., Heck, J. W., and Stanley, H. R.: Focal epithelial hyperplasia: an unusual oral mucosal lesion found in Indian children. Oral Surg 20: 201–212, August 1965.

(17) Witkop, C. J., Jr., and Niswander, J. D.: Focal epithelial hyperplasia in Central and South American Indians and Ladinos. Oral Surg 20: 213–217, August 1965.

(18) Niswander, J. D.: Biomedical challenges presented by the American Indian. Pan American Health Organization Science Publication No. 165. Washington, D.C., 1968, pp. 133–136.

(19) Salber, E. J.: Growth of South African babies in the first year of life. Hum Biol 29: 12–39, February 1957.

(20) Parsons, P. A.: Growth in a sample of Australian Aborigines from one to twenty-three months of age. Growth 29: 207–211, June 1965.

(21) Su, T. F., and Liang, C. J.: Growth and development of Chinese infants of Hunan Province. I. Body weight, standing height and sitting height during the first year of life. Chinese Med J 58: 104–112, July 1940.

(22) Meredith, H. V.: North American Negro infants: size at birth and growth during the first post-

natal year. Hum Biol 25 : 290–308, December
1952.

(23) Neel, J.V.: Some changing constraints on the human evolutionary process. *In* Proceedings, 12th International Congress of Genetics, Tokyo, 1969, vol. 3, pp. 389–403.

(24) Niswander, J. D. : Further studies on the Xavante Indians. VII. The oral status of the Xavantes of Simões Lopes. ᵀ ᵢer J Hum Genet 19 : 543–553, July 1967.

(25) Wilson, J. S. P., and Vallance-Owen, J.: Congenital deformities and insulin antagonism. Lancet No. 7470 : 940–941, Oct. 29, 1966.

(26) Nelson, W. E., editor: Textbook of pediatrics. Ed. 7. W. B. Saunders Company, Philadelphia, 1959, pp. 50–55.

Tuberculosis

ISONIAZID PROPHYLAXIS IN ALASKAN BOARDING SCHOOLS

A Comparison of Two Doses

GEORGE W. COMSTOCK,[1] LAUREL M. HAMMES, AND ANTONIO PIO

SUMMARY_____

A comparison of the effectiveness of two dosage regimens of isoniazid in preventing active tuberculosis was started in 1958 in four boarding schools in southeastern Alaska. The "standard" regimen was 5 mg of isoniazid per kg of body weight per day, and the "test" regimen was 1.25 mg per kg of body weight per day. Both were given for a period of six months.

During the ensuing ten years, active tuberculosis developed among 1.9 per cent of the students who took the standard dose for the full six months and among 5.7 per cent of those who took the test dose for six months.

Comparisons with tuberculosis case rates in another study among groups taking the standard dose of isoniazid or a placebo for six months indicated that the dose of 1.25 mg per kg of body weight per day was no more effective than the placebo. Although six months of daily isoniazid in the standard dosage may not be optimal, the reduction in tuberculosis attributable to this regimen is similar to that achieved by a full year of isoniazid in most other trials.

INTRODUCTION

Controlled trials of the ability of isoniazid to prevent tuberculosis were well under way by 1958. At that time, the Public Health Service's cooperative trials alone had enrolled nearly 70,000 participants representing a remarkably wide range of personal and social characteristics (1). It seemed certain that it was only a matter of time until a reliable answer would be obtained to the initial question, "Can the development of active tuberculosis be prevented by the administration of isoniazid for a year in a daily dosage of approximately 5 mg per kg of body weight?"

This regimen, now the standard for chemoprophylaxis against tuberculosis, had been selected on the basis of animal experiments and therapeutic experience that indicated that this dosage should fall within the effective range if the trials showed isoniazid to have real preventive capacity (2, 3). The selection of an optimal dose would be more difficult. On the one hand, isoniazid should be administered

[1] Supported by the Department of Epidemiology, School of Hygiene and Public Health, Johns Hopkins University; Public Health Service Research Career Award No. K6-HE-21,670 from the National Heart Institute; and Graduate Training Grant No. CD 00001 from the National Center for Chronic Disease Control, Public Health Service, U.S. Department of Health, Education, and Welfare.

long enough and in sufficiently large dosage to obtain maximal effectiveness; on the other, acceptability would be increased by smaller doses and shorter duration. Bringing these two opposing considerations into appropriate balance should result in the greatest public health usefulness of prophylaxis. Because the most appealing possibility lay in the chance that the optimal regimen was less than the standard, this possibility was first explored.

A population that seemed suitable for testing a new dosage regimen was found during a controlled trial of isoniazid prophylaxis among Eskimo villagers in the Bethel area of Alaska (4, 5). Most Aleuts, Eskimos, and Indians in Alaska live in small settlements, few of which contain more than 300 persons. Although nearly all villages have elementary schools covering the first eight grades, most children who wished to continue their education have had to go to high school in larger communities. For this reason, the Bureau of Indian Affairs has maintained a boarding high school at Mt. Edgecumbe in southeastern Alaska. Students arrive each year in late August and return home in May by means of a far-flung airlift. A boarding school for the first eight grades, Wrangell Institute, also is maintained in southeastern Alaska by the Bureau of Indian Affairs. This school has served children from villages too small to warrant a school of their own as well as those from villages where schools were being rebuilt, repaired, or enlarged.

In spite of an extensive BCG program throughout Alaska in the early 1950s (6) and thorough screening programs throughout the school years, tuberculosis long had been the major health problem in these boarding schools. Both schools were immediately receptive to any reasonable plan to prevent active tuberculosis among their students. Two other schools also participated—the Practical Nurse Training School, part of the Mt. Edgecumbe complex, and Sheldon Jackson High School and Junior College, located in Sitka across a narrow ship channel from Mt. Edgecumbe and operated by the Presbyterian Church.

The initial plan was to consider a daily dosage of 5 mg per kg of body weight as the standard and to compare with this the efficacy of one fourth of that daily dosage. It was appreciated that the school year was only

nine months long, but it was believed that controlled administration of medication in a school environment would result in an annual intake not too different from that achieved by the average free-living population in 12 months.

Original expectations were not completely realized. The wave of tuberculosis was receding rapidly in Alaska, even in the most heavily infected areas (7, 8). With diminishing cases, a quick answer was not forthcoming. Furthermore, medication could not be given during the entire school year for a number of administrative reasons. Consequently, this paper reports the experience with tuberculosis during a ten-year period among two groups of students, one taking 5 mg and the other taking 1.25 mg of isoniazid per kg of body weight per day, each regimen given for a period of only six months.

MATERIALS AND METHODS

The program was started in the fall of 1958. All students were invited to participate after the trial had been explained at assembly programs. Grounds for exclusion were current treatment for active tuberculosis, a history of epilepsy, previous participation in this or other trials of isoniazid prophylaxis, and failure to have the standard school medical permit on file. Only 3 students refused to participate.

Chest roentgenograms taken each fall shortly after arrival at school were read by one of the writers. School medical records were searched for a history of previous tuberculosis or epilepsy. Tuberculin testing was not done in the schools initially, largely because of the widespread belief that virtually all students would be reactors. When it became apparent that many students did not react to tuberculin on entering school and that new infections were not occurring in the school environment, tuberculin tests were added to the examinations performed before admitting students to the trial. A reaction was defined as induration of 5 mm or more in diameter 48 hours after the intracutaneous injection of 0.1 μg of PPD-S.

The Practical Nurse Training School was closed in 1961. Starting with the school year 1961 to 1962, only tuberculin reactors were admitted to the program. The trial was discontinued at Wrangell Institute in the summer of 1962 and in the two remaining schools in the summer of 1963. The numbers of tuberculin reactors in the school populations had become too small to justify the expense of continuing to add new students to the trial.

At Wrangell Institute, medication was allocated by school classroom, all members of each class taking the same dosage. It was given to the students five days each week by the teachers, together with a multivitamin capsule. The teachers also kept a simple daily record of medication consumed. In the other schools, medication was allocated by dormitory unit. These units varied considerably in size; the median number of students was 25. Medication was given out once each day by students selected for this purpose and supervised by the adult dormitory advisors. Again, simple records of daily consumption of medication were kept for each student. Complaints thought to be related to side effects of medication were referred to the school infirmaries where the decision was made to stop or continue medication.

Medication for the standard or full-dose regimen was provided in tablets containing 100 mg of isoniazid, and that for the test or quarter-dose regimen in tablets containing 25 mg of isoniazid. Both preparations were identical in all other respects. Medication allocated to each classroom or dormitory unit was identified by separate code numbers whose significance was known only to a statistician in the central office in Washington, D. C. Students at Wrangell Institute took two tablets each day, five days a week; others took three tablets once each day, a dosage approximating 5 mg per kg of body weight for the full-dose regimen and 1.25 mg per kg of body weight for the quarter-dose regimen.

Regularity in taking isoniazid was rated by dividing the total amount of medication taken during the six-month period by the amount of medication advised and expressing this ratio as a percentage. The duration of the program varied only a few days from year to year, and, as noted earlier, it lasted almost exactly six months.

A "case" of tuberculosis was defined as a person who, after admission to the trial, was found to have significant evidence of active tuberculosis that had not been present at the start. A "case" so defined represented either newly developed tuberculosis or reactivation of old disease. Items considered in this assessment were deaths certified as caused by tuberculosis, hospital or outpatient treatment for tuberculosis, bacteriologic examinations demonstrating *Mycobacterium tuberculosis*, unfavorable changes in the chest roentgenogram, and clinical diagnoses of nonpulmonary tuberculosis. This information was garnered from periodic reviews of the tuberculosis case register of the Alaska Department of Health and Welfare from September 1958 through August 1968 and from a search of death certificates of Alaskan residents through December 1966. All assessments by clinicians and investigators were made without knowledge of the regimen to which the subject had been assigned.

Slightly more than half of the study participants were admitted to the trial in 1958 and hence had ten years of follow-up observation. The remainder were followed for a period of six to nine years, depending on the year they were admitted to the trial. The average period of observation for the entire group was 8.9 years.

RESULTS

During the five years in which students entered the trial, 1,701 were given medication. As shown in table 1, 810 were assigned the standard, full dose of isoniazid (approximately 5 mg per kg of body weight per day), and 860 were given the test, quarter dose (approximately 1.25 mg per kg of body weight per day). Thirty-one students were first assigned one dose and then the other as the result of moving from one dormitory unit to another; this small group will not be considered further.

The initial characteristics of the two medication groups are shown in table 2. About half were admitted during the first year of the trial, when students at all grade levels were eligible. In subsequent years, only new students were admitted. During the fourth and fifth years (1961 to 1963), the Practical Nurse Training School no longer was in operation, and at the other schools only tuberculin reactors were offered medication. Wrangell Institute was not included in the program during the fifth year (1962 to 1963), but most of the decrease in participants during that year resulted from the rapidly declining proportion of tuberculin reactors among school entrants.

The importance of tuberculosis to this population in the years prior to the trial was shown by their initial tuberculosis status. Although students under treatment for tuberculosis were excluded from the study population, one fourth of the remainder had been diagnosed as having had tuberculosis, and nearly one-tenth had had antituberculous treatment. Students with previously known tuberculosis who had not been treated did not represent failure of the tuberculosis control program in Alaska but were persons who were considered at that time to need no treatment, mostly with diagnoses of suspected or minimal inactive tuberculosis.

Although the populations assigned the full

TABLE 1

MEDICATION ALLOCATED TO PARTICIPANTS IN STUDY

Medication	No. of Subjects	%
Full-dose isoniazid........	810	47.6
Quarter-dose isoniazid....	860	50.6
Both doses..............	31	1.8
Total..............	1,701	100.0

246

dose and the quarter dose were not identical in all respects, they were surprisingly similar considering the relatively large and varied sizes of the allocation units. The comparisons for a number of important characteristics also are shown in table 2. Of particular importance is the fact that the proportions of persons with previous diagnoses of tuberculosis, either treated or untreated, were virtually identical for both of the dosage regimens. Not all participants were tuberculin tested, but there was no reason to believe that there were important differences in the prevalence of tuberculin sensitivity between the groups of students allocated to the two regimens. The two groups were believed to be sufficiently similar to warrant direct comparisons without statistical adjustment for the minor differences observed.

More than 90 per cent of both groups com-

TABLE 2

COMPARISON OF GROUPS ASSIGNED FULL-DOSE AND QUARTER-DOSE OF ISONIAZID

Characteristics	Full-Dose		Quarter-Dose	
	No.	%	No.	%
School year of medication				
1958–59	399	49.2	459	53.4
1959–60	132	16.3	95	11.1
1960–61	126	15.6	120	13.9
1961–62	104	12.8	129	15.0
1962–63	49	6.1	57	6.6
Ethnic group				
Southeastern Alaskan Indian	177	21.9	157	18.2
Athabascan Indian	145	17.9	142	16.5
Aleut	103	12.7	121	14.1
Eskimo	345	42.6	396	46.0
Other	40	4.9	44	5.2
Sex				
Male	449	55.4	441	51.3
Female	361	44.6	419	48.7
Age, years				
5–9	27	3.3	23	2.7
10–14	238	29.4	298	34.7
15–19	505	62.3	507	58.9
20+	40	5.0	32	3.7
Initial tuberculosis status				
Previously treated tuberculosis	75	9.3	79	9.2
Untreated tuberculosis	131	16.2	143	16.6
No known tuberculosis	604	74.5	638	74.2
Total	810	100.0	860	100.0

TABLE 3

REASONS FOR DISCONTINUING MEDICATION

Reasons	Full-Dose Isoniazid		Quarter-Dose Isoniazid	
	No.	%	No.	%
Completed advised period	739	91.2	790	91.9
Illness	3	0.4	7	0.8
Medication side effects	4	0.5	1	0.1
Left school	48	5.9	27	3.1
Refused to continue	0	—	4	0.5
Not stated	16	2.0	31	3.6
Total	810	100.0	860	100.0

TABLE 4

PROPORTION OF ADVISED MEDICATION TAKEN BY STUDY PARTICIPANTS ON EACH DOSAGE REGIMEN

Percentage of Advised Medication Taken	Full-Dose Isoniazid		Quarter-Dose Isoniazid	
	No.	%	No.	%
Not stated	20	2.5	21	2.4
0–29	24	2.9	21	2.4
30–49	24	2.9	22	2.5
50–69	71	8.8	103	12.0
70–89	158	19.5	157	18.3
90+	513	63.4	536	62.4
Total	810	100.0	860	100.0

pleted the six-month period of medication. The numbers of students who stopped prematurely, and their reasons for doing so, are shown in table 3. In 10, illnesses developed that were not thought to be related to the medication but that interfered with their continuing on the program, usually because of hospitalization. Only 5 stopped because of side effects of medication. Most withdrew from the program because they dropped out of school. The reasons for discontinuing medication could not be determined for 47 students. Almost all of these withdrawals occurred at one school during the first year, and it is believed that they resulted from administrative rather than medical factors.

The proportion of medication that was recorded as taken is shown in table 4. Most of the students who took only 50 to 89 per cent of the recommended total dosage were at Wrangell Institute. Because medication could be given there for only five days each week, the highest possible proportion of medication taken was slightly more than 70 per cent. Most other lapses in taking medication occurred for various administrative reasons and not from lack of cooperation.

During the observation period, 66 cases of tuberculosis among the two groups were recorded in the tuberculosis case register of the Alaska Department of Health and Welfare. Their distribution by dosage regimen is shown in table 5. In all instances, there were more cases among students assigned the quarter dose than among those assigned the full dose. Almost all cases were pulmonary, and about one-third were confirmed by recovery of *Mycobacterium tuberculosis* from the sputum. Fifteen deaths had occurred in the two groups through 1966. No deaths from tuberculosis were recorded; all but 2 deaths resulted from violent causes, most of them accidents. This observation underscores the previously noted high frequency of accidental death in Alaska (9).

The occurrence of tuberculosis among the two study groups according to other characteristics of the populations is shown in table 6. In nearly every category, the case rates were significantly higher among persons assigned to the quarter-dose regimen. Case rates were high among Athabascan Indians and Eskimos and low among Aleuts, Indians from southeastern Alaska, and other ethnic groups. These rates presumably reflect the prevalence of tuberculosis among these ethnic groups during the past two decades. The greatest differences in case rates between the two groups of subjects were noted in persons with previously diagnosed tuberculosis and in persons who took the highest proportion of the

TABLE 5
UNFAVORABLE EVENTS OCCURRING AMONG PARTICIPANTS FROM DATE OF STARTING TRIAL TO SEPTEMBER 1, 1968

Unfavorable Events	Full Dose Isoniazid	Quarter Dose Isoniazid
Cases of tuberculosis	20	46
M. tuberculosis recovered	9	14
M. tuberculosis not recovered		
Pulmonary	10	29
Nonpulmonary	1	3
Nontuberculous deaths	6	9

TABLE 6
CASES OF TUBERCULOSIS OCCURRING DURING OBSERVATION PERIOD BY CHARACTERISTICS OF POPULATION AND DOSAGE REGIMEN

Characteristics	Full-Dose Isoniazid		Quarter-Dose Isoniazid	
	No.	Rate per 100	No.	Rate per 100
Ethnic group				
Athabascan Indian	5	3.4	11	7.7
Eskimo	12	3.4	31	7.8
Other	3	0.9	4	1.2
Sex				
Male	10	2.2	24	5.4
Female	10	2.7	22	5.2
Age				
5–14	9	3.3	12	3.7
15+	11	2.0	34	6.3
Initial tuberculosis status				
Previously treated tuberculosis	4	5.3	12	15.1
Untreated tuberculosis	4	3.0	15	10.4
No known tuberculosis	12	1.9	19	2.9
Percentage of medication taken				
Less than 50	3	4.4	2	3.1
50–79	7	3.0	13	5.0
80+	10	1.9	31	5.7
Total	20	2.4	46	5.3

advised amount of medication. In each of these instances, the case rates in persons receiving the quarter-dose regimen were three times higher than among those taking the full-dose regimen. The numbers of cases were too small, however, to conclude with confidence that the effectiveness of the full dose was truly greater among persons with evidence of previous tuberculous disease.

To take account of the variable observation periods caused by admitting subjects to the study throughout a five-year period, the cumulative probability of tuberculosis developing was calculated by applying standard life-table techniques. The results are shown for each dosage regimen in table 7. At all times after the start of the trial, the probability of active tuberculosis developing was considerably greater among students assigned the quarter-dose regimen. The tendency for active tuberculosis to decrease with the passage of time was probably related to two factors. Among those admitted to the trials, there was undoubtedly an appreciable number of newly in-

248

TABLE 7
CUMULATIVE PROBABILITY OF DEVELOPING TUBERCULOSIS DURING OBSERVATION PERIOD IN NUMBER OF CASES PER 100 PERSONS AT RISK

Years after Start of Trial	Full-Dose Isoniazid		Quarter-Dose Isoniazid	
	Cumulative No. of Cases	Cumulative Probability	Cumulative No. of Cases	Cumulative Probability
2	9	1.1	18	2.1
4	13	1.6	28	3.3
6	16	2.0	42	5.0
8	19	2.4	45	5.4
10	20	2.7	46	5.6

fected persons as well as a number of previously treated persons whose treatment had been concluded very recently. It is well known that the risks of active disease developing for both of these groups diminish rapidly with time for several years and then tend to level off (10–12). It is also known that a fair number of graduates from these schools leave Alaska; whether they return if tuberculosis develops is not known. However, there is no reason to believe that either of these factors should affect the two study groups differently.

DISCUSSION

In a previously reported trial of isoniazid prophylaxis among Eskimos in the Bethel area of Alaska, the full dose of isoniazid (5 mg per kg of body weight per day) was given to half of the participants, and placebo was given to the other half (4, 5). It was recommended that both medications be taken for one year. However, 514 persons from the isoniazid group and 494 from the placebo group took only 40 to 59 per cent of the recommended annual dose, or, in other words, took medication for only six months. Thus over a year's time, the amount of isoniazid taken by the 514 persons in the Bethel study was essentially the same as that taken by the 513 subjects in the present study who took 90 per cent or more of the full dose over a six-month period. The full dose in these two subpopulations thus may be considered as the "standard," against which the performance of placebo may be judged in the Bethel study and that of the quarter-dose regimen may be judged in the present study.

In the Bethel study, the case rate among persons who took placebo for six months of the year was 2.7 times higher than the case rate among persons taking isoniazid for six months (5). In the present study, the case rate among students taking the quarter dose for six months was 3.0 times higher than the case rate among students taking the full dose of isoniazid for six months. These two ratios, 2.7 and 3.0, are not significantly different. Their similarity indicates that isoniazid in the quarter dosage (1.25 mg per kg of body weight per day) for six months had no more effect in preventing tuberculosis than did placebo.

In the search for a regimen that is optimal from the combined criteria of effectiveness in preventing tuberculosis and acceptability to recipients, it is clear that the quarter dose should no longer be considered. The results of the present study do strengthen a suggestion put forth previously as a result of the Bethel study (5), namely, that six months of isoniazid at the daily dosage of 5 mg per kg of body weight might be sufficient to accomplish most of the preventive effect attainable with isoniazid prophylaxis.

Acknowledgments

A field study such as this depends on the cooperation of so many persons that it is impossible to thank them all. The school personnel, particularly the advisors and the clinic staffs, were always most helpful, often at the cost of considerable inconvenience to themselves. Two supervising nurses from the Arctic Health Research Center, Mrs. Merilys Porter Brown and Miss Mary Elizabeth Allen, and three members of the clerical staff, Miss Alma Waisanen, Miss Mildred Williams, and Mrs. Carol Baum, were responsible for much of the planning and the day-to-day working of the study. The dedicated work of the tuberculosis case-register staff at the Alaska Department of Health and Welfare tremendously simplified our follow-up problems. Mrs. Elise M. Chapman of the Tuberculosis Branch, National Communicable Disease Center supervised much of the machine-room work. Finally, and most importantly, we are grateful to the unsung heroes of research, the students who cooperated so well to add a small bit to human knowledge of disease prevention.

REFERENCES

(1) Ferebee, S. H., Mount, F. W., and Comstock, G. W.: The use of chemotherapy as a prophylactic measure in tuberculosis, Ann. N. Y. Acad. Sci., 1963, *106*, 151.

(2) Palmer, C. E., Ferebee, S. H., and Hopwood, L.: Studies on prevention of experimental tuberculosis with isoniazid: II. Effects of different dosage regimens, Amer. Rev. Tuberc., 1956, *74*, 917.

(3) Mount, F. W., Jenkins, B. E., and Ferebee, S. H.: Control study of comparative efficacy of isoniazid, streptomycin-isoniazid, and streptomycin-para-aminosalicylic acid in pulmonary tuberculosis therapy: IV. Report on forty-week observations on 583 patients with streptomycin-susceptible infections, Amer. Rev. Tuberc., 1953, 68, 264.

(4) Comstock, G. W.: Isoniazid prophylaxis in an undeveloped area, Amer. Rev. Resp. Dis., 1962, 86, 810.

(5) Comstock, G. W., Ferebee, S. H., and Hammes, L. M.: A controlled trial of community-wide isoniazid prophylaxis in Alaska, Amer. Rev. Resp. Dis., 1967, 95, 935.

(6) Weiss, E. S.: Tuberculin sensitivity in Alaska, Public Health Rep., 1953, 68, 23.

(7) Comstock, G. W., and Philip, R. N.: Decline of the tuberculosis epidemic in Alaska, Public Health Rep., 1961, 76, 19.

(8) Hanson, M. L., Comstock, G. W., and Haley, C. E.: Community isoniazid prophylaxis program in an underdeveloped area of Alaska, Public Health Rep., 1967, 82, 1045.

(9) Boyd, D. L., Maynard, J. E., and Hammes, L. M.: Accident mortality in Alaska, 1958–1962, Arch. Environ. Health (Chicago), 1968, 17, 101.

(10) Zeidberg, L. D., Dillon, A., and Gass, R. S.: Risk of developing tuberculosis among children of tuberculous parents, Amer. Rev. Tuberc., 1954, 70, 1009.

(11) Comstock, G. W.: Untreated inactive pulmonary tuberculosis: Risk of reactivation, Public Health Rep., 1962, 77, 461.

(12) Hilleboe, H. E.: Post-sanatorium tuberculosis survival rates in Minnesota, Public Health Rep., 1941, 56, 895.

Inactivation of isoniazid by Canadian Eskimos and Indians

C. W. L. Jeanes, M.D., O. Schaefer, M.D. and L. Eidus, M.D.

Isoniazid (INH), the most potent antituberculous drug, is acetylated and inactivated in the liver by acetyltransferase enzyme. The rate of acetylation is genetically controlled; it exhibits a bimodal pattern. Based on the elimination rate of free INH from the blood, individuals may be divided into slow and fast inactivators. Slow inactivation is inherited as a homozygous autosomal recessive trait, while fast inactivation is due to either a homo- or heterozygous dominant gene. Japanese Thais, Koreans,[1] Saame Lapps[2] and Eskimos[3] are mainly fast acetylators, while the majority of Caucasians are slow inactivators.[4-6]

Fast inactivation is of little consequence in daily treatment, particularly with triple regimen;[7] however, in intermittent chemotherapy or irregular self administration of the drugs, it may contribute to treatment failures. Therefore, investigation of INH metabolism as well as the introduction of a simple urine test for phenotyping of INH inactivators on a large scale are of great importance in the planning of an effective domiciliary treatment program particularly for the population of the Canadian Far North and for fast inactivators in general.

A study was carried out in co-operation with the Chronic Disease Control and the Northern Medical Research Unit at the Charles Camsell Hospital, Edmonton, with the following objectives:—

a) To determine the INH inactivation rate in Canadian Eskimos and Indians.

b) To establish correlation between INH inactivation (estimated in plasma specimens by the fall-off technique) and excretion of INH and its metabolite in urine in order to devise a simple urine test for mass phenotyping, avoiding thereby repeated venipunctures.

c) To assess the need for changes in INH dosage and frequency of administration or for different drug preparation (with protracted absorption rate) in order to compensate for fast acetylation.

Procedure

Twenty-six Eskimos and 46 Indian patients received 3 mg./kg. INH intramuscularly. Ten ml. blood was collected in heparinized vacutainers before, and two and four hours after drug administration. The plasma was separated by centrifugation, frozen immediately, and stored at −20°C until examination. The free INH concentrations of the two- and four-hour plasma samples were estimated in μg./ml. The values obtained were plotted on a logarithmic scale against the time in minutes registered on a linear scale and the half-life of the INH determined graphically.[8]

In 60 patients, urine specimens were also collected before drug administration, and two, four, six, eight and 10 hours thereafter. On each occasion, the patients emptied the bladder completely. The total volume of all samples voided was measured and a portion of each was stored in deep freeze at $-20°C$. In these specimens the concentrations (μg./ml.) of free INH, acetylisoniazid (Ac-INH) and isonicotinic acid (INA) were estimated and the two-hourly excretion of these compounds determined in mg. The results were then expressed as free INH, and the recovery rate of INH and its metabolite calculated in proportion to the dose administered.

Methods

For estimation of free INH in plasma, the method of Eidus and Harnanansingh[9] was used with a minor modification for urine specimens.[10] Determination of acetylisoniazid is based on colour reaction, described by Eidus and Hamilton,[11] and modified to a quantitative method by Venkataraman, Eidus and Tripathy.[12] Isonicotinic acid was estimated by the method of Nielsch.[13] During the entire study, all chemical determinations were carried out in duplicate.

Results

Patients producing half-life values (t ½) of 160 minutes or over may be regarded as slow inactivators, while the upper limit of fast acetylators is set at 110 minutes. Out of 72 patients examined in this study, only 20 were slow inactivators, with an average half-life of 288.4 minutes. The larger group (52) were fast acetylators, exhibiting a t ½ of 81.2 minutes. Three patients of the latter group, with a half-life of 111, 128 and 134 minutes, could perhaps be classified as intermediate. Such a distinction was, however, not made in this study, and for practical reasons they were included in the group of fast acetylators.

Among the 26 Eskimos examined, six were of Delta origin and the remainder belonged to the Central and Eastern Eskimos (Table Ia). Except for one patient with a half-life of 134 minutes, all Eskimos produced values under 110 minutes, exhibiting a t ½ average of 78.2 minutes. The patient producing the high half-life value (134') had, according to an unconfirmed source, a Caucasian father. One of the patient's siblings had Caucasian features but the patient himself did not show such features.

Table I

INH inactivation rates in various Eskimo and Indian groups

Ethnic origin	Tribe	Total	Fast	av. t ½	Slow	av. t ½
a) ESKIMO						
a) Delta and Alaskan		6	6	70.2	—	—
b) Central and Eastern		20	20	80.6	—	—
Total: %		26	26 100	78.2	—	—
b) INDIAN						
a) Algonquin-speaking	Northern Cree	11	5	79.0	6	306.2
	Prairie Cree	3	2	112.0	1	456.0
b) Athabascan-speaking	Loucheux Indian	4	1	95.0	3	231.0
	Slave Indian	6	2	94.0	4	251.3
	Southern Yukon Indian (Little Stick Indian)	8	4	95.5	4	291.8
	Tlingit	2	1	111.0	1	375.0
	Yellowknife Band Indian	2	2	83.5	—	—
	Dogrib Indian	2	2	74.0	—	—
	Chippewyan Indian	8	7	68.9	1	234.0
Total: %		46	26 56.5%	84.3	20 43.5%	288.4

Out of 46 Indians, 26 (56.5%) were fast, and 20 (43.5%) were slow inactivators (Table Ib). Ib). If we exclude from these calculations five Metis, all of them slow inactivators, the ratio is changed to 63.4% fast and 36.6% slow inactivators. The patients investigated can probably be divided into two major groups: Indians living along the Mackenzie fur trader's route, with a considerable white admixture. To this group belong the Algonquin-speaking Northern Cree and the Athabascan, and the Tlingit-speaking Southern Yukon Indians and Slave Indians from the Mackenzie. The second group, the Yellowknife Band, Dogrib and Chippewyan Indians, were relatively untouched until about 1930, living away from the main traffic and trade routes. In 12 patients belonging to the latter tribes, only one slow acetylator was found, while the rate of slow activators was considerably higher among the rest of the Indians. After deduction of the five Metis and 12 members of the second group, the proportion becomes 15 (51.7%) fast versus 14 (48.3%) slow inactivators. It seems that Caucasian mixture plays an important role in the outcome of the phenotyping. The number of patients is far too small and the investigation is lacking in detailed genetic markers and kinship studies, therefore no final conclusions can be drawn. Further investigations should follow this pilot study to confirm the present observations.

The results of the metabolic studies are shown in Table II. They demonstrate the two-hourly average excretion rate for INH and its metabolite in fast and slow inactivators. It may be noted that free INH rapidly decreases in urine specimens of fast acetylators, and only 12.41% of the dose administered is excreted unaltered during a 10-hour collection period. The excretion rate of free INH is two and one-half times higher in slow inactivators, namely, 27.11%. On the other hand, the average recovery rates of Ac-INH and INA in the same period are twice as high in fast as in slow inactivators. These differences are statistically significant at the $P > .001$ level.

In fast inactivators INH is rapidly metabolized and the excretion rate of the derivatives, particularly Ac-INH, is greater than that of the original compound. Therefore, six hours following drug administration 57.17% of the dose given is already excreted in the urine, while only 37.95% could be recovered in slow inactivators. During the 10-hour period the excretion of INH increases in fast acetylators to 73.93% in comparison with the 55.60% recovery rate in slow metabolizers. In the latter group approximately 50% of the recovered drug is free INH. In slow inactivators the metabolic transformation of INH occurs

254

Table II

Average excretion rate of INH and its metabolite during 10-hour period in urine specimens collected every two hours following drug administration.

Phenotype	Compound	Collection time in Hours					Total excretion rate in 10 hours
		2	4	6	8	10	
Fast	INH	6.86	3.36	1.36	0.59	0.24	12.41
	Ac-INH	10.03	11.61	9.34	6.52	3.88	41.38
	INA	3.95	5.83	4.83	3.35	2.18	20.14
Total 2-hourly excretion rate:		20.84	20.80	15.53	10.46	6.30	73.93
Slow	INH	7.10	7.66	5.55	4.28	2.52	27.11
	Ac-INH	3.28	4.58	4.05	4.08	2.64	18.63
	INA	1.32	2.39	2.02	2.40	1.73	9.86
Total 2-hourly excretion rate:		11.70	14.63	11.62	10.76	6.89	55.60

gradually, resulting in even excretion of the derivatives in the four-, six- and eight-hour collection periods.

In both groups of inactivators the rate of isonicotinic acid excretion closely follows that of Ac-INH, and is approximately half of it in the four-, six- and eight-hour collection periods. According to Peters, Miller and Brown,[15] the primary metabolic change, depending on the inactivator status, is acetylation of isoniazid. INA is a product of Ac-INH as a secondary reaction. The high excretion of INA in fast inactivators is due to the greater availability of the acetylated compound for conversion.

Earlier, an attempt was made to utilize the recovery rate of free INH in pooled overnight urine specimens for phenotyping of inactivators.[16-18] A repetition of the method in this laboratory showed that the recommended urine test is not suitable for phenotyping INH acetylators, as it does not produce a sharp division between the two groups of inactivators and overlapping values frequently occur.

Isoniazid and Ac-INH are present in reverse proportion in urine specimens of slow and fast acetylators, therefore it is more practical to use the fraction of Ac-INH versus INH concentration for phenotyping of inactivators. The proportion between the concentrations (μg./ml.) of Ac-INH and free INH in urine is termed by us "Inactivation Index". An average of these indices, calculated from the urine specimens of 40 fast and 20 slow inactivators, collected in two-hourly intervals, is shown in Table III. It may be noted that the indices of slow inactivators remained fairly even, increasing from 0.63 at 2-hour, to 1.60 at 10-hour collection times. The indices of fast inactivators increased rapidly with every collection period, from 2.14 at 2 hours to over 50 at 10 hours. In urine specimens collected between six and eight hours the average indices of fast acetylators were 19.24 times higher than those of slow inactivators.

Fig. 1 demonstrates inactivation indices of 60 patients determined in urine specimens collected in the six-hour to eight-hour period after intramuscular administration of 8

Table III

Average inactivation indices of **40** fast and **20** slow acetylators at two, four, six, eight and 10 hours after intramuscular administration of 3 mg./kg. isoniazid

| Phenotype | Collection time in hours | | | | |
	2	4	6	8	10
Fast	2.14	5.45	13.10	25.98	>50
Slow	0.63	0.86	1.05	1.35	1.60

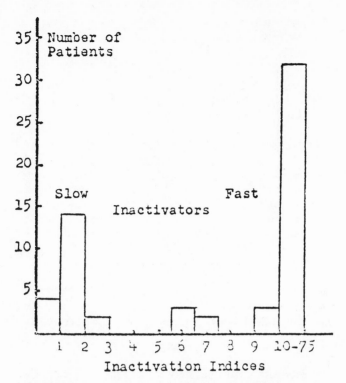

FIG. 1—Inactivation indices of urine specimens collected from 40 fast and 20 slow inactivators in the six- to eight-hour period following drug administration.

mg./kg. INH. The slow inactivators produced indices of 3 and under, while fast acetylators exhibited high indices. However, five patients in the latter group produced somewhat lower indices than the majority (5.5 to 7.5). Three of the above patients, with indices from 5.5 to 6.5, also exhibited longer plasma half-life values than the rest of the fast acetylators, namely 111, 128 and 134 min. The remaining two patients with indices between 6.5 and 7.5 showed plasma half-lives of 96 and 98 min. The rest of the fast acetylators (35), with indices between nine and 75, showed an average INH half-life of 75.6 min. The indices of the urine specimens seem to follow closely the half-life values obtained by the fall-off technique. A comparison of the t ½ values with the inactivation indices of the same patient shows that, with a decrease of the half-life values, the indices are increasing in reverse proportion (Fig. 2). This means that there is an association between t ½ and indices and that rapid elimination from the blood corresponds with high indices. The lowest indices in the group labelled as fast inactivators were produced by three

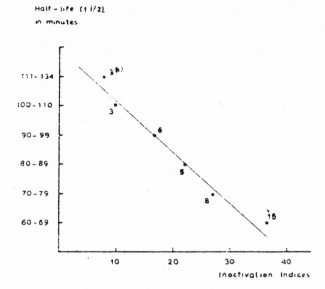

Half - life (t 1/2)
in minutes
•) Number of Patients

FIG. 2 — Relation between half-life values (t ½) and averages of corresponding inactivation indices of fast acetylators in the six- to eight-hour collection time of urine specimens.

patients with t ½ values between 111 and 134 min. while the highest indices are exhibited by 15 patients with a half-life between 60 and 69 min. This remarkable agreement between index and half-life values confirms that urine tests can be employed for phenotyping of INH inactivators.

While inactivation indices provide a distinct division between the two groups of inactivators, overlapping values were obtained when the recovery rate of free INH had been calculated in the same urine samples. In the 60 urine specimens discussed above, four slow inactivators exhibited a recovery rate which would place them into the group of fast acetylators, while one fast acetylator produced a recovery rate identical to that of slow acetylators. Thus, five erroneous groupings would be received if only the excretion rate of free INH were taken into consideration.

Discussion

The inactivation of INH was studied in Canadian Eskimos and Indians. It was found that all 26 Eskimos investigated inactivated isoniazid rapidly. Out of 41 Indians, 26 (63.4%) belonged to the fast acetylators, while five Metis, also included in this study, were slow acetylators. It seems that the white admixture plays an important role in the outcome of the phenotyping. In 216 Eskimos, Armstrong and Peart[3] found 95% rapid inactivators. In 14 American Indians, Mitchell, Bell and Riemensneider[19] observed 79% fast inactivators. Scott, Wright and Weaver[20] reported from Alaska that 79% of the Eskimos and 62% of Athabascan-speaking Indians were fast inactivators. According to Sunahara, Urano and Ogawa,[1] 89% of Koreans, 85% of Ryukyuans, 72% of Thais and 88% of Japanese are rapid acetylators. The rate of fast inactivators is considerably lower in Caucasians. Only 32% of Swedes[5] and 41% of Finns[21] are fast inactivators. In North America, Harris, Knight and Selin[4] examined whites of European descent and found that 45% were fast acetylators. Jessamine, Hamilton and Eidus[22] reported in Canada that of a small group of white patients seven out of 24 (approximately 30%) were fast acetylators.

In contrast to previous reports,[17, 23-25] it is generally accepted today that rapid acetylation of INH has no effect on the outcome of chemotherapy with daily double or triple regimens of primary antituberculous drugs. It may, however, influence unfavourably intermittent INH treatment.[26, 27] According to Tiitinen,[21] the reason for not responding to treatment and thus developing chronic tuberculosis depends either on the therapeutic mismanagement or on the patient himself. Alcoholism, psychopathic behaviour and poor social environment often play a more important role in development of drug resistance than physiological conditions. In the past, during the initiation of chemotherapy, inadequate treatment (prescription of a single drug or administration for too short a period) was one of the causes for developing chronic tuberculosis. Today, we are again at the crossroads in the treatment of tuberculosis by rationalizing it and changing over from sanatorium to domiciliary and probably to intermittent therapy. If we want to avoid the mistakes of the past, efficient and realistic principles have to be established for domiciliary treatment and the latter has to be controlled by reliable supervision. For planning and monitoring intermittent chemotherapy, it is important to possess a method for phenotyping which is relatively simple, dependable and does not require repeated venipunctures. It produces results comparable to those of the fall-off technique and can be performed on a large scale. Methods employed in the past for estimation of INH in serum often suffered from great inaccuracy; furthermore, in a number of studies the criteria for distinguishing the two groups of acetylators were arbitrarily set. Tests based on the recovery rate of free INH in urine specimens[16-18] proved to be unsatisfactory, owing to overlapping values. Tiitinen[28] determined the excretion of free INH in three-hour urine samples of 335 subjects, as a percentage of total hydrazides, following an intravenous injection of 5 mg./kg. isoniazid. The results of the urine test did not correlate with the INH half-life values estimated by the fall-off technique. Out of 192 slow inactivators, 31 fell in the group of fast acetylators, according to the urine test. Furthermore, out of 143 fast acetylators in the same study, 15 emerged as slow inactivators when phenotyped by urine specimens.

Recently, Russell[29] introduced a method for determination of acetylator phenotypes. A repetition of his test did not give satisfactory results. The method employs small INH doses (100 mg. INH taken orally three times per day), and therefore produces too low drug concentrations in urine. Furthermore it utilizes semi-quantitative procedures not suitable for this purpose. The introduction of a urine test for phenotyping should be based on detailed metabolic studies, aimed to devise optimal conditions for this procedure. The Inactivation Index recommended by us ensures a distinct division between the two groups of acetylators and is in agreement with the results of the fall-off technique. An additional simplification could be achieved by adaptation of the method to a colorimeter often available even in poorly equipped laboratories.

The introduction of the urine test for phenotyping of INH acetylators is not only useful for intermittent chemotherapy; it may also assist in studying INH-Matrix preparations with attenuated absorption, in order to compensate the fast acetylation. A double or triple dose, as mixture of isoniazid and INH-Matrix preparation, would probably ensure a similar effect in fast acetylators as that of plain isoniazid in slow inactivators. With the increased dosage of an attenuated preparation, the addition of Vitamin B$_6$ is essential. But even so, an excessively high dose may cause side effects if administered to slow inactivators. A distinct division of patients according to their inactivation status seems therefore an important prerequisite for such trials.

The authors would like to express their thanks to Mr. J. S. Mandel, Lecturer, Department of Epidemiology and Community Medicine, University of Ottawa, for carrying out the statistical analyses.

References

1. SUNAHARA S, URANO M, OGAWA M: Genetical and geographic studies on isoniazid inactivation. *Science* 134: 1530-1531, 1961

2. TIITINEN H, MATTILA MJ, ERICKSSON, AW: Comparison of the isoniazid inactivation in Finns and Lapps. *Ann Med Intern Fenn* 57: 161-165, 1968

3. ARMSTRONG AR, PEART HE: Comparison between the behaviour of Eskimos and non Eskimos to the administration of isoniazid. *Am Rev Resp Dis* 81: 588-594, 1960

4. HARRIS HW, KNIGHT RA, SELIN MJ: Comparison of isoniazid concentrations in the blood of people of Japanese and European descent. *Am Rev Tuberc* 78: 944-948, 1958

5. EVANS DAP, MANLEY KA, MCKUSICK VA: Genetic control of isoniazid metabolism in man. *Br Med J* II, 485-491, 1960

6. HANNGREN A, BORGA O, SJOEQVIST F: Inactivation of isoniazid (INH) in Swedish tuberculous patients before and during treatment with para-aminosalicylic acid (PAS). *Scand J Resp Dis* 51: 61-69, 1970

7. SUNAHARA S: Genetical, geographical and clinical studies on isoniazid metabolism. Proc. XVIth Int Tuberc Conf Excerpta Medica Amst p 513, 1961

8. JENNE JW: Studies of human patterns of isoniazid metabolism using an intravenous fall-off technique with a chemical method. *Am Rev Resp Dis* 81: 1-8, 1960

9. EIDUS L, HARNANANSINGH AMT: A more sensitive spectrophotometric method for determination of isoniazid in serum and plasma. *Clin Chem* 17: 492-494, 1971

10. EIDUS L, HARNANANSINGH AMT, JESSAMINE AG: Urine test for phenotyping isoniazid inactivators. *Am Rev Resp Dis* 104: 537-591, 1971

11. EIDUS L, HAMILTON EJ: A new method for the determination of N-acetylizoniazid in urine of ambulatory patients. *Am Rev Resp Dis* 89: 587-588, 1964

12. VENKATARAMAN P, EIDUS L, TRIPATHY SP: Method for estimation of acetylisoniazid in urine. *Tubercle* (Lond.) 49: 210-216, 1968

13. NIELSCH W: Nachweis und Bestimmung von pyridin-4 — Derivativen. Chemikerzeitung 82: 329-341, 1958

14. DUFOUR AP, KNIGHT R.A, HARRIS HW: Genetics of isoniazid metabolism in Caucasian, Negro and Japanese populations. *Science* 145: 391, 1964

15. PETERS JH, MILLER KS, BROWN P: Studies on the metabolic basis for the genetically determined capacities for isoniazid inactivation in man. *J Pharm Exp Ther* 150: 298-304, 1965

16. IWAINSKY H, GERLOFF W, SCHMIEDEL A: Die Differenzierung zwischen INH-Inaktivierern and normal abbauenden Patienten mit Hilfe eines einfachen Testes. *Beitr Klin Tuberk* 124: 384-389, 1961

17. TEICHMANN W, KOHLER R: Beitrag zur schnellen Differenzierung des individuellen INH-Stoffwechsels. *Praxis Pneumologie* 18: 535-541, 1964

18. MAIER N, MOISESCU V: Eine schnelle Methode zur Bestimmung der Konzentration des durch die Nieren ausgeschiedenen INH. *Beitr Klin Tuberk* 128: 213-217, 1964

19. MITCHELL RS, BELL JC, RIEMENSNEIDER DK: Further observations with isoniazid inactivation tests. *Vet Adm 19th Conf Chemother Tuberc Tr* 19: 62, 1960

20. SCOTT EM, WRIGHT RC, WEAVER DD: The discrimination of phenotype for rate of disappearance of isonicotinoyl hydrozide from serum. *J Clin Invest* 48: 1173-1176, 1969

21. TIITINEN H: Isoniazid inactivation status and the development of chronic tuberculosis. *Scand J Resp Dis* 50: 227-234, 1969

22. JESSAMINE AG, HAMILTON EJ, EIDUS L: A clinical study of isoniazid inactivation. *Can Med Assoc J* 89: 1214-1217, 1963

23. IWAINSKY H, KAUFFMANN GW, SIEGEL D, et al: The effect of INH metabolism on the therapy of pulmonary tuberculosis. *Beitr Klin Tuberk* 122: 324-332, 1960

24. MITCHELL RS, BELL JC: Clinical implication of isoniazid blood levels in pulmonary tuberculosis. *New Engl J Med* 257: 1066-1070, 1957

25. MYDLAK G, VOLKMANN W: The importance of analysis of INH metabolism in therapy. *Z Tuberk* 124: 44-48, 1965

26. MENON NK: Madras study of supervised once-weekly chemotherapy in the treatment of pulmonary tuberculosis. Clinical aspects. *Tubercle* (Lond.) 49: Suppl. p. 76

27. TRIPATHY SP: Madras study of supervised once-weekly chemotherapy in treatment of pulmonary tuberculosis: Laboratory aspects. *Tubercle* (Lond.) 49: Suppl. p. 78

28. TIITINEN H: Isoniazid and Ethionamide serum levels and inactivation in Finnish subjects. *Scand J Resp Dis* 50: 110-124, 1969

29. RUSSELL DW: Simple method for determining acetylator phenotype. *Br Med J* 3: 324-325, 1970

Genetically Related Disorders

Genetic Disorders in Isolated Populations

Edward M. Scott, PhD.

Four rare genetic diseases, Kuskokwim disease, serum cholinesterase deficiency, methemoglobinemia, and adrenogenital syndrome, have been found in unusually high frequency in Western Alaska. Their presence can be explained by genetic principles applicable to small populations.

To describe the genetic composition of a population one must consider those factors that significantly influence inheritance in that population. In Northern people there are three such factors— the effective size of the population, the degree of mixing of it, and the mating habits of the people.

In Alaska, the number of inhabitants was always small. The limiting factor could have been the available food resources, since famines are known to have occurred. Infectious disease may have also limited the population, since Alaskans were never wholly isolated from adjacent American and Asiatic people. In either case, very high death rates occurred periodically.

There was little mixing or migration of the population. Distances were great and most Eskimos and Indians lived in a fixed location. They established relationships with villages immediately adjacent to them, but anyone who lived more than 150 km away was "different" and a stranger. Warfare, which elsewhere was an important factor in mixing of populations, was insignificant in Alaska.

In selecting mates, matings within the immediate family were outlawed, and marriage between cousins was frowned upon. Generally, one selected a mate who was believed to be unrelated. But most people, while they knew who their cousins and

Table 1.—Polymorphic Genetic Markers in Alaskan Eskimos and Indians

Blood Groups	Serum Proteins	RBC Enzymes
ABO (no A$_2$)	Haptoglobin	Acid phosphatase (no C)
MNS	Gc	Phosphoglucomutase$_1$
Rh (no Rh—)	Gm	
P	Cholinesterase$_2$	
Le		
Fy		
Jk		

Table 2.—Homozygous Markers in Alaskan Eskimos and Indians	
Blood Groups	**RBC Enzymes***
Lu	Glucose-6-P dehydrogenase
K	6-P-gluconate dehydrogenase
Xg	Adenylate kinase
Di	Adenosine deaminase
* Hemoglobin is also homozygous.	

The genetic consequences of these factors are a high degree of homozygosity, prominent founder effects, genetic drift, and a characteristic nonrandom appearance of recessive traits.

Genetic theory of small populations predicts that the population will tend to be homozygous, and Eskimos and Indians do show little variability in many characteristics. Many of the common polymorphisms are found, as is shown in Table 1, but these are the polymorphisms that are found in all human populations. Many other markers, however, are not found. Our experience has been that if a polymorphism is present in less than 10% of other populations, it will not be present in our people. A

their grandparents were, did not know who their great-grandparents were. The number of persons available for mating was limited to those who were eligible among the 200 to 400 people in the immediate vicinity, and consequently most marriages occurred between people who were not aware that they were distantly related.

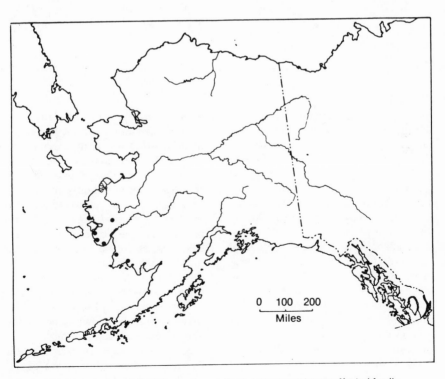

Fig 1.—Location of cases of Kuskokwim disease. Each dot represents one affected family.

Fig 2. — Origin of persons with deficiency of serum cholinesterase. Here and in Fig 3, the earliest known origin of persons affected is shown rather than their present location. Heterozygotes can be detected and were used in determining origins.

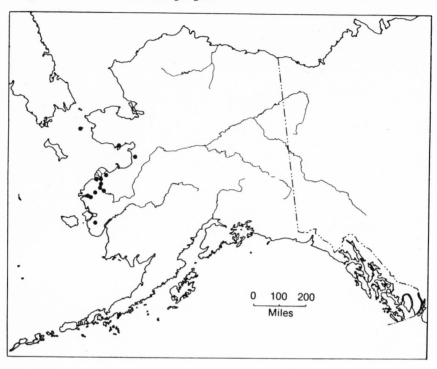

partial list of homozygous markers is shown in Table 2. Further, if you search for any one specific genetic disease, you probably will not find it.

Because of the limited size of the population and the catastrophic nature of famine or illness, the founder effect is of great importance. An inherited trait from one individual may affect a very large number of people within as few as three generations. Because of the mating pattern, a recessive gene that is introduced in this manner will not ordinarily appear in homozygous form for at least 100 years or in the fourth or fifth generation. Ultimately, and particularly if the gene is benign, it may appear with an unusually high prev-

alence or over a very wide area.

There are four Alaskan hereditary disorders that illustrate these points. The first is an arthrogrypotic syndrome called Kuskokwim disease that has been found only in Alaska.[1] This disease is characterized by multiple joint contractures affecting principally the knees and ankles. The muscles appear to be normal and motor unit function is unimpaired. Seventeen cases in seven families are known in an area of about 100,000 sq km, as shown in Fig 1. None of the seven families is known to be related, and all are Southern Eskimos.

The disease appears to be an autosomal recessive with a gene frequency of about 4%. The cause appears to

Table 3.—Persons in Eskimo Villages with the C5 variant of Serum Cholinesterase			
Village	No. Tested	No. C+5	P*
Marshall	77	0	.05
Pilot Station	99	2	...
St. Mary's	151	2	.05
Mountain Village	151	9	...
Emmonak	242	31	.01
Alakanuk	194	22	.01
Sheldon's Point	71	9	.02
Kotlik	150	13	...
King Island	43	1	...
Unalakleet	151	3	.05
Hooper Bay	357	4	.01
Chevak	225	11	...
Chefornak	99	12	.02
Total	2,010	119	

* Probability that observed number of C+5 persons differs from the average of all villages, with the χ^2 test.

be a defective attachment of tendons that is most evident in the extensor muscles under constant strain. The patients can only walk on their knees or in a duck-like waddle, and thus are easily recognized. Historically, no cases were known until the first appeared about 50 years ago.

It seems probable the gene was introduced many generations ago, that it then diffused by outbreeding throughout the people over a considerable area, and the patients represent the first instances where the homozygous condition occurred. To spread over any area this large, at least five generations seem necessary, with perhaps ten more likely.

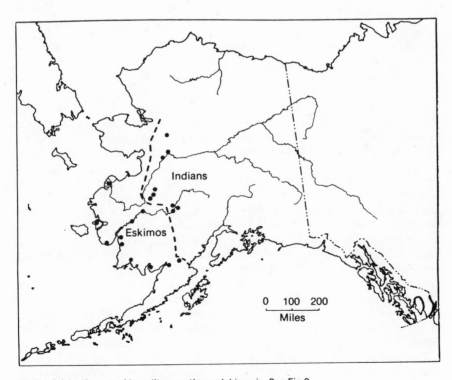

Fig 3.—Origin of cases of hereditary methemoglobinemia. See Fig 2.

Fig 4.—Location of cases of adrenal hyperplasia. Each dot represents one affected family.

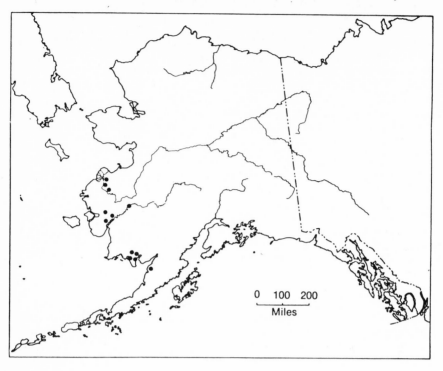

The second inherited condition is a complete deficiency of cholinesterase in serum, the so-called "silent" gene.[2] This deficiency is wholly benign ordinarily and only causes difficulty when succinylcholine is used medically as a muscle relaxant. The action of the drug is greatly prolonged in these people. The condition is readily detected biochemically, and has been found in 51 people among 29 Eskimo families. As shown in Fig 2, it is found over a considerable area of Western Alaska, but predominantly in Southern Eskimos. As much as 1% to 2% of the population may be affected.

The deficiency is an autosomal recessive with a gene frequency that may be as high as 15% in certain places. There is no way of knowing when it first appeared. To spread as far as it has, and to have as high a frequency, it must have been introduced quite long ago. A founder effect is quite possible.

As part of this study we determined the prevalence of C5, an electrophoretic variant of cholinesterase found in 5% to 10% of most populations.[3] Six percent of 2,010 Eskimos were affected, but in the 13 villages in Fig 2 the prevalence ranged from 0 to 13%. As shown in Table 3, eight of the 13 villages deviated significantly from the average of 6% Thus, random genetic drift is a significant factor in this population.

268

Hereditary methemoglobinemia is another enzyme deficiency that appears to be benign, causing only a characteristic cyanosis. Twenty-nine people among 14 families are affected, located over a very large area as indicated in Fig 3.[4] Six widely scattered families are Eskimo, while the rest are Indian. Methemoglobinemia is another autosomal recessive in which the enzyme deficiency can be easily measured. The overall gene frequency is about 4%, but in two Indian groups it is about 7%.

If this condition has a single origin, it must have been introduced very long ago. An Indian origin seems probable, since it is also frequent in the Navaho in the Southwest United States, who are related linguistically to Alaskan Indians.[5] Athabaskan Indians are believed to have moved into Alaska about 1,500 years ago, and they have maintained a limited contact with Eskimos. Methemoglobinemia has been found only in those Indians living close to Eskimos, and it is more prevalent in these Indians than in Eskimos.

Finally, 15 cases of adrenogenital syndrome have been found since 1959 in 12 Eskimo families as described by Hirschfeld and Fleshman.[6] The disease is characterized as severe congenital salt-losing adrenal hyperplasia, and is quickly fatal without treatment. The families cover a considerable area as shown in Fig 4. The disease appears to be an autosomal recessive with a gene frequency of at least 4%. This frequency is probably too low due to incomplete recognition. Over three quarters of the cases have been girls who are commonly recognized by ambiguous genitalia. Affected boys could be easily overlooked in an area where infant deaths are common and often receive no medical attention.

The specific enzyme deficiency that causes the disease has not been determined. The spread of a genetic disease over this large an area appears possible, but the attainment of this high a gene frequency for a lethal recessive is more difficult to explain. The explanation appears to be a comparatively recent introduction of the gene, a spread over a considerable area through outbreeding, followed by appearance of the homozygous form.

In conclusion, studies on Alaskan populations have shown that while most recessive inherited diseases are unknown, a few occur with uncommonly high frequency. These results are consistent with genetic theory for small populations. The advantage of studies in isolated populations are that one can usually assume a single cause for any syndrome and can find all living relatives within a reasonable distance. A curious fact is that the four diseases that have been studied in detail all occur in the same area of Alaska, while none have been found as yet in other parts of the state.

References

1. Petajan JH, et al: Arthrogryposis syndrome (Kuskokwim disease) in the Eskimo. *JAMA* 209:1481-1486, 1969.

2. Gutsche BB, Scott EM, Wright RC: Hereditary deficiency of pseudocholinesterase in Eskimos. *Nature* 215:322-323, 1967.

3. Scott EM, Weaver DD, Wright RC: Discrimination of phenotypes in human serum cholinesterase deficiency. *Am J Hum Genet* 22:363-369, 1970.

4. Scott EM: The relation of diaphorase of human erythrocytes to inheritance of methemoglobinemia. *J Clin Invest* 39:1176-1179, 1960.

5. Balsamo P, Hardy WR, Scott EM: Hereditary methemoglobinemia due to diaphorase deficiency in Navajo Indians. *J Pediatr* 65:928-931, 1964.

6. Hirschfeld AJ, Fleshman JK: An unusually high incidence of salt-losing congenital adrenal hyperplasia in the Alaskan Eskimo. *J Pediatr* 75:492-494, 1969.

PHOTODERMATITIS IN NORTH AMERICAN INDIANS: FAMILIAL ACTINIC PRURIGO

A. R.Birt, M.D., F.R.C.P. (C), and R. A. Davis, M.B., B.S., C.R.C.P. (C)

A distinctive photodermatitis of the polymorphic light eruption type has been described in North American Indians by Schenck,[1] Everett et al.,[2] and Birt.[3] In 1968, Londoño et al.[4] reported a condition of striking similarity in Colombia, South America. Individuals in both groups described in North and South America react adversely to sunlight; both tend to develop the dermatitis very early in life, often before the age of 10. The condition is more common in females and is chronic and recurrent. Frequently there is a positive family history.

Lesions on the face may be eczematous (Fig. 1, 2) or plaque-like (Fig. 3, 4). Pruriginous papules (Fig. 5) are common on the exposed areas of the arms, hands and legs. Impetiginization (Fig. 6) is frequent, and many patients have cheilitis, particularly of the lower lip. We have noted cheilitis as the sole manifestation of this disease entity.

It is our opinion, and Londoño agrees, that we are probably describing the same disease. The mediator of this photodermatitis is not known, but we suspect that it is transmitted as an autosomal dominant trait. In North America, all of the reported cases of this disease have occurred in North American Indians, or their descendents. The racial origin of those affected in Colombia is not reported. In our experience, the classical clinical picture associated with the typical history has enabled us to discover the hereditary trait even in patients with the usual Caucasian appearance.

Fig. 7, a map showing distribution of the condition, is based on personal knowledge of the situation in Canada, and on information obtained from a questionnaire sent recently to all members of the American Dermatological Association. It shows that the geographic distribution of this photodermatitis of North American Indians is confined to the central plains of Canada and the United States. If this photodermatitis is transmitted as a hereditary trait, and if the same hereditary trait accounts for the occurrence of familial actinic prurigo in Colombia, then one would also expect to find it in Mexico and Central America. We are aware that photosensitivity in Mexico fulfills the other criteria of the photodermatitis that we have described.

Psoralen Therapy

For several years we have treated these patients with antimalarial drugs and local light-screening preparations, having little success. The common secondary infection

Based on a paper presented to the First Joint Meeting of the Mexican Academy of Dermatology and the Canadian Dermatological Association, Mexico City, March 7-11, 1970.

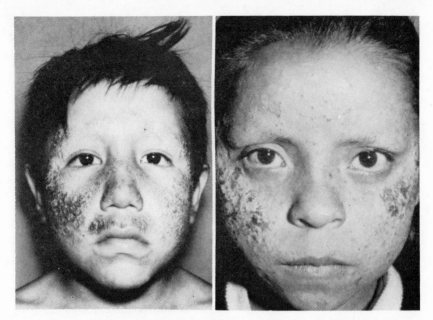

Fig.1—Left, eczematous eruption in a North American Indian boy (Winnipeg, Canada).
Fig. 2—Eczematous eruption in a South American girl (Bogotá, Colombia).

is treated with local and systemic anti-biotics. The most effective corticosteroid preparation in our experience is 0.1 per cent betamethasone valerate ointment or cream, combined with 0.5 per cent neomycin sul-fate, if secondary infection is present.

However, in no case was the dermatitis controlled by the use of these applications, although itching was relieved. Therefore, in 1968, we started a clinical trial to study the effect on the dermatitis of the oral ad-ministration of Trisoralen combined with ultraviolet light.

The psoralens[5] are furocoumarins that sensitize the skin to ultraviolet light in the area of 3600 Å. Of the several compounds available and examined, the most potent is 4-5¹-8 trimethylpsoralen (Trisoralen).[6, 7, 8] The skin becomes photosensitive about an hour after ingestion of the psoralens. Sensi-tivity is maximal in two hours and grad-ually declines and disappears at the end of eight hours.[9]

Ultraviolet light produces thickening of the stratum corneum.[10] Oral ingestion of psoralen, followed by exposure to ultra-violet light one hour later, causes a much greater thickening of the stratum cor-neum,[11] as well as producing an increase in the density of the layer. It also causes de-velopment of an eosinophilic homogenous layer at the base of the stratum corneum, which resembles the stratum lucidum of the palms and soles. These changes take two weeks to develop in normal skin and last for about six months.

In addition, the abnormal adherence of the altered stratum corneum causes in-creased retention of melanin in the layer, and melanin is found in the basal cell layer

271

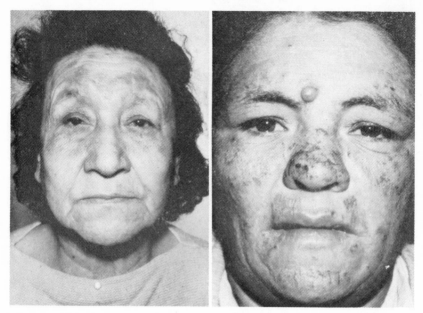

Fig 3—Left, plaque-like lesions of the face of a North American Indian woman (Winnipeg, Canada).
Fig. 4—Plaque-like lesions on the face of a South American woman (Bogotá, Colombia).

of the epidermis. It is believed that these changes, namely a thickened adherent horny layer and higher melanin pigment content in the epidermis, are responsible for the increased protection against ultraviolet rays.

The sole reference to the use of combined therapy with psoralen and ultraviolet light for this type of dermatitis is a study by Schenck[1] reported in 1960. He treated 13 Chippewa Indians suffering from solar dermatitis during July and August, using 20 mgm Methoxsalen given by mouth, followed two hours later by graduated exposure to natural sunlight for 14 days.

He attempted a controlled trial using lactone as a placebo, in place of Methoxsalen. The results showed that regardless of medication, most patients improved under limited controlled exposure to sunlight while in the hospital, whereas in the outpatients Methoxsalen caused a worsening of the conditions in six of the nine who could be evaluated. Schenck suggested that a further trial of Methoxsalen might be worthwhile in the spring before the onset of the dermatitis.

Methoxsalen in a single oral dosage of 30 mgm followed by natural sunlight exposure after two hours has been used with success by Jillson[12] to treat the persistent light reaction type of contact photodermatitis resulting from bithionol. This single treatment provided protection from the effects of sunlight for a year.

Investigation and Treatment

In 1968 and 1969 we treated 22 patients (Fig. 8), who ranged in age from 7-87 years. There were 17 patients below 30; of these six were less than 10 years old. There were

272

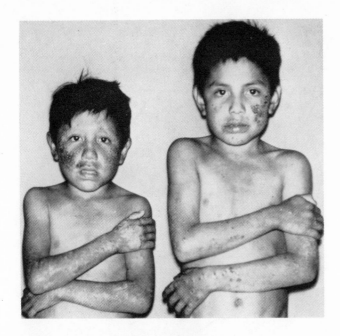

Fig. 5—North American Indian brothers with eczematous eruption on the face, and papular prurigo-like lesions on the exposed areas of the upper limbs and hands.

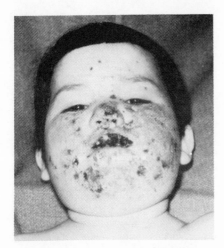

Fig. 6—Impetigenized eczematous eruption in North American Indian child.

three males and 19 females. The dermatitis had been present from two months to 40 years.

From February until May of 1968 we admitted six patients to the hospital. Physical examinations of all were normal except for the dermatitis, which was present in varying degrees. One boy of 17 was treated, whose main complaint was a severe cheilitis that had been present since infancy.

A complete blood count, erythocyte sedimentation rate, three examinations for LE cells, urinalysis, blood and urine examination for porphyrins, and bromsulphthalin retention test were performed. The results were normal.

The patients were given oral Trisoralen tablets in a dosage of 5 mgm daily if they were under 10 and 10 mgm if older. One

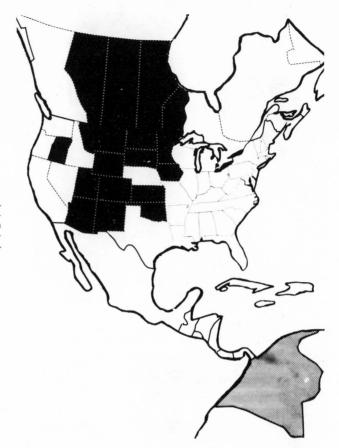

Fig. 7—Geographic distribution of known photosensitive Indians in North America, and familial actinic prurigo in Colombia.

hour later they received general ultraviolet light from an Alpine sun lamp (Hanovia) at a distance of 36 inches. The initial exposure was 45 seconds. Exposure times were gradually increased to a maximum of about 10 minutes at the end of 14 days. In no case was there an exacerbation of the dermatitis.

Erythema due to overdosage with the ultraviolet light was noted in two patients, but did not reappear with reduction of the exposure time. Two patients had dryness and peeling of the skin and follicular papules on the trunk, which we attributed to poral closure. These changes disappeared within a few days with the use of a simple emollient cream and reduction of the ultraviolet light exposure. At the end of two weeks the laboratory tests were repeated and no abnormalities found.

The patients were discharged with instructions to continue taking the tablets

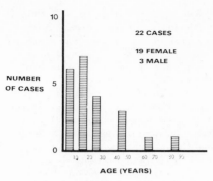

10

22 CASES

19 FEMALE
3 MALE

NUMBER
OF CASES

5

0

10 20 30 40 50 60 70 80 90

AGE (YEARS)

Fig. 8—Age and sex distribution of North American
Indians treated with Trisoralen.

one to one and one-half hours before ex-
posing themselves to the mid-day sun.

In 1969 we treated a further sampling of
16 patients—five in the hospital, five as
outpatients attending the Physiotherapy
Department, and six as outpatients, using
natural sunlight only. The same laboratory
tests were performed and no abnormalities
found. In 1969 we decided to reduce the
exposure to ultraviolet light since we hoped
to avoid erythema and skin peeling, which
reduces the thickening of the stratum corneum. Treatment was started during
March to July.

A Westinghouse Fluorescent sunlamp
(F.S. 40) was used at a distance of 36 inches
from the patient. The minimal erythema
dose (MED) was determined. One to one
and one-half hours following ingestion of
the Trisoralen, general ultraviolet light exposure was given, starting with one-half of
the MED. A daily increment in exposure
was given, depending on the patient's response to the previous day's treatment, i.e.,
the degree of itching or erythema. At the
end of a five-day course of treatment, the
patients were discharged to continue taking
the Trisoralen one to one and one-half
hours before exposure to mid-day sunlight.

Initial sunlight exposure was 30 minutes,
with daily increases of 10 minutes.

The six patients treated entirely with
natural sunlight and Trisoralen were instructed to expose themselves to the sun for
an initial period of 20 minutes with a daily
increase of 10 minutes.

In addition to the Trisoralen and ultraviolet light, the majority of the patients
were given betamethasone valerate ointment to use on the skin to relieve itching
and to combat the eczematous component
of the dermatitis.

Patients were seen in the outpatient department or in our offices, and Trisoralen
was continued throughout the summer
months, depending on the response of the
individual patient.

No side effects from the Trisoralen, such
as nausea, vomiting, vertigo or mental ex-
citation, were encountered.

Some of the patients treated in 1968 were
treated again in 1969, and follow-up was
possible in five cases over 18 months.

Results

Treatment was initiated in 22 patients.
Evaluation and follow-up was possible in
16 patients. Results were classified as good
in 13, no change in one, worse in two.

If the skin lesions cleared or were markedly reduced during the summer months,
this was considered a good result.

There was found to be little difference
in the response to treatment over the long
term, regardless of whether or not the patient was admitted to the hospital. The
conditions of those with a severe degree
of dermatitis at the onset would of course
improve more quickly while they were in
the hospital, because of low natural sunlight exposure.

It was interesting to note that the dermatitis did not flare up following exposure to
ultraviolet lamps or sunlight after ingestion

of Trisoralen. However, we discovered that the dermatitis would reappear or worsen during the summer if the tablets were discontinued. Recommencing the Trisoralen would quickly bring the dermatitis under control.

After this article was presented, one of the patients who was apparently worse with treatment improved markedly when the dosage of Trisoralen was increased from 5 mgm to 10 mgm daily. The other two patients, one of whom was not improved and one who became worse, both had cheilitis only.

From our limited experience, it appears that Trisoralen, 5 to 10 mgm daily by mouth, followed one to one and one-half hours later by exposure to sunlight is an effective and safe form of treatment for photodermatitis in North American Indians. This treatment should be continued throughout the summer, or even longer if necessary.

Discussion

The geographical distribution of the polymorphic light type of photodermatitis in North American Indians has been shown to be limited to the central plains of Canada and the United States. It is highly probable that the photodermatitis described in Colombia is the same disorder. From personal contact with dermatologists present at the Mexican-Canadian Congress of Dermatology in Mexico City in 1970, it became apparent that a type of photodermatitis that conformed remarkably well to the clinical description given above was common in Mexico,[13] Honduras,[14] and Guatemala.[15] Dermatologists in these countries found, as did we, that the use of conventional light-screening local applications was of little value in protecting affected individuals, and that porphyria was not a factor. We can speculate that long ago the Indian peoples of the central plains of North America, Mexico, Central America, Colombia and perhaps other countries in South America shared a common ancestral origin, and that some of them inherited a trait capable of manifesting itself as a distinctive form of photodermatitis. According to Josephy,[16] among others, the Indian peoples did migrate southward from the North American continent through Mexico and Central America to South America, which tends to support the theory of a possible common racial origin of patients affected by this photodermatitis. However, much more research is required into the racial background of affected patients in Mexico, Central and South America before one can prove or disprove theories concerning hereditary traits.

In our experience, the continuous daily use of Trisoralen, 5 to 10 mgm, followed by exposure to sunlight, adequately controls photodermatitis in North American Indians, and prevents relapses without producing any apparent toxic effects. However, comparable results were not obtained in our two patients in whom cheilitis was the major manifestation.

The disappointing results obtained by Schenck, who used methoxsalen and sunlight in treating Chippewa Indians, may perhaps be attributed to the short period of treatment, 14 days. We found that unless the treatment was continued for longer periods of several months, the majority of patients relapsed. It is possible that there may be a difference in the action of Trisoralen as opposed to methoxsalen. We have no personal experience of the use of methoxsalen for this condition.

Summary

A successful form of treatment for photodermatitis in North American Indians employing Trisoralen combined with sunlight or ultraviolet light is described. The geographical distribution of the dermatitis in Canada and the United States is presented, and the probable relationship of the dermatitis to familial actinic prurigo in Colombia and light sensitivity in Mexico and Central America is discussed.

Acknowledgments: We are indebted to Dr. Fabio Londoño for his kind permission to reproduce photographs of his patients shown in Fig. 2 and 4.

The authors are grateful for the kind assistance of the Paul B. Elder Company, Bryan, Ohio, who provided the supply of Trisoralen tablets used in this study.

References

1. Schenk R R: Controlled trial of Methoxsalen in solar dermatitis of Chippewa Indian. JAMA 172:1134-1137, 1960

2. Everett M A, Crockett W, Lamb J H, and Minor D: Light-sensitive eruptions in American Indians. Arch Derm 83:243-248, 1961

3. Birt A R: Photodermatitis in Indians of Manitoba. Canad Med Assn J 98:392-397, 1968

4. Londoño F, Muvdi F, Giraldo F, Rueda L A, and Caputo A: Familial actinic prurigo. Derm Ibero Lat-Am 111:61-71, 1968

5. Fowlks W L: Chemistry of Psoralens. J Invest Derm 32:249-254, 1959

6 Pathak M A and Fitzpatrick T B: Relationship of molecular configuration of activity of furocoumarins which increase cutaneous responses following long wave ultraviolet radiation. J Invest Derm 32:255-262, 1959

7. Pathak M A, Fellman J H, and Kaufman K D: Effect of structural alterations on the erythemal activity of furocoumarins: Psoralens. J Invest Derm 35:165-183, 1960

8. Pathak M A: Mechanism of Psoralen photosensitization and in vivo biological action spectrum of 8-Methoxypsoralen. J Invest Derm 37:397-407, 1961

9. Becker S W Jr: Use and abuse of Psoralens. JAMA 173:1483-1485, 1960

10. Miescher G: Das problem des lichtschutzer und der lichtgewohnung. Strahlentherapie 35:403-443, 1930

11. Becker S W Jr: Effects of 8-Methoxypsoralen and ultraviolet light in human skin. Science 127:878, 1958

12. Jillson O F: The persistent light reactors. Derm Digest 3:59-67, 1964

13. Dominguez L: Personal communication, Mexico, D.F.

14. Corrales H: Personal communication, Teguciqalpa, Honduras.

15. Cordero F A: Personal communication, Guatamala City, Guatamala.

16. Josephy Alvin M Jr: The Indian Heritage of America. New York, Alfred A. Knopf, 1968

277

NORRIE'S DISEASE IN NORTH AMERICA

FREDERICK C. BLODI & WILLIAM S. HUNTER

In 1927 NORRIE described several families in whom the male members were born blind or became blind soon after birth. He also noticed at that time that many of these affected children had defective hearing or were deaf. In some of them there was also mental retardation. He clearly recognized this entity as a sex-linked recessive trait and subsequent reports have verified this assumption.

The eye disease, in general, resembles that of Coats' disease. In both retinas there appear numerous hemorrhages and later on an organized white mass is visible behind the lens. The eyes become atrophic and a cataract and degenerative corneal changes develop.

Histologic examination of enucleated globes have only rarely been done. In general they show a hemorrhagic retinal detachment with secondary degenerative changes, rubeosis of the iris, posterior synechiae and ectropium uveae.

In a recent monograph WARBURG (1966) has accumulated all available material on this condition. The first sibship in the United States was described only a year ago by HANSEN (1968).

The relationship to Coats' disease is an obvious one. Coats' disease is also a vascular retinal lesion occurring usually in young male patients but it affects only one eye in the majority of the cases. It is also characterized by exudation and hemorrhage into and beneath the retina. The primary lesion is here a congenital retinal teleangiectasia. Leber's disease of the retinal vessels is probably only an early or minimal phase of Coats' disease. The primary lesion of Norrie's disease is unknown, though it may very well also

278

be a retinal angioma. Coats' disease has recently been reviewed and delineated by MANSCHOT & DE BRUIJN (1967) and by GOMEZ MORALES (1965). Some variations in the clinical picture and course have been described. While most cases are unilateral (WOODS & DUKE, 1963) bilateral cases do occur (GREEN, 1967). The disease may become manifest or be detected in patients who have reached middle or old age (HENKIND & MORGAN, 1966).

The congenital nature of the condition could lead one to suspect that this is a genetically determined disease. However, familial Coats' disease has been observed only extremely rarely. In one family, reported by SMALL (1968), the children also suffered from muscular dystrophy, deafness and mental retardation. This family is somewhat of a link to Norrie's disease.

We would like to describe two families with Norrie's disease, in which the condition was present in several generations. In a number of instances enucleated eyes became available for histologic examination.

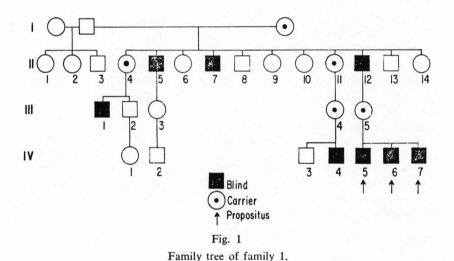

Fig. 1

Family tree of family 1.

Family 1 (fig. 1):
Our attention was drawn to this family because we saw in our clinic three brothers (IV-5, IV-6, IV-7) who were all blind since early infancy and who had defective hearing. Two of the eyes are available for histologic examination. The first eye was enucleated in 1957 and at that time the suspicion was

279

high that this could be a retinoblastoma. The other eye was enucleated because of painful, degenerative changes.

1) J.A.K. (48–4929 [IV/5]) was born on December 27, 1947. His birth weight was 9 lbs and 1 oz. Pregnancy and delivery had been normal. Soon after birth a white reflex was noticed by the mother in each eye. The child behaved like a blind infant.

He was first seen at the University Hospital in Iowa City on April 28, 1948. There was a searching nystagmus in both eyes. In the right eye the cornea was clear, but there was no anterior chamber, the brown iris being plastered against the cornea. Through the dilated pupil a white-yellow mass was seen behind the clear lens. Numerous blood vessels and few fresh hemorrhages were seen in that mass. A red reflex was seen in the periphery of the fundus. The left eye also had no anterior chamber. The pupil was irregular because of posterior synechiae and partly occluded by a membrane. Back of the lens was a similar hemorrhagic mass. No red fundus reflex could be obtained.

The child's hearing was definitely decreased. X-rays of the orbits did not show any calcifications within the globes. The child was examined under anesthesia, but nothing additional was found.

The patient was followed for several years. He attended the Iowa Braille and Sight Saving School. In 1952 both eyes became atrophic. In 1963 a band keratopathy developed in both eyes.

He graduated from high school and is gainfully employed.

2) R.H.K. (58–3124 [IV/6]) was born on February 20, 1949. His birth weight was 6 lbs and 1 oz. Pregnancy and delivery had been normal. The termination of pregnancy was on term and no supplemental oxygen was given. It soon became apparent that the child was blind. As of the age of one year he had a few tonic-clonic seizures. He was slow in growth and development. His hearing was diminished, but he spoke his first word when he was one. He did not walk until he was two. His psychomotor deficit became more apparent and his attacks more frequent. The EEG was grossly abnormal showing widespread cerebral involvement and a probable deep, midline disturbance. Skull films were negative. The cerebrospinal fluid was negative.

He was first seen in our clinic on May 1958. Both eyes were atrophic and deeply set in the orbit. Neither eye had light perception and both showed a searching nystagmus. The right conjunctiva was slightly injected. There was a band keratopathy on that side and the cornea was too cloudy to see the interior of the eye. The left cornea also had a band keratopathy and a degenerative pannus. The anterior chamber was here shallow with many peripheral anterior synechiae. The left pupil was occluded by a membrane.

The right eye became progressively painful and was enucleated on April 10, 1959.

The patient developed fairly well. He was put on medication because of chronic epilepsy with infrequent grand mal seizures. Though his hearing was defective he could attend the Iowa Braille and Sight Saving School. He died by drowning in the summer of 1963.

The histologic examination of the enucleated right globe (Path. 3791) reveals an atrophic globe (18 × 19 × 20 mm) with a flattened, opaque cornea, which is markedly thickened. Its epithelium is irregular and basophilic deposits are found beneath it. The stroma is thick and vascularized. The anterior chamber is nearly absent because of extensive anterior synechiae. The iris is thick and the pupil is occluded. The lens is partly calcified.

The retina is completely detached showing numerous old and recent hemorrhages. The retina is drawn anteriorly by a cyclitic membrane on the temporal side (fig. 2). Nummerous cysts and cholesterol clefts are seen in the atrophic

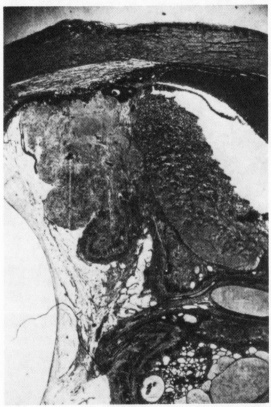

Fig. 2

Complete, hemorrhagic detachment of the right retina in case 2 (IV 6). Vascularized membrane in front of the retina and blood beneath it. Bone formation at the ora serrata. (Hematoxylin and Eosin, ×15).

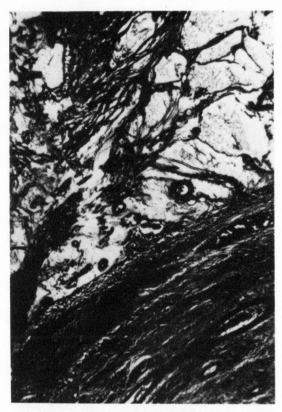

Fig. 3

Higher magnification of figure 2. Dilated blood vessels and hemorrhages in the retina; vascularized membrane on it. (Hematoxylin and Eosin, x100).

retina. On its anterior surface lies a fibrous, vascularized layer of connective tissue extending from one part of the ciliary body to the other (fig. 3). The choroid shows bone deposition and many calcified drusen.

3) M.K.K. (57–15979 [IV/7]) was born on August 30, 1957. His birth weight was 7 lbs and 5 ozs. Pregnancy and delivery had been normal. When he was two months old he was seen by his local ophthalmologist because of persistent tearing on the right side. The lacrimal duct was irrigated and at the same time a large fundus hemorrhage was noted on this side. Two weeks later a retinal hemorrhage was found in the left eye.

He was first seen in the Eye Clinic on December 5, 1957. The right eye was larger than normal, the cornea hazy and the pupil large and nasally displaced. It did not react to light. A white, elevated mass was seen in the fundus. Tension was normal to fingers. The left cornea was clear and the pupil reacted to light. A white mass was seen in the temporal periphery of the fundus. Tension was normal to fingers.

Four days later the child was examined under general anesthesia. The right eye was enucleated because a retinoblastoma could not be excluded. With the pupil dilated, the left fundus showed a marked dilatation of the temporal retinal vessels. The disc was blurred. Temporally a smooth, elevated white mass was seen with small vessels on it. A few hemorrhages were spattered over the fundus.

Three months later (2/27/68) the left anterior chamber was shallow, the pupil measured 3 mm in diameter and was fixed. A huge yellow detachment was seen in the fundus. On May 6, 1958 the left retinal detachment had become complete and hemorrhages were found behind the retina nasally. A hyphema appeared in September.

When examined in February, 1960 cholesterol crystals filled the anterior chamber and the eye was soft. He was last seen in 1964 with an atrophic left globe. At the present time he is still a student of the Iowa Braille and Sight Saving School.

The enucleated right globe (Path. 3493) is of normal size. The anterior chamber is shallow and the lens shows beginning cataractous changes. The retina is totally detached and shows severe pigmentary and glial degeneration. Numerous old, organizing and fresh hemorrhages are in and on the retina (fig. 4). The detached retina is covered by a layer of newformed blood vessels (fig. 5). In the choroid are a few inflammatory foci.

The first eye was enucleated because of the strong possibilty that it harbored a retinoblastoma. When it became evident that we were dealing with a familial hemorrhagic retinal disease we attempted to construct the family tree (fig. 1). The three brothers, who are the propositi, are IV/5, IV/6 and IV/7. All the members with the exception of II/4 and her offspring, live or had lived within the State of Iowa.

It turned out that the grandfather (II/12) of the three brothers had also been seen in the Eye Clinic.

4) Mr. L. A. (62–22577 and 44–4003) was born in 1894. He was first seen in the Eye Clinic on September 23, 1948 at the age of 54. He stated that he had been practically blind and poor of hearing since childhood.

At that time the left eye was atrophic and had no light perception. The cornea was milky white and showed a marked band keratopathy. The right eye had a visual acuity of 3/60. The cornea showed a beginning band keratopathy. The lens was completely opaque. Both eyes showed a rotatory nystagmus.

On September 29, 1948 the right cataract was extracted. The fundus could later on be seen. There was diffuse chorioretinal atrophy, gliosis and large elevated

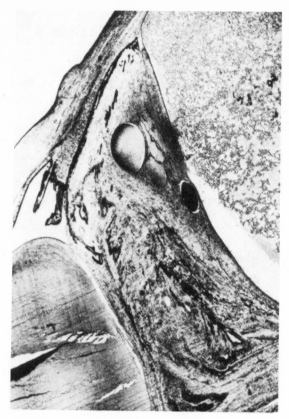

Fig. 4

Complete, hemorrhagic retinal detachment in the right eye of case 3 (IV/7).
(Hemotoxylin and Eosin, x15).

scars were seen in the temporal periphery. Vision with aphakic correction was
6/60.

The patient died in 1962 because of a bronchogenic carcinoma.

5) The cousin of the propositi, (IV/4), was examined by another ophthalmologist. He too was blind since birth and hard of hearing. Both eyes were atrophic
and the corneas opaque.

6) A similar eye report was obtained from a cousin of the mother of the propositi
(III/1).

No eye report is available on II/5 and II/7. The mother of the propositi had.

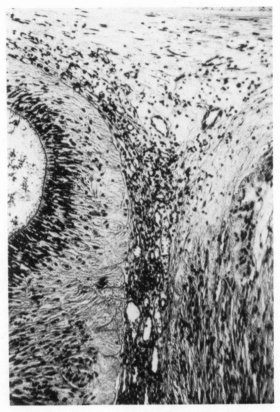

Fig. 5

Higher magnification of figure 2. A dense vascularized membrane lies on the retina. (Hematoxylin and Eosin, x 150)

however, known them and was sure that they had been blind and nearly deaf since childhood.

Family 2 (fig. 6):

The second family was originally reported 20 years ago by WILSON (1949). It is a family of Indians from the Manitoulin Island in Ontario and most of the affected males could be examined at the Hospital for Sick Children in Toronto. We could extend this family tree by one more generation. Three

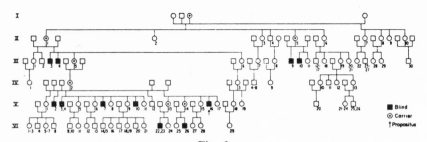

Fig. 6

Family tree of family 2.

more affected males were detected and more pathologic material could be studied.

The family tree (fig. 6) shows again that only males are affected. The defect is transmitted through the females. This is especially apparent in the offspring of IV/2 where six blind males have three different fathers but the same mother.

1) The patient who first drew the attention of the ophthalmologists to this family was W. McM (V/16). He was admitted September 9, 1947 at the age of 18 days. The eyes had been red from birth. The pregnancy was normal and delivery was on term. The birth weight was 6 lbs and 8 ozs.

On physical examination the right pupil appeared large with a green-white reflex in it. Behind the lens were blood vessels and blotches of blood in a whitish mass. Behind it smooth, dark folds were visible, apparently representing the retina. Cornea, sclera, conjunctiva and iris appeared normal. There was no light perception in this eye.

The left eye appeared essentially the same but there seems to have been some light perception.

Intraocular pressure was 21 in both eyes.

The right eye was enucleated on October 2, 1947.

The child remained mentally retarded and was brought up in an institution.

The enucleated right eye (147–47) is smaller than normal. The cornea is clear. The anterior chamber is shallow and filled with an eosinophilic, homogeneous fluid. There are peripheral anterior synechiae. The lens shows beginning cataractous changes. The retina is completely detached. The subretinal fluid contains blood and there are fresh hemorrhages in the retina. On the retina is a thin, vascularized membrane (fig. 7).

2) The oldest halfbrother (V/2) of the propositus was only seen once. The right eye showed posterior synechiae and a soft, greyish-yellow lens. The left iris was atrophic and the pupil dilated. The lens was small and the vitreous filled with a pinkish mass.

286

3) The second oldest halfbrother of the propositus is L.T. (V/3). He was admitted in August 1928 at the age of five years. At birth his eyes appeared normal. At the age of two months they became greyish and the child had never been able to see.

On psysical examination the right eye showed a dilated pupil and a small atrophic lens which was dislocated backward. The anterior chamber was deep. The eye itself was small and a large opaque mass was seen behind the lens.

The left eye showed a dense opacity of the cornea. The lens was cataractous and the pupil well dilated but did not react to light. The eye itself was small and soft.

The right eye was enucleated August 28, 1928.

The left eye became atrophic and was covered by a shell for cosmetic porposes.

The child developed with normal intelligence, but was deaf. He was well known among his tribe as a witch-doctor ('Bear walker').

Histologic examination of the enucleated right eye (2833-28) shows a phthisical globe with a deep anterior chamber and extensive peripheral anterior synechiae. An extension of Descemet's membrane and proliferating pigment epithelium cover the anterior surface of the iris. Calcium and bone are deposited at the posterior pole. The interior of the eye is filled with an organized hemorrhage, fresh blood, old blood pigment and cholesterol crystals (fig. 8).

4) The boy A.T. (V/4) is a brother of the previous patient. He was admitted to the hospital in August 1928 at the age of seven years. At that time his mother said that his eyes had been normal at birth and for the first two months of life. pregnancy had been normal and delivery on term. Later a greyish reflex appeared in the pupillary area of both eyes. Since then he has never been able to see, but could only appreciate bright light. His health was otherwise normal.

On examination the right eye appeared smaller than the left one. In the right eye numerous posterior synechiae were seen in a greyish yellow reflex in back of the lens. The left pupil was dilated and did not react to light. The lens was small and opaque and the vitreous behind it was filled with a pinkish mass. The iris was somewhat atrophic.

The child was definitely of normal intelligence, but completely deaf. He died three years later in an institution for the blind.

5) A younger brother is W.T. (V/7). He was admitted in July 1935 at the age of $2\frac{1}{2}$ months, his mother stated that at birth his eyes seemed to be normal. He could follow movements during the first few days. The pregnancy had been normal and the delivery was on term. At the age of ten days the colored part of the eye became cloudy and smoky. This condition got worse in the next two weeks.

On examination the child appeared to be blind, though there was a slight indication of some light perception. Both pupils were dilated showing an ectropion uveae and they did not react to light. The lenses were clear. A yellow, partly

287

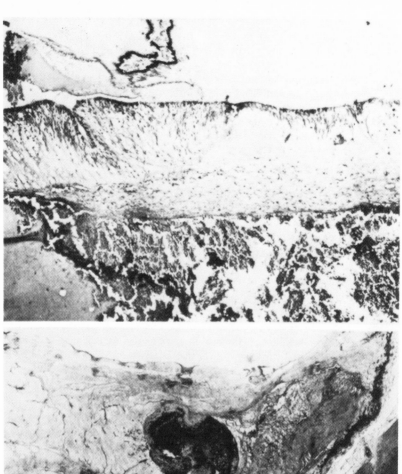

Fig. 7 and 8

Hemorrhagic detachment in the right eye of case 1 (V/16). The retina is hemorrhagic and edematous. (Hematoxylin and Eosin, x 125).

Fresh blood (center) and organized old blood fill the right eye of case 3 (V/3). (Hematoxylin and Eosin, x 15).

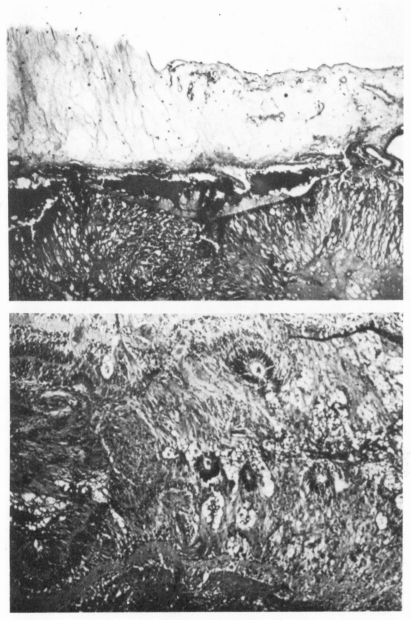

Fig. 9 and 10

Detached retina with a vascularized, preretinal membrane. Left eye of case 5 (V/7). (Hematoxylin and Eosin, x 125).

Completely disorganized detached retina filled with edema and blood in the same eye as figure 9. A few rosettes are present. (Hematoxylin and Eosin, x 125).

vascularized mass lay behind each lens. The intraocular pressure was increased in both eyes.

The left eye was enucleated on July 24, 1935.

The boy has developed with normal intelligence but has been completely deaf.

Histologic examination of the left eye (3218-35) shows extensive peripheral anterior synechiae. An extension of Descemet's membrane and proliferating pigment epithelium cover the anterior surface of the iris. There is a moderate ectropium uveae. The retina is completely detached and blood is found in the retina and beneath it. A vascularized preretinal membrane is present (fig. 9). A few small, rosette-like structures are seen in the retina (fig. 10).

6) The youngest affected halfbrother of the propositus was W. T. (V/10). He was admitted in August 1928 at the age of 2½ years.

His mother stated that his eyes appeared normal at birth but at the age of two months they became greyish. He has not been able to see since then but he could perceive bright light.

On examination both corneas were clear and the pupils dilated. They did not react to light. Numerous posterior synechiae had developed in both eyes and the lenses were opaque bilaterally. The fundus could not be seen.

The patient died at the age of six of an unknown cause.

7) The oldest affected male in the sixth generation is K.B. (VI/22), born May 31, 1961. He was admitted July 10, 1961 at the age of 41 days. The mother had noticed a white reflex in the left pupil from birth. The child was born on term and the birth weight was 7 lbs and 3 ozs.

On physical examination both eyes showed a wandering, uncoordinated nystagmus. The right retina appeared detached with a mass visible on the temporal side behind the lens.

In the left eye a white retrolental mass was seen against the posterior lens surface. This mass was infiltrated with blood vessels and had a definite concave anterior surface.

The child was examined under general anesthesia and no definite lens changes were noted, nor could any elongated ciliary processes be found at the periphery of the lens.

The left eye was enucleated on August 8, 1961.

In September, 1961 the right anterior chamber was flat. The iris appeared frayed and atrophic and was pressed against the cornea. The pupil was fixed.

In 1967 his hearing was tested and apparently he was not deaf.

Histologic examination of the left eye (AFIP Acc. 1014117) shows the iris bowing backwards with dense posterior synechiae. Newformed bloodvessels cover the anterior iris surfae. The retina is completely detached and lies in a funnel-shaped form behind the lens. In the atrophic retina are large vessels and hemorrhages (fig. 11). There is also blood in the subretinal fluid. A few rosette-like structures are seen in the retinal tissue (fig. 12).

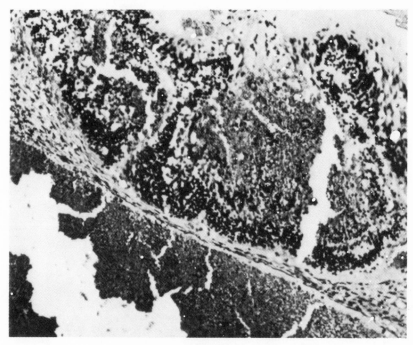

Fig. 11

Hemorrhagic retina with blood in the subretinal fluid in the left eye of case 7
(VI/22). (Hematoxylin and Eosin, x 75).

8) The younger brother of the previous patient is M.B. (VI/23). He was born on
April 10, 1962 on term after normal delivery. The mother noticed soon after
birth a whitish appearance of the pupils similar to the one seen in his brother.

The patient was examined May 4, 1962. Both fundi showed large vitreous strands
and opacities. In the left eye a hyaloid artery was present.

The patient was re-examined in November 1962. At that time the right anterior
chamber was absent and a white opaque mass was seen behind the lens. In the left
eye a similar white mass was seen nasally behind the lens. A red reflex was
obtainable temporally and the anterior chamber on that side was shallow.

The child developed with some mental retardation.

9) A cousin of the preceding two patients is K.A. (VI/26). He was born November 29, 1965 on term and after normal delivery. Soon after birth the mother had
noticed a whitish reflex in the pupils.

He was seen in the clinic in June, 1967. Both eyes showed a band keratopathy
and microphthalmos (fig. 13).

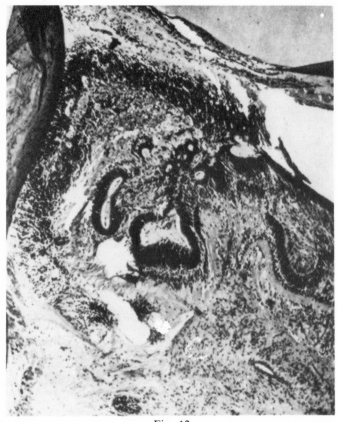

Fig. 12

Rosette-like structures in the disorganized retina. Same eye as figure 11. (Hematoxylin and Eosin, x 75).

The patient was examined under general anesthesia on October 6, 1967. The right cornea measured 8.5 x 7 and the left 9 x 8 mm. Both corneas were moderately hazy. The intraocular pressure was 2/10 gm with Schiøtz. The iris appeared dark brown in both eyes and there was an extropion uveae with posterior synechiae present bilaterally. The pupils were irregular and did not react to light. Anterior chambers were shallow and the lenses almost touched the cornea. A whitish mass was visible behind the lens in both eyes.

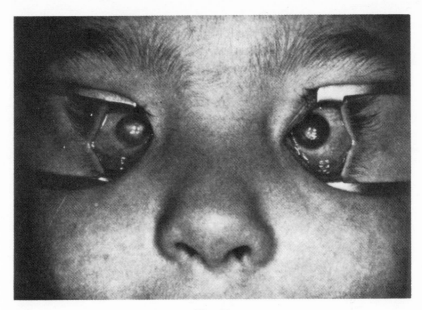

Fig. 13

Clinical appearance of the eyes in case 9 (VI/26).

CONCLUSION & SUMMARY

NORRIE's disease is a congenital or infantile, bilateral, hemorrhagic retinal detachment which is transmitted as a sex-linked recessive. Many of the affected children are poor of hearing, some are mentally retarded.

Two affected families are reported from North America. They encompass three and four generations respectively. Nineteen affected males are described clinically and six eyes could be studied histologically. The salient features of the histologic picture are: A complete retinal detachment, retinal hemorrhages and edema, a vascularized preretinal membrane and secondary degenerative change. These features are identical with those found in the usual Coats' disease.

REFERENCES

GOMEZ MORALES, A. Coats' disease. *Amer. J. Ophthal.* 60, *855–865* (1965).

GREEN, W. R. Bilateral Coats' disease. *Arch. Ophthal.* 77, *378–383* (1967).

HANSEN, A. C. Norrie's disease. *Amer. J. Ophthal.* 66, *328–332* (1968).

HENKIND, P. & G. MORGAN Peripheral retinal angioma with exudative retinopathy in adults (Coats' lesion). *Brit. J. Ophthal.* 50, *2–11* (1966).

MANSCHOT, W. A. & W. C. DE BRUIJN Coats' disease. *Brit. J. Ophthal.* 51, *145–157* (1967).

SMALL, R. G. Coats' disease and muscular dystrophy. *Trans. amer. Acad. Ophthal. Otolaryng.* 72, *225–231* (1968).

WARBURG, M. Norrie's disease. *Acta. ophthal.*, Suppl. 89 (1966).

WILSON, W. M. G. Congenital blindness (pseudoglioma) occurring as a sex-linked developmental anomaly. *Canad. med. Assoc. J.* 60, *580–585* (1949).

WOODS, A. C. & J. R. DUKE Coats' disease. *Brit. J. Ophthal.* 44, *385–412* (1963).

Departments of Ophthalmology, University of Iowa & University of Toronto.

Sex-Linked Cleft Palate in a British Columbia Indian Family

R. B. Lowry, M.B., B.Ch., F.R.C.P.(C)

In a previous paper[1] we reported on the higher frequency of the cleft lip and palate complex in the Indians as compared to the non-Indians of British Columbia. Only 15% of the Indians had an isolated cleft palate in contrast to 33% of the non-Indians. Closer examination of this entity in the Indians revealed a familial clustering which is probably explained by a single gene. In this family the cleft never involves the primary palate (lip, alveolus, and hard palate to incisive foramen) and, with one possible exception (V[63]), the secondary palate (hard palate from incisive foramen posteriorly and soft palate) was never completely cleft. In fact, the majority of those affected had a submucous cleft (i.e., intact mucosa with a cleft of the muscle).

METHODOLOGY

The family, who belong to the Kwakiutl band, was ascertained at the British Columbia Registry for Handicapped Children. A number of field trips were made to the areas involved, and detailed family histories were obtained in addition to examination of as many members as possible. Persons suspected of having a submucous cleft palate were given a complete physical examination by the author; and, with two exceptions (III[22] and V[63]), all were brought for further evaluation at the Cleft Palate Clinic at The Health Centre for Children, Vancouver General Hospital. Those not suspected of having a submucous cleft palate were given only a partial examination, which included oral structures. A total of 122 persons were examined.

RESULTS

Twelve affected persons, all male, were found in this family and are listed in Table I. In addition, two other members are listed who are possibly affected and upon whom a clear decision cannot be made at the present time. There was considerable variation in palatal morphology (Fig. 1 a–d). However, most showed either an absent uvula or a small cleft in the posterior edge of the soft palate. A palpable notch in the posterior edge of the hard palate was found in almost all of the patients; a history of regurgitation of milk and other fluids through the nose when bottle fed was very frequent. In this area no information was available concerning three older members, since their mothers were either dead or could not remember. Although nasality is a somewhat subjective observation, it was commented upon by many different observers (school teachers, public health nurses, and so forth) in each case. Of the two other members who were possibly affected, one (IV[43]) showed a bifid uvula with a short palate which elevated peculiarly. The other member (V[64]), who had an absent uvula, was evaluated at the Cleft Palate Clinic on two occasions when he had intermittent nasality and bouts of recurrent otitis media. A lateral cineradiograph of the soft palate was unsatisfactory due to the patient's lack of cooperation during the examination. The unaffected members of the pedigree (Fig. 2), particularly the parents and siblings of affected persons, were examined carefully to see if they showed any minimal signs of anatomic or physiologic palatal insufficiency.

Bifid uvula was noted in IV[1], IV[2], IV[5], and in two of the three children of IV[5]. It was also found in IV[59], V[58], and III[19] and one of her unaffected sons, IV[64]. Three unaffected males (IV[30], IV[36], and V[34]) and two mothers with affected sons (III[18] and III[21]) had extremely

TABLE I

CLINICAL FINDINGS IN THE AFFECTED AND POSSIBLY AFFECTED SUBJECTS

Pedigree Number	Regurgitation	Nasality	Palpable Notch	Bifid Uvula	Incomplete Cleft Visible	Ear Infection	Other
				Affected			
III-22	NK	+	−	−	+	NK	Morphology similar to Fig. 1a, no palatal surgery
IV-3	NK	+	+	−	+	NK	Fig. 1c, no palatal surgery
IV-8	NK	+	+	−	+	NK	Palatal repair, age unknown
IV-49	+	+	+	−	−	+	Diagnosed age 10, palatal repair age 11
IV-52	+	+	+	+	−	−	No surgery
IV-56	+	+	+	−	+	+	Made worse by T and A
IV-62	+	+	+	NK	NK	+	Palatal repair age 5
IV-65	−	−	+	−	+	+	No surgery, Fig. 1d
IV-67	+	+	+	−	+	+	Palatal repair
IV-68	+	+	+	+	−	+	No surgery, Fig. 1b
V-59	+	+	+	+	+	−	Palatal repair age 3 8/12, Fig. 1a
V-63	NK	NK	+	+	+	+	Palatal repair
				Possibly Affected			
IV-43	−	−	−	+	−	−	Short palate, elevates peculiarly
V-64	−	+	−	−	−	+	Absent uvula, intermittent nasality

+ = present; − = absent; NK = not known.

small uvulae. In this particular kindred there were no other associated malformations or mental retardation. No formal dermatoglyphic analysis was attempted, but the patterns of all affected males were noted. There was a preponderance of whorl patterns on the digits which is commonly found in British Columbia Indians. Thenar patterns were also seen in three patients, but otherwise there was nothing of note. Because the thenar patterns in IV[67] were very unusual, chromosome studies were undertaken and showed a modal number of 46 with an apparently missing No. 16 and an ad-

ditional chromosome in the C-group. No other abnormalities were detected in the karyotype. The buccal smear was chromatin negative. Further studies revealed that his affected brother (IV[68]), his mother (III[21]), and his maternal grandmother (II[7]) had the same karyotype. However, his father did not. A similar abnormal karyotype was found in III[15] and her affected son (IV[49]), but it was not found in III[18] and her affected son (IV[56]) or another affected male (V[59]). Our interpretation was that the abnormal karyotype represented a variant of the No. 16 chromosome which was con-

Fig. 1. Variation in morphology of soft palate. Pedigree numbers refer to individuals in Figure 2 and Table I. *a*, V⁹—absent uvula and minimal cleft of soft palate. *b*, IV⁶⁵—short and bifid uvula. This is stuck together with mucus but can be teased apart. *c*, IV³—more extensive cleft of soft palate than shown in *a*. *d*, IV⁶⁵—absent uvula, minimal notch in soft palate, but palpable notch in posterior edge of hard palate.

⋙→

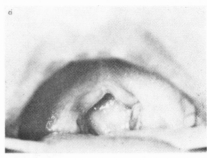

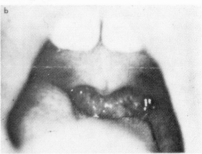

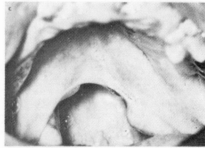

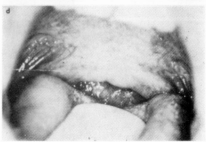

sistent with normal development and was not related to the presence or absence of cleft palate. However, other interpretations, such as a balanced translocation, are possible; and, further chromosome studies and blood group studies are pending.

DISCUSSION

There seems to be a lack of awareness among pediatricians and general practitioners of the submucous cleft palate entity. The symptoms and signs include nasal regurgitation of fluids as an infant, nasal speech with secondary articulation errors later, midline separation of the soft palatal muscle with an intact mucosa, and a notch in the posterior edge of the hard palate.[2] Imperfect speech is noted by the parents of such a child, but they are reassured by the physician that he will grow out of it. Since frequent episodes of otitis media and tonsillitis are often present, the child with a submucous cleft is often subjected to a tonsillectomy and adenoidectomy, which merely makes the speech worse. Thus, these children appear at speech and cleft palate clinics at age 5 or older when parental anxiety over future school progress has increased. The incidence of submucous cleft palate among cleft palate patients has been reported as varying between 3% and 6%[3,4] of all cleft palate patients, but this is probably an underestimate. The more minimal cases will probably not require surgery, but others will require it in order to achieve the best speech result. The references cited[2-5] should be consulted for more details on the surgical aspects of the condition. It is essential that all physicians who are performing tonsillectomy and adenoidectomy on children should be aware of and look carefully for this condition preoperatively.

The pedigree suggests that the defect in this family may be the result of a single gene, ei-

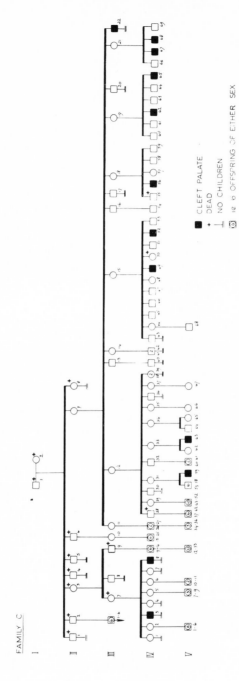

FIG. 2. Family pedigree

298

ther x-linked or sex-limited autosomal recessive. Consanguinity was found in one set of parents (first cousins) who had an affected boy, but two other mothers with affected sons have married Caucasians and the chances of both husbands being heterozygotes for this gene would seem to be remote. Therefore, it seems likely that the gene responsible is x-linked, but there are a number of features which suggest variable expressivity, for example the palatal morphology in those affected and the absent uvula and intermittent nasality in V^{64}. Possibly nonpenetrance occurs since one might expect one of the four male offspring of III^{12} to be affected. Three of these patients were examined by the author and IV^{30} and IV^{36} were both noted to have extremely broad uvulae but no nasality in speech, no history of regurgitation, and no palpable notch. IV^{28} was not examined because he was deceased, but he was not recorded as having any nasality. However, since III^{12} has at least two grandsons who are affected, we may assume that she has the gene.

Whether those individuals with bifid uvula are expressing the gene or not is impossible to say since the frequency of bifid uvula in the British Columbia Indians is about 1 in 10. The reason for thinking IV^{43} is possibly affected is he has a short palate in addition to a bifid uvula. Furthermore, his palate elevates in a peculiar fashion. In certain other Indian families who were studied by the author, bifid uvula appears to segregate as an autosomal dominant trait. However, cleft palate does not occur with any increased frequency.[7] In the family reported here, the frequency of bifid uvula is less than 1 in 10; thus, those who express this anomaly may have the x-linked gene for cleft palate. Although not all persons in the pedigree, particularly some of those still living in generation III, were examined, an opinion was obtained on their speech from either their spouses, other relatives, public health nurses, and so forth, and none apparently had obvious cleft palate speech. The majority of those unaffected in generations IV and V were examined by the author.

Sex-linked cleft palate has previously been described by Weinstein and Cohen,[7] but the present family has a different disorder because none of the other facial or somatic abnormalities described in their family were found. The only other example of single gene inheritance producing cleft lip and palate is the dominantly

inherited syndrome described by Van der Woude[8] in which there are congenital lip pits. It is generally recognized that cleft lip, with or without cleft palate, is a separate entity from isolated cleft palate; however, both groups are thought to be the result of polygenic inheritance. Because of the high frequency of the cleft lip and palate complex in the Indians of British Columbia, it would be ideal to study each family in depth in order to see if there are other examples of genetic heterogeneity.

SUMMARY

An Indian family from British Columbia is described in which 12 males have an incomplete cleft of the secondary palate, some belonging to the submucous variety. The symptoms and signs which should prompt a physician to make this diagnosis are nasal regurgitation of fluids in infancy, nasal speech, repeated attacks of otitis media, bifid uvula, and a palpable notch in the posterior edge of the hard palate. It is suggested that this type of cleft is the result of a sex-linked gene.

This study was supported by National Health Grant No. 609-7-155 and Medical Research Council of Canada Grant No. MA 3415.

The study would not have been possible without the generous cooperation and enthusiasm of the members of the Upper Island Health Unit (director, Dr. G. A. Gibson) and especially Mrs. Anne Grant, Public Health Nurse, who drew this family to my attention and arranged for many of the family interviews and examinations. The author would also like to thank Dr. Margaret J. Corey for the chromosomal analyses, Dr. A. D. Courtemanche for many helpful discussions, Dr. Carl Chisholm for information on V^{63}, and Sheila Manning for assistance with the pedigree.

REFERENCES

1. Lowry, R. B., and Renwick, D. H. G.: Incidence of cleft lip and palate in British Columbia Indians. J. Med. Genet., 6:67, 1969.
2. Calnan, J.: Submucous cleft palate. Brit. J. Plast. Surg., 5:264, 1954.
3. Porterfield, H. W., and Trabue, J. C.: Submucous cleft palate. Plast. Reconstr. Surg., 35: 45, 1965.
4. Gylling, V., and Soivio, A.: Submucous cleft

palate: Surgical treatment and results. Acta Chir. Scand., **129**:282, 1965.

5. Thaler, S., and Smith, H. W.: Submucous cleft palate. Arch. Otolaryng., **88**:184, 1968.

6. Lowry, R. B., and Pyper, J. B.: Bifid uvula in British Columbia Indians. Unpublished manuscript.

7. Weinstein, E. D., and Cohen, M. M.: Sex-linked cleft palate: Report of a family and review of 77 kindreds. J. Med. Genet., **3**:17, 1966.

8. Van der Woude, A.: Fistula labii inferioris congenita and its association with cleft lip and palate. Amer. J. Hum. Genet., **6**:244, 1954.

AUTHOR INDEX

KEY-WORD TITLE INDEX